The Vaccine Handbook™: A Practical Guide for Clinicians

The Vaccine Handbook™: A Practical Guide for Clinicians

Gary S. Marshall, M.D.

Professor of Pediatrics
Division of Pediatric Infectious Diseases
University of Louisville School of Medicine
Louisville, Kentucky

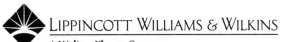

LIPPINCOTT WILLIAMS & WILKINS
A **Wolters Kluwer** Company

Philadelphia · Baltimore · New York · London
Buenos Aires · Hong Kong · Sydney · Tokyo

Acquisitions Editor: Hal Pollard and James Merritt
Developmental Editor: Karen Carter
Supervising Editor: Mary Ann McLaughlin
Production Editor: Amanda W. Yanovitch, Silverchair Science
+ Communications
Manufacturing Manager: Benjamin Rivera
Cover Designer: David Levy
Compositor: Silverchair Science + Communications
Printer: R. R. Donnelley

ISBN: 0-7817-3569-6

Care has been taken to confirm the accuracy of the information
presented and to describe generally accepted practices. However, the
authors, editors, and publisher are not responsible for errors or omis-
sions or for any consequences from application of the information in
this book and make no warranty, expressed or implied, with respect
to the currency, completeness, or accuracy of the contents of the publication. Application of this information in a particular situation
remains the professional responsibility of the practitioner.

The authors, editor, and publisher have exerted every effort to
ensure that drug selection and dosage set forth in this text are in accordance with current recommendations and practice at the time of publication. However, in view of ongoing research, changes in government
regulations, and the constant flow of information relating to drug therapy and drug reactions, the reader is urged to check the package insert
for each drug for any change in indications and dosage and for added
warnings and precautions. This is particularly important when the recommended agent is a new or infrequently employed drug.

Some drugs and medical devices presented in this publication have
Food and Drug Administration (FDA) clearance for limited use in
restricted research settings. It is the responsibility of health care providers to ascertain the FDA status of each drug or device planned for
use in their clinical practice.

10 9 8 7 6 5 4 3 2 1

For Cherie, Emily, and Cullen

Contents

Contributing Authors

Penelope H. Dennehy, M.D.
Professor of Pediatrics
Division of Pediatric Infectious Diseases
Brown Medical School
Associate Director, Pediatric Infectious Diseases
Hasbro Children's Hospital
Providence, Rhode Island
Chapters 5, 6, and 7

David P. Greenberg, M.D.
Associate Professor of Pediatrics
University of Pittsburgh School of Medicine
Division of Allergy, Immunology, and Infectious Diseases
Children's Hospital of Pittsburgh
Pittsburgh, Pennsylvania
Chapters 6, 8, and 10

Paul A. Offit, M.D.
Professor of Pediatrics
Division of Infectious Diseases
University of Pennsylvania School of Medicine
Chief, Division of Infectious Diseases
The Children's Hospital of Philadelphia
Philadelphia, Pennsylvania
Chapter 13

Tina Q. Tan, M.D.
Associate Professor of Pediatrics
Division of Pediatric Infectious Diseases
Feinberg School of Medicine
Northwestern University
Codirector, Pediatric Travel Medicine Clinic
Director, International Adoptee Clinic
Children's Memorial Hospital
Chicago, Illinois
Chapters 11 and 12

Preface

> *We, the undersigned, support immunization as the safest, most effective way to control and eradicate infectious diseases. Infectious diseases were once prevalent in the United States, inflicting widespread suffering and death on young and old, rich and poor alike. Deadly diseases such as smallpox, polio, diphtheria and measles have, for the most part, become distant memories. Most of the credit goes to vaccines, medical miracles that many take for granted.*
>
> *Vaccination eradicated smallpox but the other diseases still exist. Without immunization, they quickly can return and cause widespread harm . . . Although there are extremely rare instances of serious adverse reactions to vaccines, vaccines have a demonstrated record of safety and are held to the highest standard . . .*
>
> *Childhood and adult infectious diseases pose a real threat to personal and public health. Those who are not vaccinated leave not only themselves, but others, vulnerable to dangerous diseases. Vaccines are the most effective option for preventing and stopping the spread of infectious diseases . . .*

So begins the Open Statement on Vaccines, a declaration endorsed by many medical and public health practitioners, academicians, leaders of professional organizations, Nobel laureates, former U.S. Surgeon Generals, and the former Secretary of Health and Human Services. That this statement even exists in the year 2003 (it can be found at www.sabin.org/programs_open_vaccine.htm, accessed 02/07/03) and that so many individuals have felt compelled to sign it explains to a large extent why this book was written. Vaccination stands out as one of the greatest public health achievements of the twentieth century—we now enjoy freedom from contagious diseases that is unprecedented in human history. Paradoxically, the challenges faced by those who give vaccines to patients could not be greater, and our historic successes are threatened.

In 1982, children in the United States received one series of shots [diphtheria, tetanus, and whole-cell pertussis vaccine (DTP)], one oral vaccine series [oral poliovirus vaccine (OPV)], and one measles, mumps, and rubella vaccine (MMR) before they entered school—six shots given, seven diseases prevented. Today, they routinely receive six or seven separate series of shots [hepatitis B vaccine (Hep-B); diphtheria, tetanus, and acellular pertussis vaccine (DTaP); *Haemophilus influenzae* type b (Hib) vaccine; inactivated poliovirus vaccine (IPV); MMR; 7-valent pneumococcal conjugate vaccine (PCV-7); and, in some areas, hepatitis A vaccine (Hep-A)], as well as the varicella vaccine, and it appears that influenza vaccine may become routine as well—as many as 27 shots given, 13 diseases prevented! There are new vaccines in the pipeline to prevent other diseases. There are vaccines for persons with particular risks, and there are passive immunoprophylactics for persons in particular situations. All of these changes represent great progress, but at the same time, all of these changes have bred great anxiety. Practitioners are faced with dispensing antigens in various combinations with catchy trade names made by different manufacturers—a vaccine alphabet soup that is difficult to keep straight. Parents read on the Internet that vaccines are dangerous and that vaccine policy is driven by unscrupulous profiteers. Diseases that once reminded people of the need for vaccination have faded from memory. Shortages, changes in official recommendations, and new questions about the use of vaccines in biodefense arise frequently. There are many things happening, all at the same time.

This book has a simple purpose—to draw authoritative information about vaccines together into a simple, concise, practical resource that can be used in the office or on the wards. There are already several excellent books about vaccines. The definitive textbook is *Vaccines*, edited by Stanley A. Plotkin and Walter A. Orenstein [see Chapter 14(X) for full citation]. This book, which is encyclopedic in scope and rich in content, stands out as the essential reference for specialists and scientists. Books that coherently translate the complex world of vaccinology into terms that laypeople can understand include *Vaccinating Your Child: Questions and Answers for the Concerned Parent*, by Sharon G. Humiston and Cynthia Good, and *Vaccines: What You Should Know*, by Paul A. Offit and Louis M. Bell. In addition, books that contain authoritative recommendations include the *Red Book*, published approximately every 3 years by the American Academy of Pediatrics (AAP), and *Epidemiology and Prevention of Vaccine-Preventable Diseases (Pink Book)*, published approximately every 2 years by the Centers for Disease Control and Prevention (CDC).

The Vaccine Handbook™ differs from these books in important ways. It is intended to be concise, practical, navigable, transparent, user-friendly and focused on the use of vaccines. Unlike *Vaccines*, which is geared toward academicians, and unlike *Vaccinating Your Child* and *Vaccines: What You Should Know*, which are geared toward parents and patients, *The Vaccine Handbook™* is geared toward practicing pediatricians, family physicians, internists, nurses, nurse practitioners, physicians' assistants, and clinic staff. Residents and students might also find it useful. Unlike the *Red Book*, which is about infectious diseases, *The Vaccine Handbook™* is only about vaccines and immunoprophylactics and the diseases that they prevent. It expands on the *Red Book* by including information on vaccine policy making, the vaccine safety net, risk communication, current public concerns, adult vaccines, travel, bioterrorism, passive immunization, vaccines in development, office organization, billing, legal obligations, and logistics. It differs from the *Pink Book* as well in the extent to which these topics are covered. In addition, *The Vaccine Handbook™* will be updated yearly, a critical advantage in a field that changes so rapidly.

The Vaccine Handbook™ does not contain extensive scientific discussions or unique recommendations. Instead, it provides enough background for the practitioner to understand the recommendations and explain them to his or her patients. It should be noted that, although official recommendations are the foundation of scientific vaccine practice, they have their limitations. They take time to develop and are constrained by precedent, the need for consensus, the big public health picture, and, in some cases, politics. In addition, not all contingencies and permutations are covered. The language is sometimes definitive (*vaccine X is recommended*), sometimes not definitive (*vaccine X should be considered*), and sometimes vague (*some experts believe vaccine X should be given*). There is even disagreement among sources—the package insert, for example, and the recommendations set forth by the Advisory Committee on Immunization Practices (ACIP). Wherever possible, the authors of *The Vaccine Handbook*™ have attempted to distill the material into practical guidances. For cases in which official recommendations do not exist, reasonable suggestions are offered.

One goal we all share is to prevent disease and death without causing harm. Vaccines are a means to this end, and this handbook is intended to provide help along the way.

G.S.M.

Acknowledgments

Special appreciation goes to Dr. Richard D. Clover at the University of Louisville and Dr. Sharon G. Humiston at the University of Rochester for expert review of the manuscript, as well as Dr. William L. Atkinson at the National Immunization Program for clarification of Advisory Committee on Immunization Practices recommendations. Appreciation also is extended to the many other people who contributed to this work through conversation and comment.

General Considerations

I. **Background.** *Immunization* is the process of protecting individuals from disease by making them immune. Most often this is accomplished *actively* through *vaccination*, the delivery of antigens to the host for purposes of stimulating an immune response. It can also be accomplished *passively* by the administration of antibodies. Although not technically correct in all instances, the terms *vaccination* and *immunization* are used interchangeably throughout this book.

   A. **Active immunization.** Table 1.1 provides a schema for classifying most vaccines that have been developed to date. *Live vaccines* replicate in the host, cause mild or undetectable disease, and generate immune responses that mimic those induced by natural infection. Live viral vaccines are generally *attenuated*, or weakened, by serial passage in animal or human cell culture [the oral poliovirus vaccine (OPV) is a classic example]. Attenuation can also be achieved by altering the natural route of inoculation. For example, the adenovirus vaccines used in the military in the 1970s and 1980s were not classically attenuated, but because they were administered through the gastrointestinal tract rather than the respiratory tract, they induced immunity without inducing disease. There are also live-attenuated bacterial vaccines, such as Bacille Calmette-Guérin (BCG), which is derived from *Mycobacterium bovis* and is used for prevention of disseminated tuberculosis. Live vaccines can also be *engineered*. For example, the tetravalent rhesus rotavirus vaccine (RRV-TV) consisted of a mixture of rhesus rotavirus, which is attenuated for humans, and several rhesus-human rotavirus reassortants that were created in the laboratory. Other examples include the oral typhoid Ty21a vaccine, which was attenuated through genetic manipulation, and the intranasal influenza vaccine (licensed in June 2003), which is recreated each year by reassorting parental cold-adapted strains with the appropriate circulating wild-type strains.

     Inactivated vaccines may consist of whole, inactivated agents, as in the case of whole-cell pertussis and inactivated polio vaccines, or specific components derived from the pathogen through physical, chemical, or molecular biologic means. *Component* vaccines include toxoids, protein toxins that have been chemically modified to reduce pathogenicity but retain immunogenicity. Polysaccharide vaccines, like those for pneumococcus and meningococcus, are physically purified from the bacterial capsule.

Table 1.1.   Classification of vaccines

Live attenuated			Inactivated				
					Component		
Bacterial	Viral	Engineered	Whole agent	Toxoid	Purified subunit	Engineered subunit	Recombinant
Bacille Calmette-Guérin	Adenovirus[a] Measles Mumps Polio (OPV)[a] Rubella Vaccinia Varicella Yellow fever	Influenza (intranasal)[b] Cholera CVD 103-HgR[c] (oral) Rotavirus[a] (oral) Typhoid Ty21a (oral)	Anthrax Cholera USP[a] (parenteral) Cholera WC/rBS (oral)[c,d] Hepatitis A Hepatitis B[a] (plasma-derived) Influenza (whole virus) Japanese encephalitis Pertussis[a] (whole cell) Plague Polio (IPV) Rabies Typhoid[a] (parenteral)	Diphtheria Tetanus	Pertussis (acellular) Hib polysaccharide[a] Cholera WC/rBS (oral)[c,d] Influenza (split virus) Meningoccal polysaccharide Pneumococcal polysaccharide Typhiod Vi polysaccharide	Hib conjugate Pneumococcal conjugate Meningococcal conjugate[b]	Hepatitis B (surface antigen) Lyme disease (OspA)[a]

[a]No longer used or available in the United States.
[b]Licensed in the United States in June 2003.
[c]Available outside the United States.
[d]Contains both whole-inactivated organisms and a recombinant-derived subunit.

Components can be engineered to improve immunogenicity or change the character of the immune response. For example, the *conjugation* of capsular polysaccharides to protein carriers changes the immune response from a T-cell–independent process to a T-cell–dependent one, facilitating immunogenicity in young infants and inducing immunologic memory. Component vaccines can also be produced by *recombinant DNA technology*, as in the case of hepatitis B vaccine (Hep-B), in which the gene for hepatitis B surface antigen is inserted into yeast cells, which then produce large quantities of the protein for purification.

Table 1.2 lists general characteristics of live and inactivated vaccines. These properties have very real consequences in practice, affecting storage conditions, scheduling, expected efficacy, contraindications, and the potential for adverse reactions. Some implications of these characteristics, as well as exceptions to the generalizations, are given in the footnotes.

B. Passive immunization. Passive immunization is the process by which short-term protection from disease is conferred through the administration of antibodies. This process occurs naturally during the last 2 months of pregnancy, when large quantities of IgG are transferred across the placenta to the baby. This explains the relative protection that newborns have against invasive pneumococcal and *Haemophilus influenzae* type b (Hib) infections, among others. Passive immunization is necessary for patients with humoral immune defects who cannot synthesize their own antibodies; in these cases, *polyclonal immune globulin* is used. For example, patients with agammaglobulinemia receive monthly infusions of polyclonal immune globulin for intravenous administration (IGIV) to prevent a broad range of infections. Polyclonal immune globulin is also used to prevent certain specific infections, like measles and hepatitis A, because the titer of antibody to these agents is sufficiently high in the general population from whom the immune globulin is derived.

Passive immunization is also useful for individuals at risk for particular infections; in these cases, *hyperimmune globulins*, derived from donors with high antibody levels to the pathogen, are used. Examples include varicella-zoster immune globulin (VZIG) for prevention of chickenpox in exposed immunocompromised individuals and hepatitis B immune globulin (HBIG) for neonates born to hepatitis B–carrier mothers or other individuals exposed to acute infection. It should be understood that hyperimmune globulins also contain antibodies to pathogens besides the one they target; this occurs because the individuals from whom they derive, although selected for their high antibody titers to specific pathogens, also have antibodies to other agents. In addition, although immune globulin products are made from blood, donor screening and processing of the antibodies make the risk of trans-

Table 1.2. Generalizations about vaccines

Characteristic	Live	Inactivated
Immune response	Humoral and cell mediated	Mostly humoral[a]
Dosing	One dose usually sufficient[b]	Multiple dose series required
Adjuvant[c]	Not necessary	Usually necessary[d]
Route of administration	Subcutaneous, oral, or intranasal	Subcutaneous or intramuscular
Duration of immunity	Potentially life-long[e]	Booster doses usually required
Person-to-person transmission	Possible[f]	Not possible
Inactivation by circulating passively acquired antibodies[g]	Can occur	Does not occur[h]
Use in immunocompromised host	May cause disease	Cannot cause disease
Use in pregnancy	Fetal damage theoretically possible[i]	Fetal damage theoretically unlikely[i]
Storage requirements	Reflect need to maintain viability	Reflect need to maintain chemical and physical stability
Simultaneous administration at separate sites	Acceptable	Acceptable
Interval between *same* vaccine given in sequence	Minimum intervals apply	Minimum intervals apply
Interval between *different* vaccines given in sequence	Minimum intervals apply	No minimum intervals

[a]Some inactivated vaccines stimulate limited humoral responses. For example, polysaccharides induce short-lived IgM responses and do not result in immunologic memory. Engineering can overcome these limitations, as in the conjugation of polysaccharides to protein carriers. Protein vaccines can induce memory responses that are T–helper cell dependent.

[b]Exceptions include the varicella vaccine, which requires two doses in adolescents and adults, and live-attenuated oral vaccines such as polio.

[c]Adjuvants are substances that enhance immune responses by slowing the release of antigen, increasing uptake into antigen-presenting cells or nonspecifically stimulating lymphocytes. The most common adjuvant used in vaccines is *alum*, a generic term for a variety of aluminum salts.

[d]Hib conjugate vaccines do not contain adjuvants.

[e]A second dose of measles, mumps, and rubella vaccine (MMR) is recommended because some children do not respond to the first dose, not because immunity to the first dose wanes.

[f]This phenomenon was most relevant for oral polio vaccine (OPV), for which transmission probably contributed to immunity at the population level but also caused disease in the immunocompromised contacts of vaccinees. Transmission of varicella vaccine is extremely rare, and transmission of MMR does not occur.

[g]Passive antibodies do not affect oral live vaccines such as typhoid Ty21a. Blood products derived from the United States do not contain sufficient quantities of antibody to yellow fever to inactivate that vaccine. See Table 1.4 for recommended intervals between antibody-containing products and live vaccines.

[h]To avoid antigen–antibody interactions, antibody-containing products are not administered at the same site as inactivated vaccines.

[i]See Chapter 12(II).

Table 1.3. Generalizations about passive immunization

Characteristic	Immune globulin	Hyperimmune globulin	Engineered antibodies	Antitoxins
Derived from	Humans	Humans with high antibody titers	Laboratory	Animals
Specificity	Broad	Broad	Narrow	Narrow
Route of administration	IM or IV	IM, IV, or SC	IM	IM
Dosing	Pre- or postexposure	Pre- or post-exposure	Preexposure	Postexposure
Inactivation of live vaccines	Yes	Yes	No	No
Examples	IGIM IGIV	CMV-IGIV HBIG BIG (human) RIG RSV-IGIV TIG VIG VZIG	RSV-mAb	Botulinum antitoxin Diphtheria antitoxin

mission of bloodborne pathogens negligible. Antibodies can be *engineered* for prevention of specific diseases, as in the case of RSV-mAb (Synagis), a monoclonal antibody that has the effector region of human IgG but the combining region of a mouse monoclonal antibody specific for the RSV F protein. *Antitoxins*, or heterologous hyperimmune sera, are also used for passive immunization. These are produced in animals (e.g., horses) and target toxins such as diphtheria and tetanus.

Whether passive immunization occurs *intentionally*, as in the case of immune globulin for intramuscular administration (IGIM) for prevention of hepatitis A, or *unintentionally*, as when antibodies accompany blood products transfused for other reasons (e.g., IGIV for Kawasaki disease), passively acquired antibodies can inactivate live-attenuated viral vaccines such as measles and varicella. One exception to this is RSV-mAb [see Chapter 11(IV)], which, because of its specificity for RSV alone, does not inactivate live vaccines. Yellow fever vaccine (which is also live-attenuated) does not appear to be inactivated by commercially available immune globulin products, probably because the titer of yellow fever antibody in the donors from whom these products are derived is low.

Table 1.3 summarizes characteristics of products used for passive immunization and gives some exam-

Table 1.4.   Intervals between antibody-containing products and measles and varicella vaccines

Product	Indication/usual dose[a]	Interval (mo)
RSV-mAb	Prevention of RSV (15 mg/kg IM)	None
IGIM	Pre- or postexposure (0.02 or 0.06 mL/kg IM) prophylaxis for hepatitis A	3
	Postexposure prophylaxis for measles, standard (0.25 mL/kg IM)	5
	Postexposure prophylaxis for measles, immunocompromised (0.5 mL/kg IM)	6
IGIV	Replacement therapy for immune deficiency[b] (400 mg/kg IV)	8
	ITP (400 mg/kg IV)	8
	ITP (1 g/kg IV)	10
	Kawasaki disease (2 g/kg IV)	11
Blood transfusion	Washed RBCs	None
	RBCs, adenine-saline added (10 mL/kg IV)	3
	Packed RBCs (10 mL/kg IV)	6
	Whole blood (10 mL/kg IV)	6
	Plasma or platelet products (10 mL/kg)	7
CMV-IGIV	Prevention of CMV disease in transplant patients (150 mg/kg IV)	6
HBIG	Postexposure prophylaxis for hepatitis B (0.06 mL/kg IM)	3
RSV-IGIV	Prevention of RSV (750 mg/kg IV)	9
RIG	Postexposure prophylaxis for rabies (20 IU/kg into wound and IM)	4
TIG	Postexposure prophylaxis for tetanus (250 U IM)	3
VZIG	Postexposure prophylaxis for varicella (125 U/10 kg IM)	5

[a]Details are given in Chapter 11.
[b]Live viral vaccines may be contraindicated in these patients anyway [see Chapters 5(V), 5(VII) and 12(I)].
Adapted from CDC. General recommendations on immunization: recommendations of the Advisory Committee on Immunization Practices (ACIP) and the American Academy of Family Physicians (AAFP). *MMWR* 2002;51 (RR-2):7.

ples. Table 1.4 gives suggested intervals between receipt of immune globulin products and measles and varicella vaccines.
  II. **General rules for active immunization.** The following general rules are useful to keep in mind:
    A. **There are no contraindications to simultaneous administration of any vaccines.** Simultaneous administration of all vaccines for which a child is eligible at a given visit is encouraged for two reasons: achievement of optimal protection is not delayed, and completion of all recommended vaccine series is more likely. There are no vaccines that cannot be given at the same time, consider-

ing both reactogenicity and immunogenicity, except for smallpox and varicella vaccines [Chapter 9(I)]. However, the vaccines must be given at separate sites and should never be mixed in the same syringe unless the products are specifically labeled for this purpose. The introduction of licensed combination vaccines (see Chapter 6) will reduce the high number of shots that is now unavoidable at certain visits.

B. Live parenteral vaccines not given simultaneously should be separated by at least 4 weeks. In general, different live vaccines can be given simultaneously. However, if parenteral live vaccines are given sequentially, they should be separated by at least 4 weeks so that replication of the first vaccine does not interfere with replication of the second (this phenomenon has been demonstrated with sequential administration of measles and varicella vaccines at intervals shorter than 30 days). Any timing sequence between a live parenteral and an inactivated vaccine, or a live oral and any other vaccine, is acceptable.

C. There are no minimum intervals between doses of different inactivated vaccines. Simultaneous administration or, better yet, the use of combination vaccines, is preferred because of improved compliance. However, there is no evidence that sequential administration of *different* inactivated vaccines at any time interval interferes with immunogenicity or increases reactogenicity.

D. There are minimum intervals between doses of the same vaccine. Proper spacing of doses in a given vaccine series is essential for an optimal immune response. For this reason, every effort should be made not to give sequential doses of the same vaccine too early. The Advisory Committee on Immunization Practices (ACIP) suggests a "grace period" wherein a dose given up to 4 days before the recommended interval should be counted as valid (except for rabies vaccine). However, some states may not accept this interpretation for their school entry requirements [(see Chapter 2(VI)], and the best advice is to give the vaccine at the recommended age and minimum interval. Invalid doses should be repeated, but the minimum interval should elapse between the invalid dose and the repeat dose. There *are* circumstances in which accelerated or compressed schedules can be used, such as in catch-up vaccination or impending international travel [see Chapter 12(V)]. However, even in such circumstances, practitioners should adhere to the minimum intervals. Table 1.5 shows the recommended minimum ages and intervals for routinely used vaccines.

E. There are minimum ages for administration of almost all vaccines. For live parenteral vaccines, the issue is inactivation of the vaccine by circulating maternal antibody, which can persist for as long as a year. For

Table 1.5.   Minimum vaccination ages and intervals

Vaccine	Dose	Recom-mended age	Mini-mum age	Recommended interval to next dose	Minimum interval to next dose
Hep-B	1[a]	Birth–2 mo	Birth	1–4 mo	4 wk
	2	1–4 mo	4 wk	2–17 mo	8 wk
	3[b]	6–18 mo	6 mo[c]	—	—
DTaP	1	2 mo	6 wk	2 mo	4 wk
	2	4 mo	10 wk	2 mo	4 wk
	3	6 mo	14 wk	6–12 mo	6 mo[c,d]
	4	15–18 mo	12 mo	3 yr	6 mo[c]
	5	4–6 yr	4 yr	—	—
Hib[e]	1[a]	2 mo	6 wk	2 mo	4 wk
	2	4 mo	10 wk	2 mo	4 wk
	3[f]	6 mo	14 wk	6–9 mo	8 wk
	4	12–15 mo	12 mo	—	—
IPV	1	2 mo	6 wk	2 mo	4 wk
	2	4 mo	10 wk	2–14 mo	4 wk
	3	6–18 mo	14 wk	3.5 yr	4 wk
	4	4–6 yr	18 wk	—	—
PCV-7[e]	1	2 mo	6 wk	2 mo	4 wk
	2	4 mo	10 wk	2 mo	4 wk
	3	6 mo	14 wk	6 mo	8 wk
	4	12–15 mo	12 mo	—	—
MMR	1	12–15 mo[g]	12 mo	3–5 yr	4 wk
	2	4–6 yr	13 mo	—	—
Varicella	1	12–18 mo	12 mo	—	—
	2[h]	—	—	4 wk	4 wk
Hep-A	1	≥2 yr	2 yr	6–18 mo[c]	6 mo[c]
	2	≥30 mo	30 mo	—	—
Inactivated influenza	1	—	6 mo[c]	—	—
	2[i]	—	—	1 mo	4 wk
Pne-PS	1	—	2 yr	5 yr[j]	5 yr
	2	—	7 yr[j]	—	—

[a]Neither PRP-OMP/Hep-B (COMVAX) nor DTaP3/Hep-B/IPV (Pediarix) should be given before 6 weeks of age.
[b]The third dose of Hep-B must be given at least 8 weeks after the second dose, 16 weeks after the first dose, and at 6 months of age or older.
[c]*Months* here refers to calendar months. For example, for a child born on January 6, a 6-month interval would be July 6.
[d]The minimum interval between the third and fourth dose of DTaP is 6 months. However, occasionally it has been discovered that this rule has been violated. In such cases, if the interval was less than 4 months, the fourth DTaP should be repeated. If the interval was 4 months or more, it does not need to be repeated.
[e]If the first dose is given at 7 months or more, fewer doses are required to complete the series [see Table 1.12 and Chapters 5(II) and 5(VI)].
[f]This dose is not required if the series includes only PRP-OMP (PedvaxHIB).
[g]During an outbreak in which measles is occurring in infants less than 12 months of age, MMR can be given as early as 6 months but *should not be counted* as part of the series.
[h]Children 13 years of age or older should receive two doses separated by at least 4 weeks.
[i]A second dose is recommended only for children 6 months to 8 years of age who are receiving the vaccine *for the first time.*
[j]Revaccination *one time only* is recommended for the highest-risk individuals [see Chapters 7(II) and 12(I)].
Adapted from CDC. General recommendations on immunization: recommendations of the Advisory Committee on Immunization Practices (ACIP) and the American Academy of Family Physicians (AAFP). *MMWR* 2002;51(RR-2):3.

other vaccines, such as Hib conjugate, administration in the first 6 weeks of life might induce immunologic tolerance. The exceptions to this rule are Hep-B and BCG, which are given at birth.

F. **Partial or fractional doses of a vaccine should never be used.** In the past, some practitioners have "split" doses of vaccines [particularly diphtheria, tetanus, and whole-cell pertussis vaccine (DTP)] into multiple smaller shots to minimize potential reactions. There is no support for this practice, even in premature infants. Less than full doses of vaccines should not be counted as valid.

G. **A multidose vaccine series should not be restarted if the recommended dosing interval is exceeded.** If there is a lapse in the administration of sequential doses of a given series, simply begin where the series was suspended, keeping in mind the minimum intervals between doses. The only exception to this rule is the oral typhoid Ty21a vaccine [see Chapter 8(IX)].

H. **Vaccines made by different manufacturers are generally interchangeable.** Vaccines from different manufacturers differ in composition, formulation, and content. However, sufficient data exist to consider the following vaccines interchangeable when completing a given vaccine series: diphtheria, tetanus, Hep-A, Hep-B, and inactivated poliovirus vaccine (IPV). Hib vaccines are also interchangeable, but if HibTITER (HbOC) or ActHIB (PRP-T) are used as the first or second dose, the primary series should include three doses [an all-PedvaxHIB (PRP-OMP) schedule requires only two doses for the primary series]. Because of limited data, the ACIP has expressed a preference for the same diphtheria, tetanus, and acellular pertussis vaccine (DTaP) product for the entire series. Practically speaking, however, this recommendation is difficult to implement, and the ACIP states that vaccination *should not be deferred* if the same product is not immediately available or if the previous products are not known. The situation is complicated because only Tripedia (DTaP2) and Infanrix (DTaP3) are licensed for the fifth dose, and this labeling technically applies only if the first four doses were the same vaccine. Thus, practitioners using DAPTACEL (DTaP5) for the first four doses are faced with the choice of using this product off label to complete the series or switching to a labeled product, thereby mixing products in the series.

I. **There is no harm in vaccinating a person who has already had the disease or the vaccine.** For some diseases, vaccination is *indicated* even if the person has had the disease. For example, infants younger than 2 years of age who had invasive Hib infection should still be vaccinated, because infection at that age does not result in effective immunity. For pneumococcus, the vaccine protects against multiple serotypes, so prior infection with a particular serotype does not obviate the need for vaccine. Influenza vaccine *must* be given each year whether or not the person has had the flu in the past. Some experts even recommend pertussis vaccine for children who have had well-documented disease (culture positive or epidemiologically linked to a culture-positive case) because the duration of natural immunity is not known. Clinicians often wonder whether a child with a questionable history of chickenpox or varicella vaccination should receive the vaccine. The motto here is *when in doubt, vaccinate!* With chickenpox, as with most other diseases, there is no evidence of harm if a person who has had the disease or the vaccine receives another dose of the vaccine. Exceptions to this rule include pneumococcal polysaccharide vaccine (Pne-PS) and possibly DTaP, for which reactogenicity may increase with increasing doses.

J. **There are limited indications for pre- or post-vaccination testing for immunity.** The only reason to test for existing immunity before vaccination is the potential for cost savings. For example, as most U.S. adults have had chickenpox, testing individuals with a negative personal history of disease may be more cost effective than administering two doses of the vaccine. However, in most circumstances, vaccines should be given without testing for immunity. A good example of this might be the child with a questionable vaccination history who is adopted from overseas [see Chapter 12(III)]; it is probably simpler to reimmunize than to test for immunity to multiple antigens. For the most part, immunity is presumed to result from appropriate vaccine schedules and doses. Testing for seroconversion is indicated in rare situations, such as in high-risk health care workers or dialysis patients given Hep-B vaccine or laboratory workers receiving preexposure rabies vaccination.

III. **Vaccine handling.** Mishandling of vaccines can reduce potency and leave individuals susceptible to disease. Table 1.6 gives specific information on the handling and storage of common vaccines, and the following list provides some general rules:

- Designate one person (and a back-up person) in charge of inventory, handling, and storage
- Maintain an inventory log, including product name, manufacturer and lot number, doses received, date received, condition on arrival, and expiration date
- Inspect products on delivery, including integrity of containers and cold-chain monitoring devices
- Store immediately under appropriate conditions
- Discard mishandled and expired vaccines (vaccines can be used until the last day of the month indicated on the expiration date)

Table 1.6. Handling and storage of common vaccines

Vaccine	Storage	Approximate shelf life (yr)	Reconstitution
DTaP[a]	Refrigerate[b] Do not freeze[c]	1.5	Not required
DT and Td	Refrigerate Do not freeze	2	Not required
DTaP2/PRP-T (Tri-HIBit)	Refrigerate Do not freeze	1.5	Required (use within 30 min)
Hep-A[d]	Refrigerate Do not freeze	3	Not required
Hep-B[a,d,e]	Refrigerate Do not freeze	3	Not required
Hib conjugates[d,e]	Refrigerate Do not freeze	2	Required for PRP-T (ActHIB) (use within 24 h)
Inactivated influenza	Refrigerate Do not freeze	Current season only	Not required
IPV[a]	Refrigerate Do not freeze	1	Not required
Men-PS	Refrigerate Do not freeze	2	Required (use single dose within 30 min and multidose within 35 d)
MMR	Refrigerate Can freeze Protect from light Store diluent at room temperature or refrigerate	2	Required (refrigerate, protect from light, use within 8 h)
PCV-7	Refrigerate Do not freeze	1.5	Not required
Pne-PS	Refrigerate Do not freeze	2	Not required
Varicella	Must freeze[f] Unreconstituted vaccine can be temporarily refrigerated up to 72 h Store diluent at room temperature or refrigerate	1.5	Required (use within 30 min)

[a]Includes DTaP3/Hep-B/IPV (Pediarix).
[b]*Refrigerate* means maintaining the temperature at 35°F to 46°F (2°C to 8°C).
[c]*Freeze* means maintaining the temperature at 5°F (−15°C) or lower.
[d]Shelf life of Hep-A/Hep-B (Twinrix) is approximately 2 years.
[e]Includes PRP-OMP/Hep-B (COMVAX).
[f]Must be in a separate freezer compartment (*not a dormitory-style freezer*) without freeze-thaw cycles.
Adapted from CDC. Vaccine management: recommendations for handling and storage of selected biologicals (January 2001). http://www.cdc.gov/nip/publications/vac_mgt_book.pdf (accessed 01/26/03); AAP. Active immunization. In: Pickering LK, ed. *Red book: 2003 report of the Committee on Infectious Diseases*, 26th ed. Elk Grove Village, IL: American Academy of Pediatrics, 2003:7–53.

- Disregard and repeat doses that were inadvertently given with mishandled or expired vaccine
- Do not open more than one multidose vial at a time
- Do not prefill syringes with vaccines that are supplied in vials
- Follow these refrigerator and freezer rules:
  - Do not store food in the vaccine refrigerator or freezer
  - Store vaccines in the middle of the shelf, not on the door
  - Use clearly labeled, color-coded trays for each product and include separate compartments for unopened and opened vials (record the date of opening or reconstitution directly on the label)
  - Rotate stock (place newly received vaccines behind current supplies)
  - Post a sign that specifies which vaccines are stored in the refrigerator and which are stored in the freezer
  - Keep a thermometer in the refrigerator and freezer and record the temperatures on a log when the office opens in the morning and when it closes in the evening. Appropriate ranges are 35°F to 46°F (2°C to 8°C) for the refrigerator and 5°F (−15°C) or lower for the freezer. A recording thermometer can also be used
  - Keep water containers in the refrigerator to help maintain steady temperatures
  - Keep upside-down ice trays in the freezer to help maintain steady temperatures and to monitor for melting
  - Place a "DO NOT UNPLUG" sign near the outlet for the refrigerator and freezer units
  - Do not use an outlet with a ground fault interrupter (i.e., one with "test" and "reset" buttons) or one connected to a wall switch
  - Use plug guards to prevent accidental dislodging
  - In the event of power failure, mark exposed products and contact the manufacturer or state health department

IV. Contraindications and precautions. A *contraindication* is a condition that *increases the likelihood of a serious adverse event*; when present, the vaccine should not be given. The only true permanent contraindication for all vaccines, based on a definitive risk, is severe allergy or anaphylaxis to the vaccine or any of its components. In this regard, it should be mentioned that most vaccines contain buffers as well as excipients, which are substances other than the vaccine that are included in the manufacturing process or added to the final product. In addition, there may be contaminating substances that carry over from early steps in processing, and some vial stoppers contain latex, which can carry over to the patient during the injection. Both excipients and contaminants can be triggers for allergic reactions in sensitized patients. The best advice is to check the package insert before administering any vaccine.

A permanent contraindication to further doses of DTaP is acute encephalopathy within 7 days of vaccination, based on the theoretic possibility of exacerbation or recurrence of encephalopathy. Pregnancy is a contraindication for live vaccines based on theoretic risks to the fetus and the possibility that naturally occurring birth defects might be attributed to the vaccine [see Chapter 12(II)]. However, there is no definitive evidence of fetal damage from any live vaccine. In addition, in some circumstances, the benefits may outweigh the risks (for example, live-attenuated yellow fever vaccine can be considered for pregnant women traveling to high-risk areas). Although live vaccines are generally contraindicated in persons with immune incompetence, there may again be situations in which the benefits outweigh the risks [see Chapter 12(I)]. For example, natural varicella probably represents a greater risk to a DiGeorge syndrome patient with mildly impaired cellular immunity than does the live-attenuated vaccine.

A *precaution* is a condition that *might increase the risk* of a serious adverse event, *compromise the immunogenicity* of the vaccine, or be *mistaken for a vaccine reaction*. When a precaution is present, the vaccine may still be given if the benefits outweigh the risks. In making these judgments, the provider must balance the prevailing epidemiology of disease and the patient's personal circumstances with the possibility of a missed opportunity. For example, a provider may want to give further DTaP vaccinations to an infant who experienced high fever after his first dose if there is an appreciable amount of pertussis in the community. Likewise, the 6-month shots could be given to a child who has a moderate febrile illness *if* there is substantial risk that the child will not return for vaccination after the illness resolves.

Table 1.7 gives notable contraindications and precautions for selected vaccines, derived from recommendations of the ACIP, the American Academy of Pediatrics (AAP), and vaccine manufacturers. Issues with individual vaccines generally apply to combinations.

Misconceptions about vaccine contraindications can result in missed opportunities. Table 1.8 lists some of these erroneous contraindications; if present, vaccines can and should be given.

V. Schedules

A. Childhood immunization schedule. In January of every year, the ACIP, AAP, and American Academy of Family Physicians (AAFP) release a harmonized childhood immunization schedule that graphically summarizes the recommendations for routine immunization of children in the United States. A modified version of the 2003 schedule is given in Table 1.9. Specifics about the vaccines are given in the footnotes and the indicated chapters of this book.

B. Adult immunization schedule. In October 2002, the ACIP released the first routine vaccination schedule for individuals 19 years of age or older. This schedule was developed in conjunction with the AAFP, the American

Table 1.7. Contraindications and precautions to further vaccine doses

Vaccine	Contraindications		Precaution	
	Condition	Reason	Condition	Reason
All vaccines	Severe allergic reaction[a] or anaphylaxis to vaccine or vaccine component[b]	Anaphylaxis	Moderate to severe acute illness	Difficulty distinguishing illness from vaccine reaction
			Latex allergy	Natural rubber in syringe and stopper
BCG	Immune deficiency or immune suppression[c]	Disease from live bacterial vaccine	—	
DTaP	Encephalopathy within 7 d	Recurrent encephalopathy	Fever ≥104.9°F (40.5°C), hypotonic-hyporesponsive episode, or inconsolable crying ≥3 h within 48 h	Recurrent reaction
	Evolving neurologic disorder	Difficulty distinguishing illness from vaccine reaction	Seizure within 3 d	Recurrent reaction
DTaP, DT, or Td	—	—	Guillain-Barré syndrome within 6 wk of tetanus-containing vaccine	Recurrent Guillain-Barré syndrome
Hep-A	—	—	Pregnancy	Theoretical risk
Hep-B	Allergy to baker's yeast	Anaphylaxis	Weight <2,000 g unless mother is HBsAg-positive	Poor immunogenicity
Hib conjugate	Age <6 wk	Induction of immune tolerance	—	
Inactivated influenza	Egg allergy[d]	Anaphylaxis	Guillain-Barré syndrome within 6 wk of previous influenza vaccine	Recurrent Guillain-Barré syndrome
			Pregnancy	Theoretical risk
IPV	Allergy to neomycin, streptomycin, or polymyxin-B	Anaphylaxis		

	Pregnancy	Possible fetal effects of live vaccine	Recent receipt of antibody-containing blood product[e]	Inactivation of live vaccine
MMR	Immune deficiency or immune suppression[c]; Allergy to neomycin or gelatin	Disease from live vaccine; Anaphylaxis	History of thrombocytopenia or thrombocytopenic purpura; Tuberculosis or positive skin test; Antibiotic therapy	Recurrent thrombocytopenia; Exacerbation of disease; Poor immunogenicity
Typhoid (oral Ty21a)	Immune deficiency or immune suppression[c]	Disease from live vaccine	—	—
Varicella	Immune deficiency or immune suppression[c]; Allergy to neomycin or gelatin; Untreated tuberculosis	Disease from live vaccine; Anaphylaxis; Exacerbation of disease	Recent receipt of antibody-containing blood product[e]; —; —; —	Inactivation of live vaccine; —; —; —
YF	Egg allergy[d]; Immune deficiency or immune suppression[c]; Age <4 mo	Anaphylaxis; Encephalitis; Encephalitis	—	—

[a] Severe allergy is IgE-mediated, occurs in minutes to hours, and requires medical attention. Examples include generalized urticaria, facial swelling, airway obstruction, wheezing, hypotension, and shock. Delayed-type hypersensitivity is generally not a contraindication.

[b] Vaccines contain trace components, excipients, and residual media, and these components may differ from one manufacturer to another. The table lists particularly common components that may induce allergic reactions. Some vaccines (e.g., influenza, Japanese encephalitis, Men-PS, Pne-PS) still contain thimerosal. Patients with severe allergy to latex should not receive vaccines supplied in vials or syringes that contain natural rubber.

[c] See Chapter 12(I).

[d] Being able to eat eggs without adverse effects is a reasonable indication of a very low risk of anaphylaxis. Mild or local manifestations of allergy to eggs or feathers are not contraindications. Skin testing with the vaccine can be done according to a protocol described in the AAP Red Book.

[e] Blood products including IGIV, IGIM, and hyperimmune globulin contain various amounts of antibodies to these vaccine viruses. The suggested interval before vaccination depends on the product (see Table 1.4). This is not an issue for monoclonal antibody products such as RSV-mAb (Synagis).

Adapted from CDC. General recommendations on immunization: recommendations of the Advisory Committee on Immunization Practices (ACIP) and the American Academy of Family Physicians (AAFP). *MMWR* 2002;51(RR-2):8–11; AAP Active immunization. In: Pickering LK, ed. *Red book: 2003 report of the Committee on Infectious Diseases,* 26th ed. Elk Grove Village, IL: American Academy of Pediatrics, 2003:7–53;798–801.

Table 1.8.   Erroneous contraindications to vaccination

Mild acute illness with fever, respiratory symptoms, or diarrhea, including most cases of otitis media
Convalescent phase of illness
Antibiotic therapy[a]
Low-grade fever and/or local redness, pain, and swelling after previous dose
Prematurity[b]
Pregnant, unimmunized, or immunosuppressed household contact[c]
Exposure to an infectious disease
Positive tuberculin skin test without active disease[d]
Simultaneous tuberculin skin testing
Breast-feeding[c]
Allergy to penicillin, duck meat or feathers, or environmental allergens
Seizures, sudden infant death syndrome, allergies, or vaccine adverse events in family members
Malnutrition

[a]Except live oral typhoid (Ty21a).
[b]The birth dose of Hep-B should be delayed (because of poor immunogenicity) in infants weighing less than 2,000 g whose mothers are HbsAg negative [see Chapter 5(III)].
[c]Preevent smallpox vaccination is an exception [Chapter 9(I)].
[d]MMR is an exception,
Adapted from CDC. General recommendations on immunization: recommendations of the Advisory Committee on Immunization Practices (ACIP) and the American Academy of Family Physicians (AAFP). *MMWR* 2002;51(RR-2):8–11; AAP. Active immunization. In: Pickering LK, ed. *Red book: 2003 report of the Committee on Infectious Diseases*, 26th ed. Elk Grove Village, IL: American Academy of Pediatrics, 2003:798–801.

College of Obstetricians and Gynecologists (ACOG), the American College of Physicians–American Society of Internal Medicine (ACP-ASIM), and the Infectious Diseases Society of America (IDSA). Table 1.10 shows the basic recommendations by age group; indications, contraindications, and details regarding administration are contained in the indicated chapters of this book. Table 1.11 shows the recommended vaccines for specific medical conditions, along with chapter references. The adult immunization schedule is updated annually.

C. **Catch-up.** Unimmunized children should be caught up as quickly as possible, using simultaneous administration of all vaccines for which they are eligible at each visit and bearing in mind the minimum intervals between doses (Table 1.5). Table 1.12 gives recommended vaccines for unimmunized children by age group.

D. **Uncertain immunization status.** If immunization status cannot be ascertained through official documents (e.g., physicians' records or the patient's shot card), the child should receive all age-appropriate vaccines as if he or she had never been immunized (Tables 1.9 and 1.12).

Table 1.9.   Childhood immunization schedule, 2003

Vaccine (route)	Chapter	Birth	1 mo	2 mo	4 mo	6 mo	12 mo	15 mo	18 mo	24 mo	4–6 yr	11–12 yr	13–18 yr
Hep-B[a] (IM)	5(III)	1st dose[b]		2nd dose[c,d]			3rd dose[c,d]					Catch-up[e]	
DTaP (IM)	5(I)			1st dose[d]	2nd dose[d]	3rd dose[d]			4th dose[f]		5th dose		Td[g]
Hib (IM)	5(II)			1st dose[c]	2nd dose[c]	3rd dose[h]	4th dose[c]						
IPV (IM, SC)	5(IV)			1st dose[d]	2nd dose[d]	3rd dose[d]			4th dose[d]		4th dose		
MMR (SC)	5(V)						1st dose[i]				2nd dose[i]	Catch-up	
Varicella (SC)	5(VII)						1 dose					Catch-up[j]	
PCV-7 (IM)	5(VI)			1st dose	2nd dose	3rd dose	4th dose				High-risk groups[k]		
Hep-A (IM)	8(IV)									High-risk groups and selected regions[l]			
Influenza (IM)	7(III)						Encouraged annually for children 6–23 mo of age and recommended for high-risk groups[m]						

[a] Hep-B has very specific timing rules:
- Second dose must be at least 4 weeks after the first dose.
- Third dose must be at least 16 weeks after the first dose and 8 weeks after the second dose.
- The last dose (third or fourth) should not be given before 6 months of age.

[b] Only *monovalent* vaccine can be used before 6 weeks of age. The first dose can be given at any time between birth and 2 months of age *only* if the mother is known to be HBsAg-negative.

[c] PRP-OMP/Hep-B (COMVAX) can be used here *but not before 6 weeks of age* [see Chapter 6(III)]. Potential overimmunization with Hep-B is not a problem.

[d] DTaP3/Hep-B/IPV (Pediarix) can be used here *but not before 6 weeks of age* [see Chapter 6(V)]. Potential overimmunization with Hep-B is not a problem.

[e] A two-dose regimen of RECOMBIVAX HB is available for ages 11 to 15 years.

[f] Can be given as early as 12 months of age if child is unlikely to return. Interval between third and fourth doses must be at least 6 months.

[g] One dose at 11 to 12 years of age if at least 5 years have elapsed since last tetanus and diphtheria vaccine. Subsequent boosters are given every 10 years.

[h] This dose is not required if PRP-OMP (PedvaxHIB or COMVAX) is used for the Hib series.

[i] The second dose can be administered at any time as long as 4 weeks or more have elapsed after the first dose and both doses are received before 12 years of age.

[j] Children 13 years of age or older need two doses separated by 4 weeks or longer.

[k] Pne-PS may also be indicated for certain high-risk children [see Chapters 7(II) and 12(I)].

[l] Two doses are given 6 months or more apart.

[m] First vaccination at 8 years of age or younger requires two doses separated by 4 weeks or more. Live-attenuated intranasal vaccine can be used in children 5 to 18 years of age [see Chapter 10(VIII)].
Adapted from AAP Recommended childhood and adolescent immunization schedule—United States, 2003. *Pediatrics* 2003;111:212. See book chapters for specific recommendations.

Table 1.10. Adult immunization schedule by age, 2002–2003

Vaccine (route)	Chapter	Age group		
		19–49 yr	50–64 yr	≥65 yr
Td (IM)	7(I)	1 booster dose every 10 yr		
Influenza (IM)	7(III)	1 annual dose if medically indicated or if requested regardless of indication[a]		1 annual dose
Pne-PS (IM, SC)	7(II)	1 dose if medically indicated (revaccinate once after 5 yr for certain conditions)		1 dose (revaccinate once after 5 yr if first vaccine given at <65 yr of age)
Hep-B (IM)	5(III)	3 doses (0, 1–2, 4–6 mo) if medically indicated		
Hep-A (IM)	8(IV)	2 doses separated by 6–12 mo if medically indicated		
MMR (SC)	5(V)	1 dose if unvaccinated or vaccine history unreliable and born after 1956 (high-risk individuals should receive 2 doses separated by 4–8 wk)		
Varicella (SC)	5(VII)	2 doses separated by 4–8 wk if susceptible		
Men-PS (SQ)	8(VII)	1 dose if medically indicated		

[a]Live-attenuated intranasal vaccine can be used here [see Chapter 10(VIII)].
Adapted from CDC. Recommended adult immunization schedule—United States, 2002–2003. *MMWR Morb Mortal Wkly Rep* 2002;51:904–908. See book chapters for specific recommendations.

Table 1.11. Immunization schedule for adults with medical conditions, 2002–2003

Medical condition	Chapter	Td	Inactivated influenza	Pne-PS	Hep-B	Hep-A	MMR	Varicella
				Vaccine				
Pregnancy	12(II)	Yes	2nd or 3rd trimester during influenza season	If otherwise indicated and benefits outweigh risks	If otherwise indicated and benefits outweigh risks	If otherwise indicated and benefits outweigh risks	Contraindicated	Contraindicated
Diabetes, heart disease, chronic pulmonary disease, chronic liver disease, alcoholism	12(I)	Yes	Yes[a]	Yes[b]	If otherwise indicated	If otherwise indicated (especially liver disease)	Catch-up	Catch-up
Congenital immunodeficiency, leukemia, lymphoma, generalized malignancy, therapy with alkylating agents, antimetabolites, radiation, high-dose steroids	12(I)	Yes	Yes	Yes (revaccinate once after 5 yr)	If otherwise indicated	If otherwise indicated	Contraindicated	Persons with isolated humoral deficiency may be vaccinated
Renal failure, hemodialysis, recipients of clotting factor concentrates	12(I)	Yes	Yes	Yes (revaccinate once after 5 yr)	Yes (special dose for dialysis)	If otherwise indicated	Catch-up	Catch-up

(continued)

Table 1.11. *Continued*

Medical condition	Chapter	Td	Inactivated influenza	Pne-PS	Hep-B	Hep-A	MMR	Varicella
							Vaccine	
Asplenia, terminal complement component deficiency[c]	12(I)	Yes	Yes	Yes (revaccinate once after 5 yr)	If otherwise indicated	If otherwise indicated	Catch-up	Catch-up
HIV infection	12(I)	Yes	Yes	Yes (revaccinate once after 5 yr)	Yes	If otherwise indicated	If otherwise indicated and not severely immunosuppressed	No[d]

[a]Chronic liver disease and alcoholism are not indicator conditions per se, but give vaccine if other indications are present or if patient requests it.

[b]Asthma is not an indication for pneumococcal vaccine.

[c]These patients should receive Men-PS as well. In the case of elective splenectomy, Men-PS and Pne-PS should be given 2 weeks or more before surgery.

[d]Varicella vaccine *is* recommended for certain children with HIV infection [see Chapter 5(VII)].

Adapted from CDC. Recommended adult immunization schedule—United States, 2002–2003. *MMWR Morb Mortal Wkly Rep* 2002;51:904–908. See book chapters for specific recommendations.

Table 1.12.   Catch-up schedule for children and adolescents

		Ages 4 mo–6 yr (minimum intervals between doses are shown)			
Vaccine	Minimum age for dose 1	Dose 2	Dose 3	Dose 4	Dose 5
DTaP	6 wk	4 wk after dose 1	4 wk after dose 2	6 mo after dose 3	6 mo after dose 4[a]
IPV	6 wk	4 wk after dose 1	4 wk after dose 2	4 wk after dose 3[b]	
Hep-B	Birth	4 wk after dose 1	8 wk after dose 2 and 16 wk after dose 1		
MMR	12 mo	4 wk after dose 1			
Varicella	12 mo				
Hib[c]	6 wk	If dose 1 given at <12 mo of age: 4 wk after dose 1 If dose 1 given at 12–14 mo of age: 8 wk after dose 1 (final dose)	If currently <12 mo of age: 4 wk after dose 2[d] If currently ≥12 mo of age and dose 2 given at <15 mo of age: 8 wk after dose 2 (final dose)[d]	If currently 12 mo–5 yr of age and received 3 doses at <12 mo of age: 8 wk after dose 3 (final dose)	
PCV-7[e]	6 wk	If currently <24 mo of age and dose 1 given at <12 mo of age: 4 wk after dose 1 If currently 24–59 mo of age or dose 1 given at ≥12 mo of age: 8 wk after dose 1 (final dose)	If currently <12 mo of age: 4 wk after dose 2 If currently ≥12 mo of age: 8 wk after dose 2 (final dose)	If currently 12 mo–5 yr of age and received 3 doses at <12 mo of age: 8 wk after dose 3 (final dose)	

(continued)

Table 1.12. *Continued*

Vaccine	Dose 2	Dose 3	Booster dose
		Ages 7–18 yr (minimum intervals between doses are shown)	
Td	4 wk after dose 1	6 mo after dose 2	If currently <11 yr of age and dose 1 given at <12 mo of age: 6 mo after dose 3 If currently ≥11 yr of age and dose 1 given at ≥12 mo of age and dose 3 given at <7 yr of age: 5 yr after dose 3 If dose 3 given at ≥7 yr of age: 10 yr after dose 3
IPV[f]	4 wk after dose 1	4 wk after dose 2	
Hep-B	4 wk after dose 1	8 wk after dose 2 and 16 wk after dose 1	
MMR	4 wk after dose 1		
Varicella	If ≥13 yr of age at dose 1: 4 wk after dose 1		

[a]Not necessary if fourth dose received at 4 years of age or older.

[b]Not necessary if fourth dose received at 4 years of age or older, unless child received a mixed OPV/IPV series.

[c]If one dose is given at 15 months of age or older, no further doses are needed. Not recommended for children 5 years of age or older.

[d]If first two doses were PRP-OMP (PedvaxHIB or COMVAX), the third and final dose should be given at 12 to 15 months of age and at least 8 weeks after the second dose.

[e]If one dose is given at 24 months of age or older, no further doses are needed. Not recommended for children 5 years of age or older.

[f]Not routinely recommended 18 years of age or older.

Adapted from AAP. Recommended childhood and adolescent immunization schedule—United States, 2003. *Pediatrics* 2003;111:212. See book chapters for specific recommendations.

VI. Effective vaccine delivery

A. Missed opportunities. Standard 4 for pediatric immunization practices [see Chapter 2(II)] calls for providers to use all clinical encounters to assess immunization status and administer vaccines for which the child is eligible, as long as true contraindications do not exist. The intent of this standard is to prevent contacts with the health care system from becoming *missed opportunities* for vaccination. Common reasons for why opportunities are missed are listed below:

- Failure of providers to consider acute care visits as a time to catch up on immunizations
- Inability to determine immunization status through patient recall, shot cards, or contact with primary care providers
- Erroneous contraindications (Table 1.8)
- Failure to give all needed vaccines simultaneously

Additional barriers may exist in emergency departments and other acute care facilities, including time constraints, insurance reimbursement, and the perception that by giving routine immunizations, the patient's relationship with his primary care provider is disrupted.

B. Reminder, recall, and tracking systems. *Reminders* are messages that immunizations are due. They may be directed at parents in the form of telephone calls (by humans or computers) or mailings (simple post cards are adequate), or they may be directed at physicians in the form of chart flags indicating that vaccines are due. *Recall* messages are notices to parents or patients that vaccinations are overdue. *Tracking systems*, which can be manual or computerized, allow each child's immunization status to be followed precisely.

Studies have consistently shown improvements in immunization rates for both children and adults if these messaging systems are used. Establishment of tracking systems is called for by Standard 12 for pediatric immunization practices [see Chapter 2(II)]. In addition, the AAP released a statement in 1995 supporting the development of tracking systems in both private and public sectors, and the following guidelines were offered (among others):

- Goals should include documenting immunization status, increasing immunization rates, decreasing costs of immunization, and facilitating immunization opportunities
- There should be accurate documentation of each child's immunization status
- Confidentiality should be preserved
- Data should be available at all times to ensure that all opportunities to immunize are used
- Data should not be used to sanction health care workers
- Data input and access should be easy

Table 1.13.   Benefits of immunization registries

Ensure that children remain current with recommendations
Provide recalls and reminders
Ensure timely vaccination after changes in location or provider
Prevent unnecessary immunization
Provide official, accurate documentation of immunization history
Assess coverage rates
Identify high-risk populations
Prevent disease outbreaks
Link with other databases (e.g., newborn screening)
Streamline immunization program management
Reduce provider paperwork
Facilitate introduction of new vaccines
Integrate vaccinations with other public health services
Facilitate monitoring of adverse events

Adapted from CDC. Development of community- and state-based immunization registries: CDC response to a report from the National Vaccine Advisory Committee. *MMWR* 2001;50(RR-17):1–17.

- Incomplete immunization status should not be used to deny any child access to care or eligibility for insurance benefits
- Collaboration between public and private initiatives should include the ability to link databases

C. **Immunization registries.** Registries are confidential, population-based, centralized computerized systems that maintain information about children's immunizations. The ideal registry contains all children in a geographic area and receives vaccination data from all regional providers. The need for registries is driven by a simple fact: An increasingly complex vaccine schedule must be administered to children who frequently relocate and change health care providers. This results in vaccination histories that are incomplete and fragmented, leading to a spectrum of errors ranging from missed opportunities to unnecessary duplication. For these reasons, one Healthy People 2010 [see Chapter 2(I)] goal is for at least 95% of children less than 6 years of age to participate in fully operational population-based registries (currently, fewer than half of children have vaccinations recorded in a registry). The potential benefits of immunization registries are summarized in Table 1.13.

The CDC has supported the development of state registries since 1993 through Section 317 Public Health Service grants. In 1998, the National Vaccine Advisory Committee (NVAC) launched the Initiative on Immunization Registries to facilitate community- and state-based registries. Four major challenges were identified that have been addressed by the Centers for Disease Control and Prevention (CDC):

- *Protecting confidentiality*—The need to gather and share information must be balanced with the family's right to privacy. Minimum specifications include executing written confidentiality policies, notifying parents of the existence of the registry and allowing them to opt out, and defining who has access and for what purposes the information can be used.

- *Participation by providers and recipients*—Because the majority of vaccine delivery has shifted to the private sector, efforts to recruit private providers are essential. Part of what makes a registry attractive to providers is simplicity, minimization of administrative burden, high quality of data, and functionality (e.g., ability to generate reminders).
- *Operational challenges*—The functional capabilities of registry hardware and software differ from community to community; this is not conducive to the overall goal of seamless information exchange. For this reason, the CDC developed the following 12 operational standards:
  - Electronically store core data elements: name, birth date, sex, birth state, mother's name, vaccine type, manufacturer, lot number, and immunization date
  - Record initiation within 6 weeks of birth
  - Have information available at each health visit
  - Receive and process information within 1 month of vaccination
  - Protect confidentiality of medical information
  - Protect security of medical information
  - Exchange information using accepted communication standards (Health Level 7)
  - Automatically identify vaccines needed at each visit
  - Automatically identify persons due for immunizations and produce recall and reminder notices
  - Produce official coverage reports
  - Produce authorized shot records
  - Promote accuracy and completion
- *Resources to maintain registries*—Registries are likely to result in cost savings by reducing the manual labor involved in pulling medical records for provider visits, managed care reporting, and school system review. Additional cost savings should accrue from eliminating duplicate immunizations and reducing disease burden. It costs approximately 5 or 6 U.S. dollars per child per year to maintain a registry, and in 1999, only 40% of this cost was covered by federal sources. In 2000, the Centers for Medicare and Medicaid Services (CMS, formerly the Health Care Financing Administration or HCFA) agreed to pay 90% of the development costs for a registry for Medicaid recipients.

VII. Monitoring immunization coverage and effectiveness. Immunization coverage and the occurrence of vaccine-preventable diseases in the United States are monitored by a number of mechanisms. Contact information for these surveys and organizations is given in Chapter 14(VI).

A. National Notifiable Disease Surveillance System (NNDSS). This is the country's primary mechanism for monitoring disease activity. Reportable diseases and their

Table 1.14.   National Immunization Survey vaccination coverage levels, ages 19 to 35 months

Vaccine (doses)	1997 (%)	2001 (%)
DTP/DT/DTaP (≥ 4)	81.5	82.1
Polio (≥ 3)	90.8	89.4
Hib (≥ 3)	92.7	93.0
MMR (≥ 1)	90.5	91.4
Hep-B (≥ 3)	83.7	88.9
Varicella (≥ 1)	25.9	76.3
4:3:1:3[a]	76.2	77.2
4:3:1:3:3[b]	—	73.7

[a]4 DTP/DT/DTaP:3 IPV:1 MMR:3 Hib.
[b]4 DTP/DT/DTaP:3 IPV:1 MMR:3 Hib:3 Hep-B.
Adapted from CDC. National, state, and urban area vaccination coverage levels among children aged 19–35 months—United States, 2001. *MMWR Morb Mortal Wkly Rep* 2002;51:664–666.

respective case definitions (now numbering more than 50) are designated by the Council of State and Territorial Epidemiologists in collaboration with the CDC. Reporting occurs at the state level, and the data are forwarded to the CDC, which launches investigations when appropriate. Specific surveillance systems are in place for congenital rubella syndrome, poliomyelitis, and diphtheria, and the CDC supports surveillance efforts for measles, pertussis, tetanus, Hib, and hepatitis B. Bacterial meningitis is monitored through laboratory-based surveillance, as is influenza, supplemented by death certificate data. Increased vaccine-preventable disease activity is a marker for suboptimal immunization coverage.

B. National Immunization Survey (NIS). Conducted annually since 1994, the NIS is a random digit–dialing telephone survey of households in the United States that estimates vaccine coverage among children 19 to 35 months of age. A mail survey of providers is also conducted to validate the information obtained from families. The survey includes all 50 states and 27 urban areas; in 2001, 33,437 household interviews were completed. Data regarding the number of children who are up-to-date on DTaP, polio, measles, Hib, Hep-B, and varicella immunizations are collected. In addition, series completion is assessed. Table 1.14 shows coverage rates for 1997 and 2001. Data from the 2000 survey demonstrated that, whereas overall coverage by 24 months of age is good, nine out of ten children received at least one vaccine outside of the recommended age range.

C. National Health Interview Survey (NIHS). This survey, which covers a broad range of health issues, has been conducted by the National Center for Health Statistics at the CDC since 1957. Personal interviews are conducted in approximately 43,000 households repre-

Table 1.15.   Immunization coverage among adults 65 years of age or older

Vaccine	NHIS (%)		BRFSS (%)	
	1995	1997	1995	1997
Influenza in previous 12 mo	58	—	60	66
Tetanus in previous 10 yr	40	—	—	—
Pneumococcal ever	34	—	38	46

Adapted from CDC. Influenza, pneumococcal, and tetanus toxoid vaccination of adults—United States, 1993–1997. *MMWR Morb Mortal Wkly Rep* 2000;49:39–62.

senting 106,000 persons each year. In 1991, a child immunization supplement was added. The survey is also an important source of information about adult vaccine coverage (Table 1.15).

D. Behavioral Risk Factor Surveillance System (BRFSS). This is a random digit–dialing telephone survey of adults conducted by state health departments with assistance from the National Centers for Chronic Disease Prevention and Health Promotion at the CDC. The data obtained are very useful for issues such as influenza and pneumococcal vaccine coverage (Table 1.15).

E. Retrospective school entry surveys. This is the most common form of state and local level surveillance. Coverage data are collected from the health records of randomly selected schools, and an assessment is made of vaccine coverage. Audits are performed to validate school entry data. The data necessarily lag several years behind current performance because children are 5 or 6 when they enter school. In addition, no information on the timing of immunizations is obtained.

F. Special area and population surveys. These studies involve small geographic units, such as counties or census tracts, or specific populations in a local area, such as Medicaid participants. These studies, largely supported by federal grants, facilitate targeting of needy groups and ensure accountability within the public and private health care sectors.

G. Clinical Assessment Software Application (CASA). This software package, available from the CDC, can be used by a provider to audit immunization performance at the facility [see Chapter 2(II)].

H. Health Plan Employer Data and Information Set (HEDIS). The National Committee for Quality Assurance, an independent nonprofit organization, monitors the performance of managed health care plans through a set of standardized measures called HEDIS. Immunization rates on preschoolers, children, adolescents and adults are captured through claims made, encounter data, and chart review.

Standards and Regulations

I. Healthy People 2010 objectives. The *Healthy People 2010: Objectives for Improving Health* report, issued January 25, 2000, is a comprehensive set of health objectives for the United States to achieve over the first decade of the new century. An extension of the 1979 Surgeon General's Report entitled *Healthy People* and *Healthy People 2000: National Health Promotion and Disease Prevention Objectives*, the Healthy People 2010 initiative identifies the most significant preventable threats to health and focuses public and private efforts to address those threats. The agenda was developed over several years by scientists, federal and state agencies, and national professional organizations, with input from the public.

Healthy People 2010 has two overarching goals: to increase quality and years of healthy life and to eliminate health disparities. Twenty-eight focus areas are identified, one of which is Immunization and Infectious Diseases, wherein the following aspects of vaccines are emphasized:

- Vaccines can prevent disease and death from infectious diseases, but they do not necessarily eliminate the causative organisms; by extension, decreased vaccine coverage can lead to reemergence of disease
- Vaccines protect individuals, and vaccinated individuals protect society through herd immunity
- Vaccines provide significant cost benefits

Tremendous progress in reducing indigenous cases of vaccine-preventable diseases is noted, successes mediated by outreach to underserved populations, expansion of school entry requirements, public financing of childhood vaccinations, and the widespread use of novel, highly effective vaccines such as the Hib conjugates. However, the report highlights the persistence of underserved groups and the fact that most vaccine-preventable diseases in the United States occur in adults, who are much less likely than children to be appropriately immunized.

The following strategies to continue protecting people from vaccine-preventable diseases are outlined in the report:

- Improving the quality and quantity of vaccine delivery services
- Minimizing financial barriers
- Increasing community participation, education, and partnership
- Improving the monitoring of disease and vaccine coverage
- Developing new or improved vaccines and improving vaccine use

The report sets objectives for 2010 for prevention of disease through universal and targeted vaccination programs. These goals are summarized in Table 2.1. The report also sets the goal for coverage with universally recommended vaccines at 90%. Baseline rates for three doses of *Haemophilus influenzae* type b (Hib); one dose of measles, mumps, and rubella (MMR); and three doses of polio vaccine in 1998 actually exceeded that mark, whereas the rates for four doses of diphtheria, tetanus, and acellular pertussis vaccine (DTaP) and three doses of hepatitis B vaccine (Hep-B) were slightly below. The rate for varicella vaccine at that time was only 43%.

II. **Standards for pediatric immunization practices.** In 1992, a working group convened by the National Vaccine Advisory Committee (NVAC) created the following standards for pediatric immunization practices, largely in response to the measles resurgence of the late 1980s, which resulted from failures in many of these areas. The standards represent the most desirable practices for pediatric health care providers and immunization programs and set the benchmark for public expectations. The means to implement many of these standards are elaborated elsewhere in this book.

- *Standard 1—Immunization services are readily available*. To maximize coverage, immunizations should be provided at times convenient for parents, such as in the evening or early morning, at lunch time, and on weekends. Integration into times when other health services are offered is beneficial. An adequate supply of vaccines should be maintained so that opportunities to vaccinate are not missed.

- *Standard 2—No barriers or unnecessary prerequisites to the receipt of vaccines exist*. Walk-in services with short wait times should be in place. Prevaccination screening, including definition of current immunization status and possible contraindications, should be rapid and efficient and should be independent of other health services (standing orders can facilitate this). Physical examinations are not necessary unless the child is sick or the visit has another purpose besides immunization. If the child does not have one, the need for a primary medical home should be emphasized.

- *Standard 3—Immunization services are available free or for a minimal fee*. Money should not be a barrier to immunization. Public and private providers holding state vaccine contracts must post signs indicating that patients will not be denied immunizations because of inability to pay. Private offices can refer un- or underinsured patients to public health clinics for immunizations.

- *Standard 4—Providers use all clinical encounters to screen and, when indicated, immunize children*. All health care providers should consider a child's immunization status no matter what the nature of the encoun-

Table 2.1.   2010 Objectives for vaccine-preventable diseases

| Disease | Group | Annual cases or incidence | | Comments |
		Baseline[a]	Target	
Diphtheria	<35 yr	1	0	Disease extremely rare
Tetanus	<35 yr	14	0	Herd immunity not applicable
Pertussis	<7 yr	3,417	2,000	Adults are a major reservoir
Hepatitis A	All ages	11.3/100,000	4.5/100,000	Children are primary source of new infections in communities
				Target high-risk groups
				Universal vaccination anticipated
Hepatitis B	2–18 yr	945	9	Infection will decrease as universally immunized
(acute)	19–24 yr	24.0/100,000	2.4/100,000	infants reach adolescence and adulthood
	25–39 yr	20.2/100,000	5.1/100,000	High-risk groups should be targeted
	≥40 yr	15.0/100,000	3.8/100,000	
	Drug users	7,232	1,808	
	Heterosexuals	15,225	1,240	
	Men who have sex with men	7,232	1,808	
Hepatitis B (perinatal)	Occupational	249	62	95% of perinatal infections preventable by appropriate
	<2 yr	1,682	400	maternal screening and infant care
Hib	<5 yr	163	0	Conjugate vaccines have resulted in near elimination
Meningococcus	All ages	1.3/100,000	1.0/100,000	Target high-risk groups
				Conjugate vaccines anticipated

Disease	Age	Baseline	Target	Comment
Pneumococcus	<5 yr	76.0/100,000	46.0/100,000	Reduced penicillin-resistant infections will accompany general reduction in cases
	≥65 yr	62.0/100,000	42.0/100,000	
Meningitis (bacterial)	1–23 mo	13.0/100,000	8.6/100,000	Widespread use of Hib and pneumococcal conjugates expected
Measles	All ages	74	0	Transmission in United States interrupted multiple times since 1993
Mumps	All ages	666	0	Interruption of spread feasible with 2 doses
Rubella	All ages	364	0	Interruption of spread feasible with 2 doses
Congenital rubella	<1 yr	7	0	Focus on women of childbearing age and foreign-born adults
Polio	All ages	0	0	Eliminated in the United States
Varicella	<18 yr	4,000,000	400,000	Monitoring effect of vaccine difficult because varicella not uniformly reportable
Lyme	Endemic areas	17.4/100,000	9.7/100,000	Since withdrawal of vaccine, efforts need to focus on minimizing exposure and controlling ticks

[a]Baseline estimates derive variously from data collected between 1990 and 1998. Adapted from U.S. Department of Health and Human Services. *Healthy People 2010*, 2nd ed. With Understanding and Improving Health and Objectives for Improving Health. 2 vols. Washington, DC: U.S. Government Printing Office, November 2000, available at www.healthypeople.gov/Document/HTML/Volume1/14Immunization.htm (accessed 01/27/03).

ter is. This includes, for example, emergency room physicians, hospital-based physicians, specialists who see the patient, and even physicians who see the patient's siblings or parents. Providers should make the most of these opportunities by giving the needed vaccines or referring to the primary care provider to do so.

- *Standard 5—Providers educate parents and guardians about immunization in general terms.* Education should include the reasons why immunizations are important, description of the diseases that they prevent, and recommended schedules. Parents should know to bring their shot record to each visit, should have the opportunity to ask questions, and should be given materials that they can take home with them.

- *Standard 6—Providers question parents or guardians about contraindications and, before immunizing a child, inform them in specific terms about the risks and benefits of the immunizations their child is to receive.* Screening should include questions about adverse events after previous vaccine doses as well as any current conditions that might be classified as contraindications or precautions [see Chapter 3(II)]. Vaccine Information Statements (VISs) and Important Information Statements [see Chapter 2(IV)] serve to inform parents and patients but should be supplemented by oral or visual explanations. Some indication of understanding by the parent should be elicited.

- *Standard 7—Providers follow only true contraindications.* There are very few true contraindications to immunization [see Chapter 1(IV) and Table 1.7]. In the absence of such, providers should exercise sound judgment as to what constitutes a medical reason to defer immunization.

- *Standard 8—Providers administer simultaneously all vaccine doses for which a child is eligible at the time of each visit.* There are essentially no routine vaccines that cannot be administered at the same time at separate sites. MMR should be given rather than the monovalent components [as advocated by certain individuals who claim a relationship between MMR and autism, see Chapter 13(IV)]. When available, combination vaccines are preferred to their equivalent, separately administered components.

- *Standard 9—Providers use accurate and complete recording procedures.* This standard goes beyond the record keeping mandated by law [see Chapters 2(IV) and 2(V)]. It calls for a permanent record that parents can carry with them and verification of immunizations received from other providers. Office record keeping should facilitate rapid retrieval of the records of preschool-aged children as well as those who have missed appointments.

- *Standard 10—Providers schedule immunization appointments in conjunction with appointments for other child health services.* This standard recognizes the need for convenience and the likely effect that convenience will have on compliance. Immunizations could be given in conjunction with dental examinations or developmental screening. Linking immunizations to the Department of Agriculture's Special Supplemental Nutrition Program for Woman, Infants, and Children (WIC) was highly successful in boosting immunization rates during the 1990s.

- *Standard 11—Providers report adverse events after immunization promptly, accurately, and completely.* This standard is a critical part of the vaccine safety net [see Chapter 13(III)]. Reporting of certain events after vaccination is required by law [see Chapter 2(IV)], and reporting of all adverse events is encouraged, whether or not they are believed to be vaccine related. Parents should be encouraged to report adverse events to providers.

- *Standard 12—Providers operate a tracking system.* Computerized or manual tracking, recall, and reminder systems should be in place. Special attention should be given to children at high risk for not completing their immunization schedule.

- *Standard 13—Providers adhere to appropriate procedures for vaccine management.* Vaccines must be handled and stored properly in accordance with the manufacturer's instructions to ensure potency [see Chapter 1(III)]. Particular attention should be paid to temperature monitoring. This is best accomplished by designating a "Vaccine Tsar" in the office whose responsibilities include inventory management and refrigerator maintenance.

- *Standard 14—Providers conduct semiannual audits to assess immunization coverage levels and to review immunization records in the patient populations that they serve.* A simple random survey of patient records can yield information about coverage rates, missed opportunities, and record quality; in general, physicians will find that they grossly overestimate the proportion of their patients who are appropriately immunized. An approach used by the National Immunization Program (NIP) to audit providers and implement change is called AFIX, for Assessment, Feedback, Incentives, and eXchange of information. This program is now linked to the Vaccines for Children (VFC) program to facilitate penetration into private offices. In addition, the Centers for Disease Control and Prevention (CDC) offers a software package called Clinical Assessment Software Application (CASA) that can be downloaded free of charge from the NIP Web site. This program is a menu-driven relational database that can audit a practice's immunization performance. Reports can be individualized and can assess coverage levels for various vaccines at various critical age markers, dropout from the vaccination schedule, and missed opportunities. The program can also generate mailing lists and recall and reminder notices.

- *Standard 15—Providers maintain up-to-date, easily retrievable medical protocols at all locations where vaccines are administered.* Protocols are written or computerized algorithms, lists, or tables that detail policies and procedures such as contraindications, possible adverse events, dose, administration technique, sites, use of equipment, handling of emergencies, and personnel responsibilities. Handbooks and personal digital assistant applications can also serve this purpose.

- *Standard 16—Providers operate with patient-oriented and community-based approaches.* Providers should be responsive to the needs of their patients and their communities. This includes seeking input and publicizing information about the availability of immunizations.
- *Standard 17—Vaccines are administered by properly trained individuals.* Those administering vaccines should be trained in sterile technique and accurate record keeping. However, they do not need to be physicians or nurses. In fact, 36 states now allow pharmacists to give vaccines, and providing vaccines at nontraditional sites such as supermarkets can help remove barriers. States may differ on statutory requirements for personnel administering vaccines.
- *Standard 18—Providers receive ongoing education and training on current immunization recommendations.* Immunization recommendations change frequently. The routine childhood schedule is updated each January, and during the year, new vaccines may be released or interim recommendations made. Providers should remain abreast of these changes. One simple way to accomplish this is to receive the *MMWR Morbidity and Mortality Weekly Report* via an E-mail listserv (subscription is free at www.cdc.gov), which publishes recommendations from the Advisory Committee on Immunization Practices (ACIP) and Notices to Readers.

III. Standards for adult immunization practices. In 1990, the National Coalition for Adult Immunization offered the following standards for adult immunization practices, which have since been adopted by many other organizations (available at www.nfid.org/ncai/publications/standards, accessed 3/17/03):

- *Standard 1—*Appropriate vaccine use should be promoted through information campaigns for health care practitioners and trainees, employers, and the public about the benefits of immunizations.
- *Standard 2—*Physicians and other health care personnel (in practice and in training) should protect themselves and prevent transmission to patients by assuring that they, themselves, are completely immunized.
- *Standard 3—*All health providers should routinely determine the immunization status of their adult patients, offer vaccines to those for whom they are indicated, and maintain complete immunization records.
- *Standard 4—*All health care providers should identify high-risk patients in need of influenza vaccine and develop a system to recall them for annual immunization each autumn.

- *Standard 5*—All health care providers and institutions should identify high-risk adult patients in hospitals and other treatment centers and assure that appropriate vaccination is considered either before discharge or as part of discharge planning.
- *Standard 6*—All licensing/accrediting agencies should support the development of comprehensive immunization programs for staff, trainees, volunteer workers, inpatients, and outpatients by health care institutions.
- *Standard 7*—States should establish preenrollment immunization requirements for colleges and other institutions of higher education.
- *Standard 8*—Institutions that train health care professionals, deliver health care, or provide laboratory or other medical support services should require appropriate immunizations for persons at risk of contracting or transmitting vaccine-preventable illnesses.
- *Standard 9*—Health care benefit programs, third-party payers, and government health care programs should provide coverage for adult immunization services.
- *Standard 10*—Standard personal and institutional immunization records should be adopted as a means of verifying the immunization status of patients and staff.

IV. **National Childhood Vaccine Injury Act.** In response to growing public concern about vaccine safety and the effects that liability issues were having on the pharmaceutical industry, Congress passed the National Childhood Vaccine Injury Act of 1986 (The Act, P.L. 99-660). The Act established the National Vaccine Injury Compensation Program (VICP), which went into effect on October 1, 1988. The VICP is a no-fault alternative to the tort system for resolving claims that result from adverse reactions to mandated childhood vaccines. It is administered jointly by the Health Resources and Services Administration (HRSA) of the Department of Health and Human Services (DHHS) (see Fig. 13.1), the U.S. Court of Federal Claims, and the Department of Justice, and it is funded by an excise tax levied on every dose of vaccine that is purchased.

To receive compensation, petitioners must demonstrate injuries found on the Vaccine Injury Table (VIT), which lists specific injuries or conditions and the time frames in which they must have occurred (updated versions can be found at www.hrsa.gov/osp/vicp/table.htm). The VIT serves as a basis for presumption of causation; individuals can file claims for injuries not listed on the VIT, but proof of causation must be given. Vaccines recommended by the ACIP for routine use in children are automatically covered under the VICP. Advice regarding the VICP and recommended changes to the VIT come from the Advisory Commission on Childhood Vaccines (ACCV), which consists of nine members (three health care professionals, three members of the general public, and three attorneys) who meet at least quarterly.

Important points about the VICP include the following:

- Currently covered vaccines are diphtheria, tetanus, pertussis, measles, mumps, rubella, polio, hepatitis B, *H. influenzae* type b, varicella, rotavirus, and pneumococcal polysaccharide conjugate
- Claims can be filed by individuals, parents, legal guardians, or trustees
- Adults are covered under the program if they receive one of the above vaccines
- Claimants must first pursue compensation through the VICP for injuries related to covered vaccines; after adjudication, they are free to reject the decision of the Court and pursue civil litigation
- Compensation is available for unreimbursable medical, custodial, and rehabilitation costs and lost earnings. There are no limits on compensation for attorney's fees for cases filed after 1988. Compensation for pain, suffering, and emotional distress and compensation to the estate in the case of death are capped at $250,000

The Act also established the Vaccine Adverse Event Reporting System (VAERS), a passive surveillance program that collects and analyzes postmarketing information about adverse vaccine events that has been in operation since 1990. Any event after vaccination can be reported, with no restriction on the interval between vaccination and the onset of illness and no requirement for medical care having been rendered. Anyone can submit a report, including health care professionals, pharmaceutical companies, parents, and patients. However, health care providers are *required* to report events that are listed by the manufacturer as a contraindication to subsequent doses as well as events listed in the Reportable Events Table (RET, Tables 2.2 and 2.3), which is similar but not identical to the VIT used by the VICP. Reports can be submitted directly on the Internet, or forms can be printed and mailed in. VAERS data are available to the public (at www.vaers.org, accessed 01/25/03), but anonymity is preserved.

The Act also required providers to give vaccine recipients or their parents or guardians a VIS for each vaccine received. A VIS is a concise description of the risks and benefits of a given vaccine written for lay people and published by the CDC. Controversy erupted in late 2002 when it was discovered that the Homeland Security Act of 2002 (P.L. 107-296) contained language that defined the word *vaccine* to include all components and ingredients listed in the product license application and product label. As such, claims alleging that thimerosal, a preservative used in vaccines until 1999, was a cause of autism would be required to be adjudicated through the VICP first rather than through the civil courts. Because VICP damages are capped, this provision was interpreted as a liability protection for the manufacturers of thimerosal, most notably Eli Lilly. To make matters worse, legislators were slow to take responsibility for introducing the provision, fueling concerns about conflicts of interest. Due to public pres-

Table 2.2. Reportable Events Table (effective August 26, 2002)

Vaccine	Event[a]	Interval from vaccination
Note: For all vaccines in the table, events listed in the package insert as contraindications to additional doses are considered reportable events.		
Tetanus in any combination	Anaphylaxis or anaphylactic shock	7 d
	Brachial neuritis	28 d
Pertussis in any combination	Anaphylaxis or anaphylactic shock	7 d
	Encephalopathy or encephalitis	7 d
Measles, mumps and rubella in any combination	Anaphylaxis or anaphylactic shock	7 d
	Encephalopathy or encephalitis	15 d
Rubella in any combination	Chronic arthritis	42 d
Measles in any combination	Thrombocytopenic purpura	7–30 d
	Vaccine-strain measles virus infection in an immunodeficient recipient	6 mo
OPV	Paralytic polio	Immunocompetent: 30 d Immunocompromised: 6 mo
	Vaccine-strain polio virus infection	Immunocompetent: 30 d Immunocompromised: 6 mo
IPV	Anaphylaxis or anaphylactic shock	7 d
Hep-B	Anaphylaxis or anaphylactic shock	7 d
Hib conjugate, varicella, PCV-7	No condition specified	
Rotavirus	Intussusception	30 d

[a]See Table 2.3 for event definitions. Any sequelae of these events, including death, are also reportable.
Adapted from the Vaccine Adverse Event Reporting System, available at www.vaers.org/reportable.htm (accessed 01/25/03).

sure, the provision was repealed, even though there remains no evidence that thimerosal was a cause of autism in children [see Chapter 13(IV)].

Certain legal obligations, listed in Table 2.4, are now binding on vaccine providers. Technically speaking, the law only covers vaccines included in the National Childhood Vaccine Injury Act, but the ACIP recommends these same procedures for all vaccines. Although the law references

Table 2.3.   Description of events for Reportable Events Table (effective August 26, 2002)

Event	Description
Anaphylaxis and anaphylactic shock	Acute, severe, potentially lethal systemic allergic reaction Begins minutes to a few hours after exposure Death can result from airway obstruction due to laryngeal edema, bronchospasm, or cardiovascular collapse
Brachial neuritis	Dysfunction limited to the upper extremity nerve plexus without involvement of other peripheral or central nervous system structures Usually preceded by deep, steady, often severe aching pain in the shoulder and upper arm Pain followed in days or weeks by weakness and atrophy of upper extremity muscle groups Sensory loss may occur but is generally a less notable feature

Encephalopathy	Must have acute encephalopathy followed by chronic encephalopathy persisting for >6 mo after vaccination
	Acute encephalopathy: severe enough to require hospitalization (whether hospitalization occurred or not) with symptoms lasting ≥24 h:
	    Children <18 mo of age without seizures: significantly decreased level of consciousness (see below)
	    Children <18 mo of age with seizures: significantly decreased level of consciousness (see below) not attributed to a postictal state or medication
	    Children ≥18 mo of age and adults: at least two of the following:
	        Significant change in mental status that is not medication related (confusional state, delirium, or psychosis)
	        Significantly decreased level of consciousness (see below), independent of seizures and not attributable to medication
	        Seizure associated with loss of consciousness
	Increased intracranial pressure may be a feature at any age
	Significantly decreased level of consciousness: at least one of the following for ≥24 h:
	        Decreased or absent response to environment (responds, if at all, only to loud voice or painful stimuli)
	        Decreased or absent eye contact (does not fix gaze on family members or other individuals)
	        Inconsistent or absent responses to external stimuli (does not recognize familiar people or things)
	Alone or in combination, the following do not demonstrate acute encephalopathy or significant change in mental status or level of consciousness:
	        Sleepiness
	        Irritability
	        High-pitched and unusual screaming

(continued)

Table 2.3. *Continued*

Event	Description
	Persistent inconsolable crying
	Bulging fontanel
	Isolated seizures
	Chronic encephalopathy
	Change in mental or neurologic status persisting for ≥6 mo after vaccination
	Exclusions:
	Return to a normal neurologic state after the acute encephalopathy
	Any subsequent chronic encephalopathy
	Genetic, prenatal, or perinatal factors
	Other exclusions: infectious, toxic, metabolic, structural, genetic, or traumatic causes of encephalopathy
Chronic arthritis	No history of arthropathy in the past 3 yr
	Joint swelling (documented within 30 d of onset) that occurred 7–42 d after a rubella vaccination
	Persistent objective signs of intermittent or continuous arthritis (documented within 3 yr of onset) lasting >6 mo
	Antibody response to rubella virus
	Exclusions:
	Musculoskeletal disorders including diffuse connective tissue diseases (e.g., rheumatoid arthritis, juvenile rheumatoid arthritis, systemic lupus erythematosus, systemic sclerosis, mixed connective tissue disease, polymyositis/dermatomyositis, fibromyalgia, necrotizing vasculitis and vasculopathies, and Sjögren's syndrome)
	Degenerative joint disease
	Infectious agents other than rubella
	Metabolic and endocrine diseases
	Trauma
	Neoplasms
	Neuropathic disorders
	Bone and cartilage disorders
	Arthritis associated with ankylosing spondylitis, psoriasis, inflammatory bowel disease, Reiter's syndrome, or blood disorders
	Joint pain or stiffness without swelling

Adapted from www.vaers.org/reportable.htm (accessed 01/25/03).

childhood vaccines, it applies to any recipient of covered vaccines regardless of age. Keep in mind there may also be state laws that supplement these national requirements.

V. **Occupational Safety and Health Administration (OSHA).** Because most vaccines are injected percutaneously, vaccine providers and their employees are at risk for needlestick injuries. As such, all facilities where vaccinations are given, including doctors' offices, public health clinics, and hospitals, fall under OSHA regulations

Table 2.4.   Federal requirements regarding vaccination

Give VIS	Give *current, take-home* copy of relevant VIS to parent, legal representative, or adult recipient with *each* dose of *each* vaccine
	Use VIS published by the CDC[a]
	Covered vaccines: DTaP, DT, Td, MMR, IPV, Hep-B, Hib, varicella, PCV-7, RRV-TV (no longer in use)
	VISs for other vaccines (e.g., influenza) are encouraged but *mandatory* if the vaccine was purchased through a federal contract
	Provide VIS for each component of a combination vaccine if there is no VIS for the combination
	Use visual or oral supplements to the VIS for illiterate or blind patients
Document in permanent medical record or office log	Publication date of the VIS and date it was given to recipient[b]
	Name and title of individual who administered vaccine
	Address where permanent record is kept
	Date of administration
	Manufacturer
	Lot number
Report to VAERS	Any event listed by manufacturer as a contraindication to subsequent doses of the vaccine
	Any event listed in the Reportable Events Table (Table 2.2) that occurs within the specified time period after vaccination

VAERS, Vaccine Adverse Event Reporting System; VIS, Vaccine Information Statement.
[a]Available at www.cdc.gov/nip/publications/VIS. No official translations are available from the CDC, but two state immunization programs (California and Minnesota) have independently translated the VISs into several languages. These documents are available from the Immunization Action Coalition (www.immunize.org). The CDC considers these *de facto* equivalents of the English versions.
[b]The patient's signature is *not* required, and the VIS should not be construed as informed consent, which may be required in certain states.

designed to minimize occupational exposure to bloodborne pathogens. Some states may have OSHA plans that exceed the federal requirements discussed below, but those plans cannot be less stringent.

In 1991, under authority of the Occupational Safety and Health Act of 1970, OSHA promulgated the Bloodborne Pathogens Standard (29 CFR 1910.1030), which mandated that employers establish and implement an exposure control plan for their employees. This plan had to include work practice controls, procedures for handling exposures, personal protective clothing and equipment, training, medical surveillance, Hep-B vaccinations, signs, and labels. In addition, engineering controls designed to isolate or remove hazards, such as sharps disposal containers, self-sheathing needles, and plastic capillary tubes, were to be used. In 2000, recognizing that occupational exposure to bloodborne pathogens was a continuing concern and that newer preventive technologies were available, Congress passed the Needlestick Safety and Prevention Act (P.L. 106-430), which directed OSHA to revise the bloodborne pathogens standard. This act called for more detail in the requirements for engineered devices; added new elements to the exposure control plan, including documentation of employee input; and required the creation of a sharps injury log. OSHA published the revised standard in the Federal Register on January 18, 2001, and it went into effect on April 18, 2001. Despite concerns expressed by the American Academy of Pediatrics (AAP) that enforcement of these standards might put the nation's immunization program at risk, OSHA does not grant exemptions.

The basic elements of the Bloodborne Pathogens Standard, as revised, are listed below. With respect to vaccinations, the most important element is the use of engineered sharps protections on needles and the proper disposal of sharps. However, most physicians' offices perform other procedures such as phlebotomy, wound cleansing, and suturing, necessitating attention to many other areas of the standard.

- *Exposure control plan*—A *written* plan needs to be in place that details all of the elements listed below. In addition, the procedures and job classifications in which exposure to blood might occur should be delineated. An annual review and update must be conducted that takes into account innovations in medical procedures and new technologic developments that reduce the risk of exposure.
- *Sharps injury log*—Employers must maintain a log of percutaneous injuries from contaminated sharps. It must include, at a minimum, the type and brand of device, department or work area where the incident occurred, and an explanation of how the incident occurred (including, for example, the procedure being performed and the body part affected). In addition, it must protect the confidentiality of the injured employee. The log should serve as a tool to identify high-risk areas and evaluate devices.
- *Engineered sharps protections*—Devices with built-in safety features or mechanisms that effectively reduce the risk of exposure must be used for procedures that have contact with blood. Such features should be an integral part of the device, allow the worker's hands to remain behind the needle at all times, remain in effect after the procedure and during disposal, and be as simple as possible. Examples pertinent to immunizations include syringes with sheaths that slide forward by a single-handed operation to cover the attached needle after use, retractable needles, and needleless systems such as jet injectors. Documentation must be provided in the exposure control plan that appropriate, commercially

available, engineered devices are evaluated each year, and justification must be provided for selecting a particular device (*not* selecting an engineered device is *not* an option). In addition, it must be documented that non-managerial, front-line employees with direct patient care responsibilities had input into the selection (this can take the form of meeting minutes or written evaluations filled out by employees). Selected devices must not jeopardize patient or employee safety or be medically inadvisable. Because sheaths and the like are considered temporary measures, even sharps with engineered protections must be disposed of in an approved container.

- *Universal precautions*—All blood and body fluids must be treated as if infectious for hepatitis B, hepatitis C, and human immunodeficiency virus (HIV), even if they are from low-risk individuals. Facilities for handwashing and personal protective equipment (e.g., gloves, gowns, masks, mouthpieces, and resuscitation bags) must be available at no cost to employees. Lab coats and scrubs, if used as protective equipment, must be laundered by the employer at no cost; home laundering is not permitted. Gloves (hypoallergenic if necessary) must be available, and handwashing is required after use. However, the use of gloves is *not* required when administering intramuscular or subcutaneous injections as long as bleeding is not anticipated.

- *Procedures*—Detailed protocols must be given for all procedures with risk, including decontamination of equipment, handling of sharps disposal containers and other regulated waste, broken glassware, and laundry. Routine cleaning of worksites should be described.

- *Sharps handling*—A protocol for handling of sharps must be in the exposure control plan. Recapping contaminated needles is prohibited, but this should not be an issue, as needles will have engineered controls. If recapping is necessary for uncontaminated needles, such as those used to draw vaccine from a vial into a syringe, the cap should be scooped up from a flat surface using the hand that is holding the syringe and needle. Disposal containers should be closable, puncture resistant, leak-proof, labeled appropriately, and located where procedures are performed. The protocol should specify how the containers are handled once they are filled.

- *Warning labels*—Orange or orange-red biohazard labels must be affixed to containers of regulated waste and refrigerators and freezers containing blood or infectious materials (labeled bags may also be used).

- *Hep-B vaccination*—Vaccination should be available at no cost to all employees with potential blood contact. The employee's health insurance cannot be used to pay this expense unless the employer routinely pays the entire premium. Employees must sign a declination form if they choose to opt out.

- *Postexposure evaluation*—Specific procedures should be outlined for handling of exposures. Baseline and follow-up laboratory tests should be done after consent is obtained and must be provided free of charge. Provisions for confidential medical follow-up must be made. Postexposure HIV prophylaxis should be offered if indicated in accord with current guidelines. The source individual's blood should be tested for bloodborne pathogens after consent is obtained; if consent is not given, this needs to be documented. Medical records on employees must be kept for the duration of employment plus 30 years.
- *Training*—Training that includes background information and the exposure control plan must be provided on assignment and annually thereafter. Documentation of training sessions, including the dates, content, trainer, and attendees, must be maintained.

Checklists, model exposure control plans, and lists of commercially available safety-engineered sharp devices can be obtained from the International Health Care Worker Safety Center at the University of Virginia at www.med.virginia.edu/medcntr/centers/epinet (accessed 01/25/03). In addition, many vaccines are now available from manufacturers in prefilled syringes and needles with engineered protections.

VI. **School mandates and state legislation.** There are no federal laws specifying which vaccines civilians must receive, and, at the present time, there are no vaccine laws for international travel. There are, however, state laws specifying which vaccines must be received before attendance at day care, preschool, school, or college is allowed. These requirements have been instrumental in the eradication or near-eradication of many diseases. The courts have repeatedly upheld the legal basis for these statutes, which include the societal mandate to protect nonenfranchised individuals (children who do not have a vote) and the rights of others to be protected from harm (transmission of disease from unimmunized individuals). There are few laws that apply to adults other than college students, those entering military service, and immigrants. However, some states, employers, or institutions might require certain vaccines or proof of immunity for selected individuals. Examples include influenza and Hep-B vaccines for health care workers, influenza and pneumococcal vaccines for residents and employees of long-term care facilities, vaccines for laboratory workers who work with specific pathogens, and rabies vaccine for animal handlers.

The CDC recommends a 4-day grace period for specific age requirements. For example, a child who receives the MMR 3 days before his first birthday should be considered as having been effectively immunized. However, some local school districts may not accept this, so the best advice is to give vaccines at the recommended ages. Practitioners may have to balance the liabilities of giving a vaccine before the exact specified age with the risk that the patient may not return to be vaccinated at the appropriate time.

All states allow exemption from school immunization requirements for medical reasons. However, states differ with regard to whether they grant religious and philosophic exemptions. The AAP emphasizes the need for sensitivity and flexibility in dealing with parents' religious beliefs. Although it also supports the repeal of religious exemption laws, it does not advocate the stringent application of medical neglect laws when parents refuse the recommended childhood immunizations. Philosophic exemptions are more problematic because the level of proof can be minimal (it may be minimal for religious exemptions as well), amounting simply to parents' being "opposed to immunization." In some cases, parents request philosophic exemptions as a matter of convenience when their children's immunizations are not up-to-date. Physicians, public health providers, and school officials should not grant philosophic exemptions in such circumstances and, in general, should work toward the repeal of philosophic exemption laws.

Because state laws are not uniform and change frequently, it is difficult to maintain an active roster of state requirements. However, the following generalizations can be made:

- All states require diphtheria, measles, rubella, and polio vaccination
- Tetanus, pertussis, and mumps vaccination, if not specifically required, are usually covered through the near-universal use of combination vaccines
- Hib requirements usually apply only to day care and preschool, as Hib disease is rare after 5 years of age
- Hep-A requirements vary geographically and are concentrated in southwestern states
- As of 2003, 48 states have requirements for Hep-B, 38 for varicella, five for meningococcal polysaccharide vaccine (Men-PS) (for college students), and three for PCV-7
- As of 2003, 47 states allow religious and 18 allow philosophic exemptions

For parents considering exemption, physicians should emphasize that disease rates among exemptors are unequivocally higher than among vaccinated individuals; in addition, large numbers of exemptors in a community put everyone at risk, including vaccinated children. The best centralized sources for information about state requirements are the National Network for Immunization Information (www.immunizationinfo.org/vaccineInfo) and the Immunization Action Coalition (www.immunize.org/laws). For the most up-to-date information, it is best to contact your state health department via Internet or telephone; Table 14.1 lists these phone numbers and Web sites.

The Immunization Encounter

I. **Communicating about vaccines.** Scientists, public health officials, and providers tend to think about vaccines in terms of probability and expected utility. The health value of getting a vaccine, and presumably the basis for decision making, is the difference between two things, illustrated in Figure 3.1: (a) the probability of avoiding the disease times the utility, or value, of avoiding the disease, and (b) the probability of a vaccine side effect times the disutility of that side effect (this simplistic analysis does not take into account opportunity costs). For example, the probability of avoiding measles through vaccination is nearly 100%, and the utility of avoiding measles for any given individual is very high, as 1 in 100 patients develops pneumonia and 1 in 1,000 dies. Thus, the first part of the equation has a high value. On the other hand, the probability of getting fever and rash from measles, mumps, and rubella vaccine (MMR) is low, approximately 5%, and the disutility of fever and rash is low, as it is self-limited. Thus, the value of the second part of the equation is low and does not detract appreciably from the value of the first part. In other words, the overall utility model overwhelmingly favors vaccination.

   Patients and the lay public, however, think differently. At the societal level, the value of vaccines paradoxically decreases as their effectiveness increases; when disease is eliminated, the public perceives no benefit from vaccines. Another way to look at this is that when vaccines work, nothing (as opposed to disease) happens. This fact, combined with widespread attention given to rare adverse events, leads to the perception that vaccines do more harm than good. At the individual level, several thought processes might be operative in a parent's reluctance to have his or her child vaccinated. Some of these represent heuristics, short-cut ways of thinking or rules of thumb that people use to simplify complex decision making. To communicate effectively, physicians should understand these thought processes and be prepared to address them, armed with information that is presented in more detail in Chapter 13. The goal of communication is not to convince doubtful parents to accept vaccination, but rather to provide enough accurate information for parents to make informed decisions. The following are examples of heuristic thought processes and suggested responses:
   - *Anchoring*—This is the tendency to interpret new risks in light of previously presented risks.

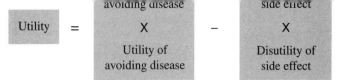

Utility	=	avoiding disease		side effect
		X	−	X
		Utility of avoiding disease		Disutility of side effect

Figure 3.1. Probabilistic thinking regarding health risks and benefits of vaccination

> *Example*: Knowing that 1,000 people die from electrocution each year tends to lower a person's estimate of the annual number of influenza deaths.
>
> *Response*: Factual information regarding disease risks can be offered; for example, patients should understand that there are more than 50,000 influenza-associated deaths in the United States each year.

- *Availability*—The ease with which a person remembers something represents the probability that it will occur.

  > *Example*: A vivid, frightening news story about vaccine-associated polio might make a parent think that this side effect was more common than it really was.
  >
  > *Response*: Factual information about side effects can be offered; for example, patients should know that vaccine-associated polio occurred once for every 2.4 million doses distributed.

- *Avoidance of ambiguity*—A known risk is more acceptable than an unknown risk.

  > *Example*: The serious sequelae of chickenpox seem more acceptable than the potential risks of the relatively new vaccine.
  >
  > *Response*: Convert the unknown risk to a known one by reviewing safety data pertaining to the vaccine and describing the rigorous pre- and postlicensure evaluation process that ensures safety (see Chapter 13).

- *Compression*—Rare risks are overestimated and common risks are underestimated.

  > *Example*: Anaphylaxis from MMR is a likely risk, but fever and rash from the measles component are rare.
  >
  > *Response*: Anaphylaxis probably occurs in fewer than 1 in one million doses, but self-limited fever and rash occur in as many as 5% of vaccinees.

- *Do-no-harm and omission bias*—A bad outcome is more tolerable if it occurs from inaction rather than action.

  > *Example*: Hospitalization with influenza is more tolerable than side effects of the vaccine because the

vaccine is something you actively choose, whereas the disease is something that happens to you.

Response: Emphasize that nothing in medicine (or life for that matter) has zero risk, and that not taking a vaccine is actually an action to accept vulnerability to the disease.

- *Exposure*—People underestimate the cumulative effect of multiple exposures.

  Example: My child is not exposed to chickenpox that much.

  Response: Contact between a school-aged child and contagious cases of chickenpox occurs almost daily in late winter and early spring.

- *Framing*—The context in which a decision is made affects the decision.

  Example: A parent may be reluctant to take on the risks of vaccination because doing so involves making a decision on behalf of his or her child.

  Response: Reframe the vaccination discussion around the viewpoint of the child, who would likely choose protection from disease if given the chance.

- *Freeloading*—Herd immunity protects unvaccinated children.

  Example: Because other children get the MMR, my child will not get measles, and there is no reason for him or her to take the risk of the vaccine.

  Response: The risk of measles is actually 35-fold higher in exemptors, even in communities in which over 90% of children are immunized.

- *Maintaining the status quo*—This is an aversion to taking on one risk to reduce another.

  Example: I'm more comfortable just taking the risk of the disease, because that's how things are now, and so far my child has been fine.

  Response: The status quo (i.e., susceptibility to disease) is not the optimal position to be in, because protection from disease is available.

- *Representativeness*—The probability that something will occur correlates with similarity of circumstances.

  Example: A dreaded vaccine side effect is likely because it happened to a child who lives in my community.

  Response: Personal anecdotes about treating children with vaccine-preventable diseases can be offered.

People do not undertake a risk-control measure such as vaccination unless they believe that they can effectively control the risk. In other words, they need to understand that the vaccine really does prevent the disease. In addition, the risk should be personally relevant and serious. Although there are thought processes that tend to favor vaccination, such as *bandwagoning* (the tendency for individuals to choose the decision of the majority as what might be wise for themselves) and *altruism* (a willingness to take on personal risks if it is for the benefit of others),

Table 3.1.   Focusing on what parents want to hear

Describe which vaccines the child will receive today
Explain why these vaccines are important
Review contraindications to each vaccine
Give a detailed account of the common, mild side effects and how to
    manage them
Give a brief account of any severe risks
Place today's vaccinations in the context of the overall schedule

nothing substitutes for a straightforward discussion with patients and parents about risks and benefits.

There is a clear disconnect between what physicians do and what parents want. For example, parents want personal verbal communication from their physicians that conveys a sense of trust and respect. Time-motion studies, however, show that physicians spend less than 2 minutes discussing vaccines with their patients. Physicians are sometimes reluctant to mention risks for fear of opening a can of worms, but parents are interested in relevant, practical information that can be easily understood. Table 3.1 gives some tips on getting to the point of what parents want to know.

In addition, the following suggestions regarding risk communication in the office setting can be made:

- *Begin the discussion early*—One of the advantages of the birth dose of hepatitis B vaccine (Hep-B) is that it opens the door to discussing vaccines immediately after parenthood has begun. In those initial discussions before hospital discharge, vaccines should be portrayed as part of the routine care that the child will receive as he or she grows up. Parents who express doubt or concern should be targeted for further discussion and should receive printed materials and other resources well before the 2-month visit.
- *Use a team approach*—Communication should be a coordinated effort between doctors, nurses, and other office personnel. Even the receptionist can provide an introduction to the vaccination visit, give Vaccine Information Statements (VISs), and direct the parent to informational materials in the waiting room. Office nurses (who are often trained in risk/benefit communication) are accessible and highly invested in immunization and can have a great impact on parents. Each member of the team should be empowered and should know his or her function during the vaccination visit.
  - *Organize the visit effectively*—Face-to-face time with the doctor can be increased by building efficiencies into the visit, beginning with a preparatory phone call to remind the parent to bring the child's shot record. Use of a screening questionnaire for contraindications [see Chapter 3(II)] can be helpful. Development of simple, direct messages and easy-to-understand printed materials can eliminate some questions and help focus the

discussion. Ultimately, the use of combination vaccines (see Chapter 6) may increase office efficiency and allow more time for communication.

- *Understand individual backgrounds*—Many factors affect risk perception, including educational, emotional, religious, psychological, spiritual, philosophic, and intuitive bases. Families differ in their orientation toward the medical establishment—some are traditional and trusting, whereas others are cautious, challenging, and oriented toward alternative practices. Vaccine messages should be delivered with these differences in mind.
- *Layer information appropriately*—Information should be presented with sensitivity to individual needs. Providers should be aware of the patient's cognitive foundation and begin with information appropriate to that level. Parents who want to know more will ask.
- *Engage patients in a decision-making partnership*—Research repeatedly shows that parents trust their physicians more than anyone else for accurate, honest information. Building on this trust, the approach should be nonjudgmental, empathetic, and mutually respectful.
- *Remove barriers*—Insufficient time is the most important barrier to effective communication. Consider scheduling vaccination visits at off-peak hours.
- *Be aware of pitfalls*—Avoid the tendency to extrapolate from limited data and to fit equivocal data into preconceived notions. Risk comparisons (e.g., the chances of a severe reaction are the same as being struck by lightning) can backfire. Consciously avoid being paternalistic and belittling.
- *Check for understanding*—Make sure parents understand what you've told them and ask whether they have any questions.

Finally, there are ten truths that are useful to keep in mind as you address the issue of vaccination with parents:

1. *Vaccines are good*—No public health intervention short of sanitation has meant more good for more people.
2. *Public concern is pervasive*—Articles in magazines, discussions on television talk shows, sound bites on the evening news, debates on Capitol Hill, and conversations in the grocery store check-out line all attest to it.
3. *Fear of vaccines can lead to public harm*—Unfounded fears can lead to decreased immunization rates and the return of disease. Many vaccine-preventable diseases are just a plane flight away, and the only thing between those diseases and our children is the collective immunity imparted by vaccination.
4. *Vaccines are not 100% safe*—Although this is true, the risks of vaccines are much less than the risks of disease (see Chapter 13).
5. *Parents want what is best for their children*—Unfortunately, some parents have become convinced that responsible parenting means protecting children from the vaccines rather than the diseases.

6. *Vaccinology is difficult to understand*—The effort involved in understanding pathogenesis, determining immunologic correlates of protection, testing vaccine candidates in animals, establishing safety, conducting field trials, and collecting data that can lead to licensure is underappreciated. Moreover, the processes by which policy and recommendations are made are confusing. Parents' lack of understanding of these processes contributes to their reluctance to vaccinate.

7. *Risk perception is critical*—The same parents who would volunteer to receive the smallpox vaccine might take their children to "chickenpox parties" to get natural chickenpox rather than the vaccine. They need to understand that children still die from chickenpox and that (without minimizing the spectre of bioterrorism) the last death from smallpox in the United States was a half-century ago.

8. *There are vaccine antichampions*—Just as there are vaccine champions, there are individuals and organizations whose agenda is to convince parents that vaccines are dangerous or unnecessary. Many of these organizations have Web sites, and it is important for practitioners to be familiar with the misinformation that is offered on them [see Chapter 14(XII)].

9. *Many questions remain unanswered*—Among these is how to approach vaccine advocacy without perceived conflicts of interest.

10. *The decision not to vaccinate is an active decision to accept the risks of disease.*

   Sometimes parents refuse vaccination even after extensive discussion with their physicians. For these situations, the American Academy of Pediatrics (AAP) Section on Infectious Diseases has developed a Refusal to Vaccinate form (available at www.cispimmunize.org/pro/pdf/RefusalToVaccinate.pdf, accessed 11/27/02) that can be signed by the parent. The form is not intended to be a legal document, and it is not clear what legal protection it would afford the practitioner. Its main purpose is to encourage parents to rethink the issue. Ultimately, practitioners may need to decide whether to retain patients who refuse all vaccinations in their practices. Retention provides continued opportunities to break down the barriers to immunization and protects the child from seeking care from chiropractors and alternative medicine practitioners. Alternatively, asking the family to leave the practice sends a powerful message regarding the importance of vaccinations in preventive medicine; this alone might be enough to change some people's minds.

II. Screening. An important part of preventing adverse events is screening patients for contraindications, precautions, and other problems before every dose of a vaccine. This can be effectively accomplished by asking the simple questions shown in Table 3.2, which are applicable to both children and adults. Standardized forms for this purpose can be downloaded free of charge from the Immunization Action

Table 3.2.   Screening questions

Question	Issue Addressed
Is the patient sick today?	Concurrent moderate to severe illness
Does the patient have severe allergies to medicines, foods, drugs, or vaccines?	Severe allergy or anaphylaxis to vaccine components or eggs
Has the patient had serious reactions to previous vaccinations?	Encephalopathy, high fever, persistent inconsolable crying, or hypotonic-hyporesponsive episode after pertussis vaccine
	Anaphylaxis or severe allergic reaction
Has the patient had a seizure, brain, or neurologic problem?	Evolving neurologic disorder
	Susceptibility to febrile seizures
	Guillain-Barré syndrome after previous vaccination
Does the patient have cancer, leukemia, a blood disorder, human immunodeficiency virus infection (HIV), acquired immune deficiency syndrome (AIDS), tuberculosis, or any problem with the immune system?	Contraindications to live vaccines
	Thrombocytopenia from MMR
	Tuberculosis (a contraindication for varicella vaccine)
In the last 3 months, has the patient received any treatments that might weaken his or her immune system, such as steroids, cancer chemotherapy, or radiation?	Contraindications to live vaccines
Are there any family members who have problems with their immune system?	Hereditary immune deficiencies
	Contacts who might be susceptible to horizontal transmission of live vaccines
Has the patient received blood transfusions or immune globulin in the past year?	Inactivation of live vaccines by passively transferred antibodies
	Discovery of undisclosed serious underlying illness
Is the patient pregnant or is there a chance she could become pregnant in the next 3 months?	Avoidance of live vaccines during pregnancy
Has the patient received any other vaccines in the last 4 weeks?	Interference between MMR and varicella vaccines
	Interval between doses of same vaccine too short for effective immunogenicity

Coalition Web site (www.immunize.org). The issues addressed by these questions are also indicated in Table 3.2.

III. **Technique**

A. **General issues.** It is probably most efficient to bring the vaccines to the examination room rather than have the patient move to a designated shot area. Young infants may do better if held on the parent's lap, whereas older children may prefer to sit on the edge of the examining table and hug their parent. Health care workers should wash their hands before treating each patient, and sterile technique should be used, including swiping of the injection site with alcohol and allowing it to dry. Gloves are *not* required unless the individual administering the vaccine has open skin lesions and is likely to come in contact with body fluids. The needle should not be changed after withdrawing the vaccine from the vial and before injecting it into the patient. A direct, rapid plunge of the needle through the skin is recommended. Aspirating back on the syringe after penetration to look for blood return is controversial. There are no data to suggest that this is necessary, but many nurses feel uncomfortable injecting before they can confirm that the needle is not resting in a vessel. Multiple vaccines can be given in the same limb but should be separated by 1 to 2 in. The AAP suggests that multiple injections can be given simultaneously by different personnel to minimize anticipatory anxiety.

There are some important differences for smallpox vaccine [see Chapter 9(I)]. This is a live vaccine that is administered intradermally with a bifurcated needle that punctures the skin and draws a small amount of blood. As such, gloves *should be worn* and the site should be covered with gauze and a semipermeable dressing. In addition, alcohol should *not* be used because it might inactivate the virus.

B. **Oral administration.** Oral administration is usually best accomplished with the child in a feeding position using a needleless syringe to deliver the vaccine. In general, vomiting within 10 minutes is an indication to repeat the dose.

C. **Intramuscular administration.** The needle should enter the skin at a 90-degree angle, penetrating deep enough to hit the muscle (Fig. 3.2). To minimize pain, traction can be applied to the skin and subcutaneous tissue before injection and released after injection. Preferred sites, which differ by age, include the anterolateral aspect of the upper thigh (vastus lateralis muscle) and the upper, outer part of the arm above the armpit and below the acromion (deltoid muscle). The required needle length also varies by age. The buttocks should not be used, because the fat layer is too thick and damage to the sciatic nerve is possible. An exception can be made for large-volume passive immunization (e.g., immune globulin), but in this case the site should be the upper, outer mass of the gluteus maximus, and the needle should be

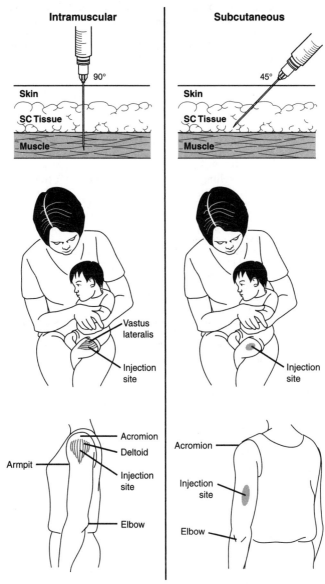

Figure 3.2.   Technique of vaccine administration [Redrawn from The Minnesota Department of Health. How to administer IM and SC injections. Available at www.immunize.org/catg.d/free.htm (accessed 11/4/02).]

directed perpendicular to the table while the patient is lying prone. Alternatively, the injection can be given in the center of the triangle formed by the anterior superior iliac spine, the tubercle of the iliac crest, and the upper border of the greater trochanter. No more than 5 mL should be given to an adult at a single site.

D. **Subcutaneous administration.** For subcutaneous injections, the skin and subcutaneous tissue should be pinched up and the needle directed at a 45-degree angle (Fig. 3.2). The preferred sites and needle length vary with age (Table 3.3).

E. **Intravenous administration [polyclonal immune globulin for intravenous administration (IGIV) products].** Some patients who receive IGIV regularly have indwelling central venous catheters. For those who do not, a temporary peripheral catheter should be inserted; for short infusions, a butterfly needle may suffice (the antecubital vein should be used for more concentrated solutions). In-line filtering is acceptable, but pore sizes greater than 15 μm should be used so as not to impede flow. Patients can be premedicated with acetaminophen, 10 to 15 mg/kg orally, and diphenhydramine, 1.00 to 1.25 mg/kg orally, intramuscularly, or intravenously, to avoid systemic reactions. Infusions are usually started slowly and the rate is increased if tolerated, but protocols differ based on the product, concentration, and total volume infused. If flushing or changes in heart rate or blood pressure occur, slowing the infusion rate usually ameliorates these symptoms. Initial infusions should be done in a medical observation unit in case anaphylaxis or other severe reactions occur. Table 3.4 gives one protocol for infusion of IGIV.

IV. **Dealing with anxiety, pain, and fever.** Vaccinations induce significant levels of stress and anxiety in children. To some extent, this can be ameliorated by truthfully informing them of what to expect before the visit occurs and by parental endorsement of vaccination as being valuable. A variety of methods have been used in an attempt to reduce pain during injection, including hypnosis, oral sucrose administration, refrigerant topical anesthetics, ice, eutectic mixture of local anesthetic (EMLA) cream, application of pressure before injection, and lidocaine iontophoresis. The efficacy of these interventions has been variable, and many require extensive training and planning. The most reasonable approach for young children is to allow parents to comfort their children (rather than assist in restraining them) and to try distraction techniques such as telling stories, listening to music, or having them blow into pinwheels or imaginary candles. It is reasonable to administer acetaminophen, 10 to 15 mg/kg orally, at the time of vaccination and at 4 and 8 hours afterward. This is particularly true for diphtheria, tetanus, and acellular pertussis (DTaP) vaccination. Samples should be kept in the office, and prescriptions should be on

Table 3.3. Vaccine administration

| Age | Intramuscular | | Subcutaneous | |
---	Site	Needle	Site	Needle
0–12 mo	Anterolateral aspect of upper thigh	$7/8$–1 in., 22- to 25-gauge	Fatty area of anterolateral thigh	$5/8$–$3/4$ in., 23- to 25-gauge
12–36 mo	Anterolateral aspect of upper thigh unless deltoid well developed	$7/8$–1 1/4 in., 22- to 25-gauge ($5/8$ in. can be used for deltoid region, 12–15 mo only)	Fatty area of anterolateral thigh or upper outer triceps area of arm	
36 mo–adult	Deltoid	1–1 1/2-in., 22- to 25-gauge	Upper outer triceps area of arm	

Adapted from the Immunization Action Coalition (www.immunize.org, document P2020, accessed 11/2/02); CDC. General recommendations on immunization. *MMWR* 2002;51(RR-2).

Table 3.4.   Protocol for infusion of polyclonal immune globulin for intravenous administration (IGIV)

	5% Solution		10% Solution	
Time (min)	Rate calculation (mL/kg/h)	Rate for 20-kg child (cc/h)	Rate calculation (mL/kg/h)	Rate for 20-kg child (cc/h)
0–15	0.6	12	0.3	6
16–30	1.2	24	0.6	12
31–45	2.4	48	1.2	24
46–end	4.8	96	2.4	48

hand for patients who must purchase drugs through medical assistance.

V. Dealing with emergencies

  A. Preparation. Acute emergencies after vaccine administration are rare. Whereas the AAP suggests observation in the office for 15 to 20 minutes after vaccination, the Advisory Committee on Immunization Practices (ACIP) has never recommended a specific waiting period. In actual fact, life-threatening emergencies such as anaphylaxis usually occur within minutes, when the patient is still likely to be within reach of medical personnel. The benefits of rapid, mass vaccination programs, such as "drive-by" influenza vaccine clinics, probably far outweigh the risks of curtailing any medical observation period. Standing orders for emergencies should be in place in the office, and Table 3.5 lists supplies that should be available, just in case.

  B. Syncope. Vasovagal reactions are most common in adolescents and young adults, particularly females. Approximately 60% occur within 5 minutes of vaccination, and approximately 90% occur within 15 minutes. Between 1990 and 2001, slightly more than 2,200 reports of syncope were made to the Vaccine Adverse Event Reporting System (VAERS). Approximately 12% of cases resulted in hospitalization, and there are some reports of serious injury such as skull fracture. Health care workers should be aware of predisposing conditions such as needle phobia and presyncopal symptoms, such as light-headedness or dizziness. At-risk individuals should be encouraged to sit or lie down. If syncope does occur, the patient should be protected as much as possible from fall injury and should be placed supine with the legs raised until symptoms abate.

  C. Anaphylaxis. Anaphylaxis occurs rapidly and is a medical emergency. Signs and symptoms include the following:

Table 3.5. Emergency office supplies for vaccination

Equipment	Drugs
Oxygen	Epinephrine 1:1,000 (aqueous)
Ventilation masks with one-way valve and ambu-bag	for subcutaneous injection
Laryngoscope	Corticosteroids (methylprednisolone, prednisone, hydrocortisone)
Face mask and nasal cannula	
Pediatric and adult airways	H_1 antihistamines (diphenhydramine, hydroxyzine)
Scalpel and 11-gauge needle for cricothyroidotomy	
Stethoscope	H_2 antihistamines (cimetidine, ranitidine)
Sphygmomanometer with appropriate cuffs	Beta-2 agonists (albuterol)
Tongue depressors	
Tourniquets	
Flashlight	
Tuberculin syringes with 5/8-in. needles	
3-cc syringes with 1-in. needles	
IV fluids, tubing, and arm boards	

Adapted from Sapien R, Hodge D. Equipping and preparing the office for emergencies. *Pediatr Ann* 1990;19:659–667; and Kagy L, Blaiss MS. Anaphylaxis in children. *Pediatr Ann* 1998;27:727–734.

- Flushing, warmth, urticaria, erythema, soft tissue edema, pruritus
- Dry mouth, swelling of the lips, tongue and throat, sneezing, congestion, rhinorrhea
- Hoarseness, stridor, cough, dyspnea, chest tightness, wheezing, cyanosis
- Tachycardia, hypotension, weak pulse, dizziness, shock, cardiovascular collapse
- Crampy abdominal pain, nausea, vomiting, diarrhea

The initial approach is to administer epinephrine 1:1,000 (aqueous) at a dose of 0.01 mL/kg subcutaneously. This dose can be repeated every 10 to 20 minutes, and a dose can be given at the vaccine injection site to slow absorption. In addition, an antihistamine such as diphenhydramine can given at a dose of 1 to 2 mg/kg (maximum, 100 mg per dose) every 4 to 6 hours orally, intramuscularly, or intravenously. The patient should be observed for several hours and, if improved and stable, can be given a long-acting epinephrine injection and sent home on an oral antihistamine for the next 24 hours.

For more severe cases, the emergency medical system should be activated immediately. Patients may require intensive emergency management, including airway maintenance, oxygen, and blood pressure support with isotonic intravenous fluids. Epinephrine can be given intravenously using 0.1 mL/kg of a 1:10,000 dilution [1:1,000 (aqueous) diluted tenfold with physiologic saline]. If repeated doses are needed, a continuous infusion is preferred [1 mL of 1:1,000 (aqueous) added to 250 mL of 5% dextrose in water (final concentration 4 μg/mL), initially infused at a rate of 0.1 μg/kg or 0.025 mL/kg per minute, increasing to 1.5 μg/kg or 0.375 mL/kg per minute]. Additional therapy may require inotropes, steroids, and H_1- and H_2-receptor blockers.

4

The Business of Vaccines in Practice

I. **Coding and billing.** Billing third-party payers for immunization services (and all other health services) is based on two systems:

- *Current Procedural Terminology (CPT) Codes*—These describe the *procedures* or *services* performed during a visit. The *visit itself* usually falls under evaluation and management codes for preventive medicine services performed in the outpatient setting, provided that the immunization occurs in the context of a comprehensive "check-up." These codes, which vary by age and whether the person is new to the practice or established as a patient, are given in Table 4.1. There are corresponding codes for the *vaccines or immune globulins themselves*, which are given in Table 4.2, and there are codes for the *administration* of the vaccines or immune globulins, given in Table 4.3. If the visit is *only* for immunization (e.g., before travel), most offices bill only for the vaccine and administration using the specific codes listed in Table 4.2. If other services are performed in addition, 99211 (office or other outpatient services, established patient) can be used for the visit along with the appropriate International Classification of Diseases, Ninth Revision (ICD-9) code describing the reason for that service (the presence of a physician is not required for this level of service).
- *ICD-9 Codes*—These describe the *reason* for the service. The *visit itself* usually falls under V20.2 (health supervision of infant or child, routine infant or child health check; 0 to 17 years of age) or V70.0 (general medical examination, routine general medical examination at a health care facility; adults). Most *vaccines themselves* have specific ICD-9 codes that are given in Table 4.2. Immune globulins generally fall under one ICD-9 code, V07.2 (need for prophylactic immunotherapy).

Table 4.2 includes some vaccines that are no longer available and some that are not yet licensed in the United States.

A routine visit for a privately insured 6-month-old infant might be coded as shown in Table 4.4. The rules for particular insurance programs may vary. If the practice receives vaccines free of charge through the Vaccines for Children (VFC) program, it cannot bill for the *vaccine itself*, but it can bill for *administration of the vaccine* and for the *visit itself*. In this case, the modifier –52 (reduced services) could potentially be added to the CPT code for the

Table 4.1.   2003 Codes for preventive medicine services

Age (yr)	New patient		Established patient	
	CPT	ICD-9	CPT	ICD-9
<1	99381	V20.2	99391	V20.2
1–4	99382	V20.2	99392	V20.2
5–11	99383	V20.2[a]	99393	V20.2[a]
12–17	99384	V20.2[a]	99394	V20.2[a]
18–39	99385	V70.0	99395	V70.0
40–64	99386	V70.0	99396	V70.0
≥65	99387	V70.0	99397	V70.0

CPT, Current Procedural Terminology; ICD-9, International Classification of Diseases, Ninth Revision.
[a]If the visit is for a school physical, V70.3 (general medical examination for adoption, camp, school admission, etc.) can be used.

Table 4.2.   2003 Codes for vaccines and immune globulins

Product	CPT	ICD-9
Vaccines		
Adenovirus, type 4, live PO	90476	V05.8
Adenovirus, type 7, live PO	90477	V05.8
Anthrax, SC	90581	V03.89
BCG, live, percutaneous	90585	V03.2
Cholera, injectable	90725	V03.0
Diphtheria, IM	90719	V03.5
Td, ≤7 yr, IM or jet injection	90718	V06.5
DT, <7 yr, IM	90702	V06.5
DTaP, IM	90700	V06.1
DTaP/Hep-B/IPV (Pediarix), IM	90723	V06.8
DTaP/Hib (TriHIBit), IM	90721	V06.8
Hep-A, adult, IM	90632	V05.3
Hep-A, pediatric/adolescent (2 dose), IM	90633	V05.3
Hep-A, pediatric/adolescent (3 dose), IM	90634	V05.3
Hep-A/Hep B (Twinrix), adult, IM	90636	V06.8 or V05.3
Hep-B, adolescent (2 dose), IM	90743	V05.3
Hep-B, adult, IM	90746	V05.3
Hep-B, dialysis or immunosuppressed (3 dose), IM	90740	V05.3
Hep-B, dialysis or immunosuppressed (4 dose), IM	90747	V05.3
Hep-B, pediatric/adolescent (3 dose), IM	90744	V05.3
Hep-B/Hib (COMVAX), IM	90748	V06.8
Hib, HbOC conjugate (HibTITER; 4 dose), IM	90645	V03.81
Hib, PRP-D conjugate (ProHIBit; booster only), IM	90646	V03.81
Hib, PRP-OMP conjugate (PedvaxHIB; 3 dose), IM	90647	V03.81
Hib, PRP-T conjugate (ActHIB, OmniHIB; 4 dose), IM	90648	V03.81
Influenza, split virus, 6–35 mo, IM or jet injection	90657	V04.8
Influenza, split virus, ≥3 yr, IM or jet injection	90658	V04.8

(continued)

Table 4.2. *Continued*

Product	CPT	ICD-9
Influenza, whole virus, IM or jet injection	90659	V04.8
Influenza, live, intranasal	90660	V04.8
IPV, SC	90713	V04.0
Japanese encephalitis, SC	90735	V05.0
Measles, live, SC or jet injection	90705	V04.2
Measles and rubella, live, SC or jet injection	90708	V06.8
MMR, live, SC or jet injection	90707	V06.4
MMRV, live, SC or jet injection	90710	V06.8
Mumps, live, SC or jet injection	90704	V04.6
Men-PS (Menomune–A/C/Y/W-135), SC or jet injection	90733	V03.89
Plague, IM or jet injection	90727	V03.3
PCV-7 (Prevnar), polyvalent, age <5 yr, IM	90669	V03.82
Pne-PS (PNEUMOVAX 23), adult or immunosuppressed, ≥2 yr, SC or IM	90732	V03.82
Rabies, IM	90675	V04.5
Rabies, intradermal	90676	V04.5
Rubella, live, SC or jet injection	90706	V04.3
Smallpox	90749[a]	V04.1
Tetanus, IM or jet injection	90703	V03.7
Typhoid, acetone-killed, dried, SC or jet injection	90693	V03.1
Typhoid, heat- and phenol-inactivated, SC or intradermal	90692	V03.1
Typhoid, live, PO	90690	V03.1
Typhoid, Vi capsular polysaccharide, IM	90691	V03.1
Varicella, live, SC	90716	V05.4
Yellow fever, live, SC	90717	V04.4
Unlisted vaccine/toxoid	90749	
Other specified vaccination against single bacterial disease		V03.89
Unspecified single bacterial disease		V03.9
Other specified single disease		V05.8
Unspecified single disease		V05.9
Other combinations		V06.8
Unspecified combined vaccine		V06.9

Immune globulins (IGs)

IGIM, human	90281	V07.2[b]
IGIV, human	90283	V07.2
Botulinum antitoxin, equine, any route	90287	V07.2
Botulinum IGIV, human	90288	V07.2
CMV-IGIV (CytoGam), human	90291	V07.2
Diphtheria antitoxin, equine, any route	90296	V07.2
Hepatitis B IG, human, IM	90371	V07.2
Rabies IG, human, IM and/or SC	90375	V07.2
Rabies IG, heat-treated, human, IM and/or SC	90376	V07.2
RSV-mAb (Synagis), IM	90378	V07.2
RSV-IGIV (RespiGam)	90379	V07.2
Tetanus IG, human, IM	90389	V07.2
Vaccinia IG, human, IM	90393	V07.2
Varicella IG, human, IM	90396	V07.2
Unlisted IG	90399	V07.2

[a]Unlisted vaccine/toxoid (there is currently no specific CPT code for smallpox vaccine).
[b]Indicates prophylactic immunotherapy.

Table 4.3.   2003 Current Procedural Terminology (CPT) codes for administration of vaccines and immune globulins

Procedure	Code	Example
Immunization administration (includes percutaneous, intradermal, SC, IM and jet injections); one vaccine (single or combination vaccine/toxoid)	90471	DTaP
Each additional parenteral vaccine (single or combination vaccine/toxoid); list separately in addition to code for primary procedure; use in conjunction with 90471	+90472	MMR plus varicella vaccine in same visit
Immunization administration by intranasal or PO route; one vaccine (single or combination vaccine/toxoid)	90473	Salmonella Ty21a
Each additional PO or intranasal vaccine (single or combination vaccine/toxoid); list separately in addition to code for primary procedure; use in conjunction with 90473	+90474	Not currently applicable in United States
Intravenous infusion for therapy/diagnosis, administered by physician or under direct supervision of physician; up to one hour	90780	RSV-IGIV
Each additional hour, up to 8 h; list separately in addition to code for primary procedure; use in conjunction with 90780	+90781	Prolonged IGIV infusion
Therapeutic, prophylactic or diagnostic injection (specify material injected); SC or IM	90782	RSV-mAb IM

vaccine to recognize the fact that it was provided to the practice free of charge.

II. **Costs and accounting.** Table 4.5 provides cost information for commonly used vaccines. The public sector cost is the contracted price between the Centers for Disease Control and Prevention (CDC) and the manufacturer, which changes from year to year. The private sector cost is based on the direct purchase price from the manufacturer. Because contractual and buying arrangements may vary for individual practices, Table 4.5 is most useful in highlighting relative differences between products.

III. **Funding vaccine services.** The majority of Americans have private health insurance. By 1999, 28 states had laws requiring insurers to cover childhood immunizations, at least to some degree. Some mandate coverage in accord with the recommended childhood immunization schedule, whereas others make reference only to "appropriate pediatric vaccines." Other states prohibit deductibles and coinsur-

Table 4.4. Coding for routine 6-month-old infant visit

Procedure	Visit		Vaccine		Vaccine administration	
	CPT	ICD-9	CPT	ICD-9	CPT	ICD-9
Check-up	99391[a]	V20.2[b]	—	—	—	—
DTaP	—	—	90700	V06.1	90471	V06.1
PRP-T Hib conjugate	—	—	90645	V03.81	90472	V03.81
PCV-7	—	—	90669	V03.82	90472	V03.82
Hep-B	—	—	90744	V05.3	90472	V05.3

CPT, Current Procedural Terminology; ICD-9, International Classification of Diseases, Ninth Revision.
[a]Established patient, periodic comprehensive medicine, less than 1 year of age.
[b]Routine infant or child health check.

ance. Self-insured employers are generally exempt from such regulation. However, federal statutes prohibit employers providing vaccine coverage as of May 1, 1993 from reducing that coverage; these statutes are aimed at preventing reductions in coverage since enactment of the VFC program. Insurance plans vary in terms of which vaccines they cover. In general, managed care plans are more likely than indemnity plans to cover vaccines and promote their use.

The VFC program, created in 1993 by the Omnibus Budget Reconciliation Act, constitutes a federal entitlement to immunization services for children 18 and younger who are (a) Medicaid eligible, (b) uninsured, (c) underinsured and receiving immunizations at federally qualified health centers or rural health clinics, or (d) Native American or Alaskan Native. Through this program, vaccines are purchased by the CDC at reduced rates and made available to eligible children free of charge. Any private provider who sees eligible children can participate in the program. Vaccines are provided at no cost to the practice, and the practice is prohibited from charging the patient for the vaccine. Patients *can*, however, be charged administration fees within limits established by the Centers for Medicare and Medicaid Services (CMS). However, patients cannot be denied vaccine if they cannot pay the fee (claims for these fees can still be submitted to Medicaid). There are no regulations regarding charges for the office visit itself.

Vaccines recommended by the Advisory Committee on Immunization Practices (ACIP) are automatically included in the VFC program. However, significant delays can occur in securing a federal contract. For example, the varicella

Table 4.5.   Vaccine costs

Vaccine	Trade name	Manu-facturer	How supplied (no. in package)	CDC cost/dose (U.S. $)	Private sector cost/dose (U.S. $)
DTaP	Tripedia	AP	1-dose vial (10)	11.75	19.65
	DAPTACEL	AP	1-dose vial (5)	12.75	20.24
	Infanrix	GSK	1-dose vial (10)	11.75	19.65
			Syringe with needle (25)	12.00	19.65
DTaP2/PRP-T	TriHIBit	AP	1-dose vial (5)	23.40	38.21
DTaP3/Hep-B/IPV	Pediarix	GSK	1-dose vial (10)	31.97[a]	58.99[a]
			Syringe (5–25)		
IPV	IPOL	AP	10-dose vial (1)	8.80	22.53
			Syringe (10)	8.80	23.31
PRP-OMP/Hep-B	COMVAX	Merck	1-dose vial (10)	21.83	42.81
Hep-A Pediatric	VAQTA	Merck	1-dose vial (10)	11.15	29.62
	Havrix	GSK	1-dose vial (10)	11.15	29.73
			Syringe (5–25)	11.40	29.73
Hep-A Adult	VAQTA	Merck	1-dose vial (5)	17.75	28.34
	Havrix	GSK	1-dose vial (1)	17.75	59.45
			Syringe w/needle (5)	17.75	59.45
Hep-A/Hep-B	Twinrix	GSK	1-dose vial (10)	36.16	77.67
			Syringe (5)	36.16	77.67
Hep-B pediatric	Engerix-B	GSK	1-dose vial (10)	9.00	24.20

Hep-B adolescent (2 doses)	RECOMBIVAX HB	Merck	Syringe (5–25)	9.25	24.20
	RECOMBIVAX HB	Merck	1-dose vial (10)	9.00	23.20
Hep-B adult	RECOMBIVAX HB	Merck	1-dose vial (10)	24.25	59.09
	Engerix-B	GSK	1-dose vial (10)	24.25	59.09
			1 dose (1)	24.25	51.73
			Syringe w/needle (5–25)		51.73
Hib	PedvaxHIB	Merck	1-dose vial (10)	8.32	21.52
	HibTITER	Wyeth	1-dose vial (5)	7.33	15.88
	ActHIB	AP	1-dose vial (5)	7.51	21.78
Influenza	Fluzone	AP	10-dose vial (1)	5.525	6.50
MMR	M-M-R$_{II}$	Merck	10-dose vial (1)	15.64	34.73
PCV-7	Prevnar	Wyeth	1-dose vial (5)	45.99	58.75
Varicella	VARIVAX	Merck	1-dose vial (10)	41.44	58.11

AP, Aventis Pasteur; GSK, GlaxoSmithKline.

[a] Estimates as of 03/17/03.

Adapted from www.cdc.gov/nip/vfc/cdc_vac_price_list.htm (accessed 01/24/03).

vaccine was recommended by the ACIP in June 1995 but was not in the VFC program until May 1996. During such delays, state Medicaid programs are still bound to cover ACIP-recommended vaccines. Overall, VFC provides vaccines for 35% of the national birth cohort, and the majority of delivery sites are private offices. This shift toward the private sector for vaccine delivery has had the positive effect of identifying a medical home for many at-risk children.

States also purchase vaccines using their own funds or block grants obtained through Section 317 of the Public Health Service Act. Some states purchase vaccines and provide them free of charge to all children, regardless of insurance status, through participating providers (who may still charge administration fees). In the year 2000, there were 15 such "universal purchase states." These programs clearly increase immunization rates, but detractors argue that public funds should not be used to pay for vaccines that insurers would otherwise cover. In addition, manufacturers are concerned that all vaccines in these states are purchased at contract rather than private-market rates. However, universal purchase is popular among providers because it eliminates the need for office-based eligibility checks and, thereby, minimizes the administrative burden.

Another public funding mechanism for immunizations is the State Children's Health Insurance Program (SCHIP), enacted in 1997. This is a block grant program targeted to low-income children who are not eligible for Medicaid and are otherwise uninsured. States can use SCHIP funds to expand Medicaid or create separate, freestanding children's insurance programs. Medicare, a completely federal insurance program, entitles adults over 65 years of age, disabled individuals, and those with end-stage renal disease to preventive vaccinations. Pneumococcal and influenza vaccines are covered without deductibles or coinsurance, and hepatitis B vaccine (Hep-B) is covered for any beneficiaries who are at risk for the disease. Vaccine administration fees are also covered.

IV. **Vaccine shortages.** The 1990s saw unique and unprecedented shortages in the supply of many routinely used vaccines. The impact of these shortages included frequent and sometimes confusing changes in the recommended immunization schedule, temporary revision of state school entry requirements, parental frustration, and a burden placed on providers to track interrupted schedules and recall patients when vaccines became available. To date, there is no evidence that the shortages resulted in disease outbreaks.

The shortages resulted from a convergence of factors:

- *Business decisions*—Vaccines are high-risk, high-cost, low-profit products compared to other pharmaceuticals. Compounding this is the fact that there are relatively few companies that produce vaccines. In fact, only four main manufacturers distribute vaccines in the United States (Aventis Pasteur, GlaxoSmithKline, Merck, and Wyeth), so disruption in one manufacturer's production can have a major effect on supply. In the late 1990s, Wyeth decided to cease production of tetanus-containing vaccines, including the diphtheria, tetanus, and acellular pertussis (DTaP) vaccine ACEL-IMMUNE, as it geared up to distribute Prevnar [pneumococcal polysaccharide conjugated to mutant diphtheria protein CRM_{197}, 7-valent (PCV-7)]. In the same year, Baxter (formerly North American Vaccines) ceased producing the DTaP vaccine CERTIVA, leaving only two DTaP manufacturers in the United States (Aventis Pasteur and GlaxoSmithKline).

- *Production problems*—Some production problems had a biologic basis. For example, the influenza A (H3N2) strain used for the 2000 to 2001 vaccine grew slowly in culture. Others were due to lengthy routine physical plant maintenance activities. When there is only one major manufacturer, as in the case of varicella and measles, mumps, and rubella (MMR) vaccines (VARIVAX and M-M-R$_{II}$, both produced by Merck), such delays can seriously affect national supplies.
- *Underestimated demand*—The recommendation in April 2000 to decrease the age for routine influenza vaccination from 65 to 50 years compounded production problems by increasing demand. Similarly, greater-than-expected demand for Prevnar (PCV-7) after it was first recommended for universal use in October 2000 contributed to shortages of that vaccine.
- *Good Manufacturing Practices (GMPs)*—GMPs require regular upgrades to production facilities, and this takes time and money. Some facility upgrades were done voluntarily in response to issues raised during routine GMP inspections. In other instances, FDA citations for violations of GMPs temporarily halted vaccine production by some companies.
- *Changes in manufacturing process*—The recommendation in 1999 to remove thimerosal from childhood vaccines [see Chapter 13(IV)] forced manufacturers to change to single-dose vials without preservatives. Besides the ramp-up time needed, single-dose vials needed to be overfilled so that providers could extract a full dose, necessitating increased production of the vaccines.

The timetable of recent vaccine shortages is best summarized by reviewing successive CDC recommendations, listed in Table 4.6. These recommendations also serve as a response reference point, should particular shortages continue or recur. In all instances when deferral was recommended, providers were asked to keep lists of patients who should be recalled once supplies improved. Information about vaccine supply can be found at www.cdc.gov/nip/news/shorgates. As of January 2003, Prevnar (PCV-7) was still in short supply. HibTITER (PRP-HbOC), made by Wyeth, was expected to be in short supply until late summer or early fall, and orders for PedvaxHIB (PRP-OMP) from Merck were taking 4 to 6 weeks to fill. In addition,

Table 4.6.   Centers for Disease Control and Prevention notices regarding vaccine shortages

Statement date (reference)	Issue	Principal recommendations
July 14, 2000 (*MMWR* 2000;49:619–622)	Potential influenza vaccine shortage	Delay implementation of organized campaigns until November Continue high-risk vaccinations Develop contingency plans

November 17, 2000 (*MMWR* 2000;49:1029–1030)	Shortage of Td	Priority given to
		    Travel to diphtheria-endemic areas
		    Wound management
		    Incomplete primary series
		    If no booster in last 10 yr:
		        Pregnancy or occupational risk
		        Adolescents
		        Adults

September 14, 2001 (*MMWR* 2001;50:783–784)	Delayed delivery of Prevnar	Defer vaccination of children >2 yr except those 2–5 yr who are high risk

December 21, 2001 (*MMWR* 2001;50:1140–1142)	Duration and severity of Prevnar shortage worse than anticipated	For severe shortage:
		    <6 mo: defer 3rd and 4th doses
		    7–12 mo: defer 3rd dose
		    12–23 mo: defer 2nd dose
		    >24 mo: no vaccination unless high risk
		Report invasive pneumococcal disease in vaccinees

Date (Reference)	Event	Recommendation
March 16, 2001 (*MMWR* 2001;50:189–190)	Wyeth Lederle and Baxter Hyland stopped production of DTaP	Defer 4th dose for infants if necessary
May 25, 2001 (*MMWR* 2001;50:418–427)	Continued Td shortage	Continue dose at 4–6 yr to provide protection during school years Defer all routine Td boosters in adults and adolescents
January 4, 2002 (*MMWR* 2002;50:1159)	Continued DTaP shortage	Give priority to primary series in infants Defer 4th and 5th doses if necessary
March 8, 2002 (*MMWR* 2002;51:190–193)	Shortages of VARIVAX and M-M-R$_{II}$	Delay varicella until 18–24 mo Further prioritize varicella to Health care workers, contacts of immunocompromised persons, adolescents, adults, high-risk children Susceptible children 5–12 yr Children 2–4 yr Defer second MMR if necessary
June 21, 2002 (*MMWR* 2002;51:529–530)	Td supply sufficient	Resume routine Td boosters
July 12, 2002 (*MMWR* 2002;51:598–599)	DTaP and MMR supply sufficient	Resume routine DTaP and MMR schedules
August 2, 2002 (*MMWR* 2002;51:679)	Varicella supply sufficient	Resume routine varicella schedule
May 16, 2003 (*MMWR* 2003;52:446)	Prevnar supply sufficient	Resume routine PCV-7 schedule

Wyeth stopped producing Pnu-Imune 23 (Pne-PS), leaving Merck as the sole supplier of Pne-PS (PNEUMOVAX 23).

Historically, approaches to potential shortages have included creating a national vaccine stockpile (better referred to as *storage and rotation contracts*), a mechanism whereby the CDC can purchase vaccine from manufacturers over and above the national need. In addition, the establishment in 1986 of a no-fault vaccine injury compensation program for individuals injured by vaccines [see Chapter 2(IV)] reduced the liability disincentives for manufacturers. The strategies for dealing with current shortages have been to prioritize immunizations for the most vulnerable individuals and to prioritize the primary series over booster doses. In the future, improved stockpiling, better liability protection, increased financial incentives, and a streamlined regulatory process may be needed. There is also talk of establishing a National Vaccine Authority to oversee production and distribution of all vaccines and to manufacture vaccines where there are gaps.

Universal Vaccines for Children and Adolescents

I. Diphtheria, tetanus, and pertussis

Corynebacterium diphtheriae is an aerobic, pleomorphic, gram-positive bacillus that produces a potent exotoxin. *Clostridium tetani* is a nonencapsulated, gram-positive, obligately anaerobic bacillus that produces a potent neurotoxin. *Bordetella pertussis* is a tiny, aerobic, gram-negative coccobacillus that produces a complex toxin as well as other virulence factors.

A. Diseases
- *Diphtheria*

  Diphtheria most often presents as *membranous nasopharyngitis* or *obstructive laryngotracheitis* associated with low-grade fever. Less commonly, cutaneous, vaginal, conjunctival, or otic infection can occur. Serious complications include upper airway obstruction caused by extensive membrane formation, myocarditis, and peripheral neuropathy.

- *Tetanus*

  Tetanus is caused by a neurotoxin produced by the anaerobic bacterium *C. tetani* in a contaminated wound. Most cases occur within 14 days of injury. Shorter incubation periods have been associated with more heavily contaminated wounds, more severe disease, and worse prognosis. *Generalized tetanus* (lockjaw) is manifest by trismus and severe muscle spasms. Onset is gradual, with progression to generalized muscle spasms over 1 to 7 days. Severe spasms, which are often aggravated by external stimuli, persist for 1 week or more and subside over a period of weeks in those who recover. *Neonatal tetanus* results from contamination of the umbilical stump. *Localized tetanus* manifests as muscle spasms in areas contiguous to an infected wound. *Cephalic tetanus* refers to cranial nerve dysfunction associated with infected wounds on the head and neck. Both localized and cephalic tetanus may precede generalized tetanus.

- *Pertussis*

  Whooping cough begins with mild upper respiratory tract symptoms (*catarrhal stage*) that progress to severe paroxysms of cough (*paroxysmal stage*), often with a characteristic inspiratory whoop that is frequently followed by vomiting. Fever is minimal or weeks. Complications include seizures, pneumonia, and encephalopathy. Disease in infants younger than 6 months of age may be atypical, with prominent apnea and absent whoop. Pertussis is most severe during the first year of life, particularly in preterm infants. Older children and adults can have atypical disease, manifesting solely as persistent cough. Infection in immunized children and older persons is often mild.

B. Epidemiology and transmission

- *Diphtheria*

Humans are the only known reservoir of *C. diphtheriae*. Patients excrete the organism for 2 to 6 weeks in nasal discharge, from the throat, or from eye or skin lesions. Antibiotic treatment shortens communicability to less than 4 days. Transmission results from intimate contact, and illness is more common in crowded living situations. Although *infection* can occur in immunized persons, *disease* is most common and severe in persons who are incompletely or not immunized. Respiratory diphtheria is most common in autumn and winter; summer epidemics can occur in warm, moist climates where skin infections are prevalent.

- *Tetanus*

Disease occurs worldwide but is more frequent in warmer climates and during warmer months, in part because contaminated wounds are more common. In the United States, fewer than 60 cases have been reported annually for the past 5 years. Spores of *C. tetani* are ubiquitous in the environment, especially where there is soil contaminated with excreta. Wounds, recognized or unrecognized, are where the organism multiplies and elaborates toxin. Contaminated wounds, those that result from deep puncture, and those with devitalized tissue are at greatest risk. Neonatal tetanus is rare in the United States but common in developing countries where women are not immunized and nonsterile umbilical cord–care practices are followed. Tetanus is not transmissible from person to person.

- *Pertussis*

Humans are the only known hosts for *B. pertussis*. Transmission occurs by close contact with respiratory secretions, and transmission rates approach 90% in nonimmune household contacts. Patients are most contagious during the catarrhal stage before the onset of paroxysms; communicability then diminishes rapidly but may persist for 3 or more weeks after onset of cough. Erythromycin therapy decreases infectivity and may limit spread. Nasopharyngeal cultures usually become negative for *B. pertussis* within

5 days of initiating therapy. Asymptomatic infection has been demonstrated but is unlikely to be a factor in transmission. Pertussis occurs endemically, with 3- to 5-year cycles of increased disease. Approximately 29% of reported cases from 1997 to 2000 occurred in children younger than 1 year of age, and approximately 41% of reported cases occurred in children younger than 5 years of age. Hospitalization of young infants with pertussis is common, as are complications such as pneumonia (12%), seizures (1%), and encephalopathy (0.2%). Adolescents and adults with unrecognized disease are important sources of transmission to children.

C. Rationale for vaccine use

- *Diphtheria*

  The introduction of diphtheria toxoid vaccines in the United States in the 1940s led to a dramatic reduction in disease incidence. High levels of vaccination have made diphtheria rare in the United States, and most cases today occur in unvaccinated or inadequately vaccinated persons. However, immunization does not completely eliminate the potential for transmission, because it does not prevent carriage of the organism in the nasopharynx or on the skin. The consequences of inadequate immunization at the population level were demonstrated in Russia and other former Soviet countries in the early 1990s, where epidemic disease caused nearly 48,000 cases in 1994 alone, and case fatality rates ranged from 3% to 23%. Diphtheria also continues to be a significant cause of morbidity and mortality in developing countries.

- *Tetanus*

  After the introduction of tetanus toxoid vaccines in the United States, the incidence of tetanus declined from 0.4 per 100,000 in 1947 to 0.02 per 100,000 in the late 1990s. The overall case-fatality rate declined from 91% to 11% during the same period. The majority of tetanus cases reported between 1989 and 1997 occurred in persons who had not completed a three-dose primary series or who had uncertain vaccination histories; no tetanus deaths occurred in persons who had received the primary series. Because naturally acquired immunity to tetanus toxin does not occur, universal primary vaccination with appropriately timed boosters is the only way to protect persons in all age groups.

- *Pertussis*

  Without vaccination, the World Health Organization (WHO) estimates that approximately 1 million deaths would occur worldwide from pertussis. In the United States, the number of cases has been reduced by approximately 95% in the vaccine era. Nevertheless, between 5,000 and 8,000 annual cases have been reported in recent years, and the incidence has increased since the early 1980s. Large outbreaks of 100 or more cases have also occurred. For example, in the

United Kingdom, immunization rates for 2-year-old children fell from 77% in 1974 to 30% in 1978, the result of unfounded adverse publicity about the whole-cell vaccine. This was followed almost immediately by an epidemic of 102,500 cases. Similarly, 13,105 cases and 41 deaths occurred in Japan in 1979, 4 years after routine immunization was temporarily suspended. These experiences, the severity of pertussis in young infants, and the benign and self-limited nature of pertussis vaccine side effects (particularly with the acellular vaccine) provide clear justification for continued routine childhood immunization. Effective primary preventive programs beginning at 2 months of age are critical, but immunization beyond infancy may further reduce the risk to infants by decreasing household exposures.

D. Vaccines. Diptheria, tetanus, and whole-cell pertussis vaccine (DTP), which was used for many years, contains diphtheria and tetanus toxoids (chemically modified forms of the respective toxins) combined with a suspension of whole, inactivated *B. pertussis*. The vaccine had a high rate of local and systemic reactions, prompting the development of acellular vaccines [DTaP(n), where *n* indicates the number of pertussis antigens], which include one or more purified components of *B. pertussis*. The currently available DTaP vaccines (Table 5.1) are sterile suspensions of pertussis antigens and diphtheria and tetanus toxoids adsorbed to alum in an isotonic sodium chloride solution. All of them contain chemically modified pertussis toxin (pertussis toxoid, or PT). In addition, most have one or more of the following antigens: filamentous hemagglutinin (FHA), pertactin (PRN, a 69-kd outer membrane protein) and fimbrial proteins (FIM, previously called *agglutinogens*). Two vaccines are no longer available in the United States: ACEL-IMMUNE (DTaP3, Wyeth) and Certiva [DTaP1, Baxter (formerly North American Vaccine)].

DTaP vaccines are labeled for active immunization against diphtheria, tetanus, and pertussis in infants and children 6 weeks through 6 years of age (before the seventh birthday), but the indications differ from product to product (Table 5.1). There is also a diphtheria and tetanus toxoid vaccine (DT, no trade name) produced by Aventis Pasteur for children who cannot receive pertussis vaccine. This vaccine is preservative free and is packaged in single-dose vials (ten per package).

E. Storage, handling, and administration
- Maintain temperature at 35° to 46°F (2° to 8°C)
- Freezing can cause the vaccine to lose potency
- Shake well before use
- Each dose is 0.5 mL given intramuscularly [see Chapter 3(III)]
- Reduced or fractional doses are not recommended, even for premature or low-birth-weight infants

F. Schedule. DTaP is routinely recommended for infants at 2, 4, and 6 months of age, followed by a fourth dose at 12

Table 5.1.   DTaP vaccines currently used in the United States

Trade name (abbreviation)	Manufacturer	Pertussis antigens	Adjuvant/ contaminants/ excipients	Preservative	Labeling	Packaging
Tripedia (DTaP2)	Aventis Pasteur	PT (23.4 μg) FHA (23.4 μg)	Alum Formaldehyde Gelatin Polysorbate 80	None	5-dose series[a]	Liquid 1-dose vial (10/pk)
Infanrix (DTaP3)	GlaxoSmith-Kline	PT (25 μg) FHA (25 μg) PRN (8 μg)	Alum Formaldehyde Polysorbate 80	2-Phenoxyethanol	5-dose series[a]	Liquid 1-dose vial (10/pk) Prefilled Tip-Lok syringe (25/pk)
DAPTACEL (DTaP5)	Aventis Pasteur	PT (10 μg) FHA (5 μg) PRN (3 μg) FIM-2 and FIM-3 (5 μg total)	Alum Formaldehyde Glutaraldehyde	2-Phenoxyethanol	First 4 doses	Liquid 1-dose vial (1, 5, or 10/pk)

pk, package.
[a]The fifth dose indication technically applies only if the four previous doses were the same vaccine.

to 18 months of age and a fifth dose at 4 to 6 years of age. For those not immunized in the first year of life, DTaP is given at 0 (initial dose), 1, 2, and 8 months, followed by a single booster at 4 to 6 years of age, just before school entry. If pertussis vaccine is contraindicated, DT should be used. After completion of childhood immunization, booster doses of Td are recommended every 10 years beginning at 11 to 12 years of age. Children who have had pertussis, even culture-proven or epidemiologically linked disease, should still probably receive DTaP because the duration of protection from natural infection is not known. See Chapter 7(I) for use of DTaP in wound management.

G. Efficacy. The immunogenicity of DTaP vaccines is similar to that of DTP. However, because antibody responses do not correlate with protection against disease, field and other epidemiologic studies are necessary to demonstrate efficacy. Household contact studies in the United States indicated efficacy of 80% or greater for the whole-cell vaccine. In prelicensure studies of several different acellular vaccines, efficacy ranged from 58% to 93%, a range that overlaps with the efficacy of whole-cell vaccines. Comparing efficacy between products is difficult because of differences in study design, vaccine schedule, case definitions, and other confounding variables. The duration of protection after DTaP has not been established.

In 1998, efficacy was estimated using data from the National Health Interview Survey (NHIS) and the National Immunization Survey (NIS). At that time, both DTP and DTaP were in use, although two-thirds of the doses were given as DTaP. Efficacy for children 7 to 18 months of age who had received three doses of vaccine was 88%.

H. Official recommendations. All infants should receive DTaP (DTP is no longer recommended) vaccine according to the above schedule. Immunization can be started as early as 4 weeks of age if pertussis is prevalent in the community, and the interval between the three doses of the primary series can be as short as 4 weeks. Pertussis immunization is not indicated for children 7 years of age or older because of the diminished risk of disease and its complications and because no vaccine in the United States is licensed for use in that age group. The Advisory Committee on Immunization Practices (ACIP) states that children who have had well-documented pertussis (culture positive for *B. pertussis* or epidemiologic linkage to a culture-positive case) do not need further pertussis immunization and should complete the series with DT. However, the American Academy of Pediatrics (AAP) notes that some experts recommend continuing acellular pertussis vaccination despite well-documented disease because the duration of natural protection is unknown. Practically speaking, it makes sense to continue the DTaP series in these patients unless there are contraindications. Patients who have had diphtheria or tetanus

Table 5.2. Reactogenicity of DTP and DTaP vaccines

Reaction	DTP (%)	Tripedia (DTaP2) (%)	Infanrix (DTaP3) (%)	DAPTACEL (DTaP5) (%)
Local reactions				
Pain	40	10	11	11
Swelling	61	20	30	5
Erythema	73	33	39	22
Systemic reactions				
Fever >101°F	16	5	3	2
Fussiness	42	19	15	9
Drowsiness	62	42	47	33
Anorexia	35	22	19	16

Note: Data from package inserts.

should still be immunized, because natural infection does not confer immunity (the amount of toxin is too small to induce effective immune responses).

The ACIP and the AAP view the licensed DTaP vaccines as equally efficacious, and neither organization has a preference for which one is used. Although they favor using the same DTaP product for the entire series given the paucity of data on interchangeability, they also caution *against* withholding vaccine if the same brand of DTaP is not available or not known. Practically speaking, providers should give whatever DTaP brand they have available rather than run the risk of missing immunization opportunities. This may include using a product off label, as only two DTaPs are licensed for the fifth dose. DTaP vaccines may be given concomitantly with any other childhood vaccines.

I. **Safety.** Local and systemic reactogenicity of DTP and DTaP products are summarized in Table 5.2. See Chapter 7(I) for safety of the Td vaccine.

The rate of local reactions increases with each subsequent dose of DTaP. Booster doses in particular may be associated with extensive local swelling, especially swelling of the entire limb in which the vaccine was given. These types of reactions are *not* contraindications to further doses. Febrile seizures from DTP, usually on the day of vaccination, were estimated to occur in 6 to 9 per 100,000 vaccinees and were not associated with subsequent seizures or neurodevelopmental disabilities. Febrile seizures from DTaP are presumably much less frequent.

The more serious reactions that occurred with whole-cell vaccines are of historic interest. They included
- Prolonged crying of 3 hours or longer (3% of DTP recipients in one large study)
- Unusual, distinctive, high-pitched cry (0.1%)
- Fever of 104.9°F (40.5°C) or higher (0.3%)
- Hypotonic-hyporesponsive episodes (1 in 1,750 immunizations)

- Seizures (occurring in 1 in 1,750 immunizations)
Severe reactions such as the above are much more rare with acellular vaccines.

J. Contraindications
- Anaphylactic reaction to a prior dose of DTaP or any of its components
- Encephalopathy within 7 days of a previous dose of DTP or DTaP

K. Precautions
- Moderate or severe acute illness
- Underlying unstable, evolving neurologic disorder
- Any of these conditions after a previous dose of DTP or DTaP
  - Fever of 104.9°F (40.5°C) or higher unexplained by another cause (within 48 hours)
  - Collapse or shocklike state (within 48 hours)
  - Persistent, inconsolable crying lasting 3 hours or longer (within 48 hours)
  - Seizure or convulsion (within 72 hours)
  - Guillain-Barré syndrome (within 6 weeks)

L. Comments. Future strategies for enhanced control of pertussis must include periodic revaccination of adolescents and adults with acellular vaccines to reduce the reservoir of infections in the community. Combination vaccines that use DTaP as the "backbone" have already been licensed, and others are in the pipeline.

KEY CONCEPTS: DIPHTHERIA, TETANUS, AND PERTUSSIS

- Diphtheria and tetanus are rare in the United States
- 5,000 to 8,000 cases of pertussis occur each year in the United States
- Tetanus differs from other diseases that are preventable by routine vaccines in that it is not transmitted from person to person
- DTP is no longer recommended because of reactogenicity
- DTaP vaccines marketed in the United States are viewed as equivalent in efficacy
- Vaccination should not be deferred if the same product that was given earlier is not available
- The primary series is three doses in infancy
- Boosters are given at 12 to 18 months and 4 to 6 years

II. *Haemophilus influenzae* type b

Haemophilus influenzae is a pleomorphic gram-negative coccobacillus that produces an antiphagocytic, serotype-specific polysaccharide capsule.

A. Disease. The most common forms of invasive *H. influenzae* type b (Hib) disease are *meningitis, bacteremia,* *epiglottitis, pneumonia, arthritis,* and *periorbital* and *buccal cellulitis.* Meningitis is the most common clinical manifestation, accounting for 50% to 65% of cases in the prevaccine era. Hallmark presenting features include fever, altered mental status, and stiff neck. The mortality rate is 2% to 5%, even with appropriate antimicrobial therapy, and neurologic sequelae occur in 15% to 30% of survivors. Osteomyelitis and pericarditis are less common. Otitis media and acute bronchitis due to *H. influenzae* are generally caused by nontypable strains.

B. Epidemiology and transmission. The organism is harbored in the upper respiratory tract, and person-to-person transmission presumably occurs by direct contact or through inhalation of respiratory droplets. Asymptomatic colonization was seen in 2% to 5% of children in the prevaccine era, but widespread use of Hib conjugate vaccines since the early 1990s has resulted in much lower colonization rates. Invasive disease now is extremely rare, and when it *is* reported, one has to be careful to verify that the strain is indeed type b. Hib disease was more frequent in boys, African Americans, Alaskan Eskimos, Apache and Navajo Indians, child care center attendees, children living in overcrowded conditions, and children who were not breastfed. Unimmunized children, particularly those younger than 4 years of age who were in prolonged close (e.g., household) contact with an infected child, were at high risk. Other factors predisposing to invasive disease included sickle cell disease, asplenia, human immunodeficiency virus (HIV) infection, certain immunodeficiency syndromes, and malignant neoplasms.

C. Rationale for vaccine use. Before the introduction of routine childhood immunization, Hib was a major cause of invasive bacterial infection in the United States, with an estimated 12,000 cases of meningitis and 8,000 other invasive syndromes annually. A striking 1 out of every 200 children in the first 5 years of life developed invasive Hib infection, with peak incidence in 6- and 12-month-old infants. In high-risk populations, disease rates were even higher. The first conjugate vaccine, ProHIBit (PRP-D, Aventis Pasteur) was licensed in 1987 for use in 18-month-old children. In 1991, after the efficacy of several conjugate Hib vaccines was demonstrated and these products were licensed for use in infants, universal Hib vaccination beginning at 2 months of age was initiated; by 1995, Hib disease had declined by more than 95%. This remarkable reduction in disease burden was partly due to the ability of conjugate vaccines to reduce nasopharyngeal carriage, leading to reduced rates of exposure and infection even in those not immunized. This is an example of herd immunity.

D. Vaccines. Conjugate Hib vaccines contain the capsular polysaccharide polyribosylribitol phosphate (PRP), linked to protein carriers. This converts *T-cell–independent* responses, characterized by short-term antibody production, poor immunogenicity in infants, and no memory, to *T-cell–dependent* responses, which are robust in infants and result in memory. Three conjugates are currently available in the United States (Table 5.3), and all are labeled for use in infants 2 months of age or older. ProHIBit (PRP-D) was withdrawn from the market in June of 2000. Hib conjugates are labeled for active immunization of infants and children 2 months through 5 years of age for the prevention of invasive disease caused by Hib.

E. **Storage, handling, and administration**
   - Maintain temperature at 35° to 46°F (2° to 8°C)
   - Freezing can cause the vaccine to lose potency
   - ActHIB (PRP-T) only: shake well after reconstitution and use within 24 hours
   - Each dose is 0.5 mL given intramuscularly [see Chapter 3(III)]

F. **Schedule.** The primary series for HibTITER (HbOC) and ActHIB (PRP-T) is three doses given at 2, 4, and 6 months of age. For PedvaxHIB (PRP-OMP), the primary series is two doses given at 2 and 4 months of age. A booster dose of any licensed product is recommended at 12 to 15 months of age, regardless of which regimen was used for the primary series. Immunization of healthy children beyond 5 years of age is not necessary, because the risk of Hib disease is small. The schedule for children not immunized in the first 6 months is given in Table 5.4.

G. **Efficacy.** Studies using the poorly immunogenic unconjugated PRP vaccine established antibody levels of 0.15 μg/mL as predictive of short-term protection and 1.0 μg/mL as predictive of long-term protection. It is not clear how applicable these levels are to conjugate vaccines which, unlike purified PRP, induce anamnestic responses. Children 15 months of age or older respond well to a single dose of any of the conjugate vaccines. In infants younger than 6 months of age, PedvaxHIB (PRP-OMP) is the only vaccine that induces significant antibody levels after a single injection. However, all three vaccines licensed for use in this age group result in high rates of seroconversion after two or three doses.

Placebo-controlled trials of both HibTITER (HbOC) and PedvaxHIB (PRP-OMP) in infants in the United States demonstrated nearly 100% protection and provided the basis for the initial licensure of these vaccines. In a northern California study, efficacy of HibTITER (HbOC) was 100% for infants receiving doses at 2, 4, and 6 months of age. In Navajo infants vaccinated at 2 and 4 months of age with PedvaxHIB (PRP-OMP), efficacy was 100% at 1 year of age and 93% at 18 months of age (these children did not receive a 12- to 18-month booster). Randomized, placebo-controlled trials of ActHIB (PRP-T) were terminated before completion when the U.S. Food and Drug

Table 5.3. Hib conjugate vaccines used in the United States

Trade name (abbreviation)	Manufacturer	Carrier protein	Polysaccharide	Adjuvant/ contaminants/ excipients	Preservative	Packaging
HibTITER (HbOC)	Wyeth	CRM$_{197}$ (cross-reactive material, a mutant diphtheria toxin)	Oligosaccharides	—	10-dose vial: thimerosal	Liquid 1-dose vial (4 or 5/pk) 10-dose vial
PedvaxHIB (PRP-OMP^a)	Merck	*Neisseria meningitidis* outer membrane protein	Large PRP	Alum	None	Liquid 1-dose vial (10/pk)
ActHIB^b OmniHIB (PRP-T)	Aventis Pasteur	Tetanus toxoid	Large PRP	Sucrose	None	Lyophilized 1-dose vial (5/pk) with vial of diluent

pk, package; PRP, polyribosylribitol phosphate, the capsular polysaccharide of Hib.
^{a}PRP-OMP is also available as a combination with Hep-B [COMVAX; see Chapter 7(II)].
^{b}ActHIB (PRP-T) can be combined in the same syringe with Tripedia (DTaP2) at the time of administration for the fourth dose only [this product is marketed by Aventis Pasteur as TriHIBit, whereas the PRP-T and DTaP2 vials are packaged together; see Chapter 7(I)].

Table 5.4. Hib vaccination for children not initiated by 6 months of age[a]

Age (mo)	First dose	Second dose	Third dose
7–11	Initial visit	2 mo later	Age 12–15 mo and at least 2 mo after second dose
12–14	Initial visit	2 mo later	Not necessary
15–59	Initial visit	Not necessary	Not necessary

[a]Any currently available Hib conjugate vaccine can be used for any dose.

Administration (FDA) approved HibTITER (HbOC) and PedvaxHIB (PRP-OMP) for use in infants. Licensure of ActHIB (PRP-T) was therefore based on comparable immunogenicity to that of the other two products.

Since 1988 when Hib conjugates were first introduced, the incidence of invasive disease in infants and young children has declined by more than 99%. In fact, the incidence of invasive infection caused by all other encapsulated types combined is now similar to that caused by type b (recent data suggest that, because laboratories are now relatively inexperienced in identifying Hib, many isolates that are labeled as such turn out to be other serotypes or non-typable strains). Today, invasive Hib disease is seen primarily in underimmunized children and infants too young to have completed the primary series.

H. **Official recommendations.** All children should receive Hib vaccine beginning at 2 months of age. Previously unimmunized children 15 to 59 months of age should receive a single dose, and those 5 years of age or older should be immunized only if they have an underlying condition predisposing to Hib disease (e.g., asplenia, IgG2 deficiency, or HIV infection). HibTITER (HbOC), ActHIB (PRP-T), and PedvaxHIB (PRP-OMP) are considered interchangeable for all doses. However, if either the 2-month or 4-month dose is HibTITER (HbOC) or ActHIB (PRP-T), a dose of any product must be given at 6 months. In contrast, if the first two doses are Pedvax-HIB (PRP-OMP), the 6-month dose is omitted. Hib vaccine may be given concomitantly with any other vaccines. Hib conjugates should not be given at younger than 6 weeks of age because of the possibility of inducing immunologic tolerance to further doses.

I. **Safety.** Local reactions occur in approximately 25% of recipients but typically are mild and last less than 24 hours. Systemic reactions (e.g., fever and irritability) are infrequent. Serious adverse events (e.g., anaphylaxis) have not been reported.

J. **Contraindications**
   • Severe allergic reaction to a previous dose or vaccine component
   • Age younger than 6 weeks

K. **Precautions.** Moderate or severe acute illness.
L. **Comments.** Early attempts to combine Hib conjugates with DTaP vaccines for the infant series were hampered by low PRP antibody responses. However, there are several combinations that are licensed in other countries, and it is likely that some will be introduced in the United States in the next few years.

KEY CONCEPTS: HAEMOPHILUS INFLUENZAE TYPE B

- Hib was leading cause of bacterial meningitis in the pre-vaccine era
- Invasive disease reduced by greater than 99% through universal vaccination
- Hib conjugates reduce nasopharyngeal carriage
- Available vaccines interchangeable but number of doses in the primary series differs by product
- PRP-OMP/Hep-B combination available for primary series
- DTaP2/PRP-T combination available for the fourth dose only

III. Hepatitis B

Hepatitis B virus is a nonenveloped, partially double-stranded DNA virus that is tropic for the liver, can establish chronic infection, and has oncogenic properties.

A. **Disease.** The incubation period ranges from 6 weeks to 6 months and averages 120 days. The clinical course of acute infection is indistinguishable from that of other types of viral hepatitis. Although infants and children are usually asymptomatic, clinical signs and symptoms occur in approximately 50% of adults. The prodromal phase usually lasts 3 to 10 days and is characterized by the insidious onset of malaise, anorexia, nausea, vomiting, right upper quadrant abdominal pain, fever, headache, myalgias, rash, arthralgia, arthritis, and dark urine. The icteric phase, which usually lasts from 1 to 3 weeks, is characterized by jaundice, elevated hepatic transaminases, light or gray colored stools, hepatic tenderness, and hepatomegaly (splenomegaly is less common). During convalescence, malaise and fatigue may persist for weeks to months, whereas jaundice, anorexia, and other symptoms disappear. Most acute hepatitis B infections in adults result in complete recovery, with elimination of hepatitis B surface antigen (HBsAg) from the blood and the production of anti-HBsAg antibody, which provides for lasting immunity. Fulminant hepatic failure occurs in less than 1% of individuals. However, 6% to 10% of adults and 90% of infants with acute infection become chronic carriers, with persistence of HBsAg in the blood.

B. Epidemiology and transmission. The virus can be transmitted by contact with contaminated secretions, including semen, vaginal secretions, blood, and saliva; through percutaneous inoculation (e.g., accidental needlesticks or sharing of needles with infected people); or perinatally from mother to infant. A human reservoir of persistently infected persons is present in nearly all communities of the world. In the United States, the reservoir is concentrated in parenteral drug abusers, sexually promiscuous individuals, those with occupationally acquired infection, and travelers returning from high-prevalence areas. In other countries with a high prevalence of infection in women of childbearing age, chronically infected children are a significant reservoir. An estimated 200 to 300 million people worldwide are chronic hepatitis B carriers. In the United States, approximately 5% of individuals have evidence of past infection, and 0.4%, or approximately 1,000,000, are chronically infected.

C. Rationale for vaccine use. Although acute hepatitis B can cause significant morbidity and death, a major rationale for immunization is to prevent chronic carriage. This is because chronic carriers can infect others over long periods of time and are at increased risk of developing cirrhosis and primary hepatocellular carcinoma. In fact, chronic hepatitis B may be the single most important factor for development of this form of cancer, and approximately 6,000 deaths each year in the United States can be blamed on the consequences of chronic hepatitis B infection. Data from Alaska show that universal childhood immunization can decrease the prevalence of chronic carriage, and data from Taiwan and Korea demonstrate that universal hepatitis B immunization can decrease the incidence of hepatocellular carcinoma. Thus, hepatitis B vaccine (Hep-B) is the first legitimate human vaccine against cancer.

Selective vaccination of high-risk populations in the 1980s failed to impact hepatitis B disease burden in the United States. Universal immunization at birth is feasible because the vaccine is immunogenic in infants. The rationale for vaccinating this early includes the following:
- Prevents the newborn encounter from becoming a missed opportunity
- Increases the likelihood that the entire three-dose series will be completed
- May reduce the number of concurrent injections that must be given at the 2-month visit
- Protects infants born to carrier mothers whose HBsAg status is not known at delivery
- Emphasizes the importance of immunization for new parents and lays the groundwork for the routine schedule in infancy

The relatively long incubation period of hepatitis B allows for postexposure prophylaxis through vaccination. In most instances, passive immunoprophylaxis with hepatitis B immune globulin (HBIG) is given concomitantly [see Chapter 11(II)].

D. Vaccines. The first Hep-B vaccines, introduced in the early 1980s, consisted of HBsAg purified from the plasma of chronically infected individuals. The recombinant vaccines introduced in the late 1980s consist of purified HBsAg. In this case, however, the protein is produced by common baker's yeast (*Saccharomyces cerevisiae*) cells that are engineered to carry the gene for HBsAg. Recombinant vaccines contain greater than 95% HBsAg protein in quantities ranging from 5 to 40 μg/mL; contaminating yeast proteins constitute up to 5% of the final product, but no yeast DNA is detectable in the vaccine. It is impossible to get hepatitis B infection from recombinant vaccine, because no viral DNA or complete viral particles are produced by the yeast cells.

Whereas plasma-derived vaccines are widely used in other parts of the world, only recombinant vaccines are used in the United States. Two products are available: RECOMBIVAX HB (Hep-B; Merck) and Engerix-B (Hep-B; GlaxoSmithKline). Each of these is available in pediatric and adult formulations, and there are special formulations for immunosuppressed patients and those on dialysis (Table 5.5). Combination vaccines containing HBsAg are also available: COMVAX [PRP-OMP/Hep-B, Merck; see Chapter 6(II)], Twinrix [Hep-A/Hep-B, GlaxoSmithKline; see Chapter 6(III)], and Pediarix [DTaP3/Hep-B/IPV, GlaxoSmithKline; see Chapter 6(V)]. Hep-B vaccines use alum as adjuvant.

RECOMBIVAX HB (Hep-B) and Engerix-B (Hep-B) are indicated for vaccination against all known subtypes of hepatitis B virus. Both are available in pediatric/adolescent and adult formulations; these formulations differ in the total amount of antigen and total volume but not in concentration. Thus, the pediatric/adolescent formulation of RECOMBIVAX HB (Hep-B) contains 5 μg of antigen in 0.5 mL, whereas the adult formulation contains 10 μg in 1.0 mL. The pediatric/adolescent formulation of Engerix-B (Hep-B) contains 10 μg in 0.5 mL, and the adult formulation contains 20 μg in 1.0 mL. For RECOMBIVAX HB (Hep-B), a child can receive one-half (0.5 mL) of the adult formulation, and an adult can receive two full pediatric/adolescent doses (0.5 mL each) given at the same site; however, for the two-dose regimen in adolescents 11 to 15 years of age, only the adult formulation at full-dose (1.0 mL) is acceptable. For Engerix-B (Hep-B), the pediatric/adolescent formulation is not labeled for use in adults, and the adult formulation is not labeled for use in children; however, the adult formulation (1.0 mL) may be used in adolescents 11 to 19 years of age.

E. Storage, handling, and administration
- Maintain temperature at 35° to 46°F (2° to 8°C)

Table 5.5. Usual dosing of Hep-B[a]

Patient group	Schedule (mo)	Formulation	
		RECOMBIVAX HB	Engerix-B
Infant of HBsAg-negative mother	Birth, 1–4, 6–18	Pediatric/adolescent[b,c]	Pediatric/adolescent[d,e]
Infant of HBsAg-positive mother[f]	Birth, 1, 6	Pediatric/adolescent[b,c]	Pediatric/adolescent[d,e]
1–10 yr	0, 1, 6	Pediatric/adolescent[b]	Pediatric/adolescent[d]
11–19 yr	0, 1, 6	Pediatric/adolescent[b]	Adult[g,h]
11–15 yr	0, 4–6[i]	Adult[j]	—
≥20 yr	0, 1, 6	Adult[j]	Adult[g,h]
Dialysis, immunocompromised	RECOMBIVAX HB: 0, 1, 6 Engerix-B: 0, 1, 2, 6	Dialysis[k]	Dialysis[l]

[a]Alternate schedules are available (consult the package insert).
[b]5 μg in 0.5-mL dose, supplied as liquid in one-dose vial (one or ten) or prefilled Luer-Lok syringe (ten), preservative free [one-half (0.5 mL) of the adult formulation may be used].
[c]COMVAX (PRP-OMP/Hep-B) can be used at 2, 4, and 12 to 15 months of age. It should not be given before 6 weeks of age [see Chapter 6(III)]. The birth dose of monovalent Hep-B should still be given.
[d]10 μg in 0.5-mL dose, supplied as liquid in one-dose vials (one or ten) or prefilled Tip-Lok syringe (5 or 25, with or without SafetyGlide needles), preservative free.
[e]Pediarix (DTaP3/Hep-B/IPV) can be used at 2, 4, and 6 months of age. It should not be given before 6 weeks of age [see Chapter 6(V)]. The birth dose of monovalent Hep-B should still be given.
[f]These infants should also receive HBIG, 0.5 mL intramuscularly, at a separate site [see Chapter 12(II)]; both vaccine and HBIG should be given within 12 hours of birth.
[g]20 μg in 1.0-mL dose, supplied as liquid in one-dose vial (1 or 25), prefilled Tip-Lok syringe (5 or 25, with or without SafetyGlide needles), preservative free.
[h]Twinrix (Hep-A/Hep-B) can be used in individuals 18 years of age or older who have indications for both Hep-A and Hep-B immunization (the usual schedule is 0, 1, and 6 months) [see Chapter 6(IV)].
[i]Children who begin the series with the pediatric (5-μg) formulation should complete the three-dose series rather than switch to the two-dose regimen (if it is not known which formulation was received first, the three-dose regimen should be used).
[j]10 μg in 1.0 mL, supplied as liquid in one-dose or three-dose vials (one or ten), preservative free.
[k]40 μg in 1.0 mL, supplied as liquid in one-dose vial, preservative free.
[l]Two adult doses (20 μg in 1.0 mL each) are given at the same site.

- Freezing can cause the vaccine to lose potency
- Shake well before use
- Each dose is 0.5 mL given intramuscularly; it may be given subcutaneously in patients at risk for hemorrhage after intramuscular injection [see Chapter 3(III)]

F. Schedule. Primary vaccination consists of three doses, given at 0, 1, and 6 months. Table 5.5 shows the two available products and their respective dosing schedules.

G. Efficacy. The three-dose series induces protective antibody levels in more than 95% of individuals younger than 40 years of age. In field trials, efficacy has been 80% to 95% and has correlated well with immunogenicity. Protection against disease is virtually 100% for persons who develop antibody concentrations 10 mIU/mL or higher. The combination of active and passive immunization at birth for infants of HBsAg-positive mothers is more than 90% effective in preventing transmission to the infant. Children immunized at birth seem to be protected for at least 10 years, and immunologic memory has been demonstrated for at least 12 years after vaccination. At the present time, there is no indication of a need for routine booster doses. Exceptions are hemodialysis patients and possibly other immunocompromised patients (see Official recommendations).

In immunogenicity studies of adolescents aged 11 to 15 years, antibody concentrations and seroprotection rates were similar between the two-dose and three-dose schedules, and the rate of decline in antibody levels over 2 years was similar. No data are available to assess long-term protection or immune memory after the two-dose schedule, and it is not known whether booster doses of vaccine will be required.

After implementation of universal infant immunization in Taiwan, the overall prevalence of hepatitis B in children 1 to 10 years of age decreased from 9.8% in 1984 to 1.3% in 1994. In the United States between 1986 and 2000, the rate of hepatitis B among children aged 1 through 9 years declined more than 80%.

H. Official recommendations. All infants should receive the Hep-B series by 18 months of age. Initiating the series at birth (before hospital discharge) is *strongly favored*, regardless of maternal HBsAg status (this is *mandatory* if the mother is HBsAg positive). In populations in which infection is highly endemic, such as Alaskan Natives, Pacific Islanders, and immigrant or refugee groups, the schedule should be completed by 12 months of age. For infants weighing less than 2 kg who are born to HBsAg-negative mothers, the first dose should be given at 1 to 30 days of age, followed by three more doses at 1 to 2, 2 to 4, and 6 to 18 months of age. All 11- to 12-year-old children who have not been previously immunized should also receive the vaccine, as should children younger than 11 years of age who are Pacific Islanders or who reside in households of first-generation immigrants from countries where hepatitis B is of high or intermediate endemicity.

Vaccination is also recommended for those with one or more of the following risk factors:

- Sexually active heterosexual adolescents and adults who have a recently acquired sexually transmitted disease, are identified as prostitutes, or have had one or more sex partners in the previous 6 months
- Men who have sex with men
- Household contacts of sexual partners of HBsAg-positive persons
- Injecting drug users
- Persons at occupational risk of infection through exposure to blood or blood-contaminated body fluids, such as health care and public safety workers
- Residents and staff of institutions for the developmentally disabled
- Hemodialysis patients (vaccination of those with early renal failure is encouraged before they require hemodialysis)
- Patients who receive clotting factor concentrates
- Members of households with international adoptees who are HBsAg-positive
- Travelers (especially children) to areas with high and intermediate rates of hepatitis B infection who have close contact with the local population or are likely to have contact with blood (such as in a medical setting) or sexual contact with residents
- Inmates in long-term correctional facilities

Passive immunoprophylaxis with HBIG (in addition to vaccination) is recommended within 12 hours of birth for infants of HBsAg-positive mothers. HBIG is indicated for other exposures as well [see Chapter 11(II)].

Booster doses are not recommended except in the case of hemodialysis and possibly other immunocompromised patients, in whom the need should be assessed by annual antibody testing. An additional dose should be given if the serum anti-HBsAg antibody concentration falls below 10 mIU/mL. The only other individuals who should routinely be tested for antibody responses after the primary series is given are health care workers who are at ongoing risk for sharps injuries. Those who are seronegative after three doses should receive another three-dose series one time only. Those who remain seronegative after this should be tested for HBsAg, as chronic carriage is one explanation for failure to respond to the vaccine.

For purposes of completing the series and achieving complete immunization, the licensed products are viewed as equivalent and interchangeable, except for the two-dose schedule for adolescents aged 11 to 15 years [only the adult formulation of RECOMBIVAX HB (Hep-B) is approved for this schedule]. Hep-B may be given concomitantly with any other vaccines.

I. **Safety.** The most common adverse reaction after Hep-B vaccination is pain at the site of injection, reported in 13% to 29% of adults and 3% to 9% of children. Mild systemic complaints such as fatigue, headache, and irritability have been reported in 11% to 17% of adults and up to 20% of children. Low-grade fever is seen in 1% of adults and up to 6% of children. It should be noted that well over 1,000,000,000 doses of Hep-B have been given worldwide since the 1980s, and serious systemic adverse events and allergic reactions have rarely been reported. Anaphylaxis is estimated to occur in 1 in 600,000 doses distributed.

J. Contraindications. History of anaphylaxis to a previous dose or any of its components.

K. Precautions. Moderate or severe acute illness.

L. Comments. A combination containing Hep-B, Pediarix (DTaP3/Hep-B/IPV), was licensed in late 2002 [see Chapter 6(V)]. This will find use in the infant immunization series.

KEY CONCEPTS: HEPATITIS B

- 1,000,000 Americans chronically infected
- 6,000 deaths each year from consequences of chronic infection
- First legitimate vaccination strategy against a form of cancer (hepatocellular)
- Vaccines made by recombinant technology using yeast cells to produce HBsAg
- Hep-B vaccines are interchangeable except for the two-dose schedule for adolescents
- Often given concomitantly (separate site) with HBIG for postexposure prophylaxis
- Booster doses not recommended for healthy persons
- Booster doses may be necessary for dialysis patients

IV. Polio

Polioviruses are small, nonenveloped, single-stranded RNA viruses that are neurotropic.

A. Disease. Approximately 95% of poliovirus infections are asymptomatic. Minor, nonspecific illness with low-grade fever and sore throat occurs in 4% to 8% of infected people; aseptic meningitis, sometimes with paresthesias, occurs in 1% to 2% of patients a few days after these symptoms resolve. In less than 1% of patients, destruction of anterior horn cells and lower motor neurons leads to rapid onset of asymmetric flaccid paralysis and areflexia, and residual paralytic disease occurs in 1 per 250 infections. Cranial nerve involvement and paralysis of respiratory muscles can occur. Findings in the cerebrospinal fluid are characteristic of viral meningitis, with mild pleocytosis and lymphocytic predominance. Adults who contracted paralytic poliomyelitis during childhood may develop postpolio syndrome, characterized by muscle pain and exacerbation of weakness 30 to 40 years later.

B. Epidemiology and transmission. Poliovirus infections occur only in humans. Spread is predominantly by the fecal-oral route, but pharyngeal secretions may be involved as well. Communicability is greatest shortly before and after onset of clinical illness; however, patients may be contagious in the absence of symptoms, and fecal excretion may persist for weeks. Immunodeficient patients can excrete virus for more than 6 months.

Infection is more common in infants and young children and occurs at an earlier age among children living in poor hygienic conditions. The risk of paralytic disease increases with age. In temperate climates, poliovirus infections are most common during the summer and autumn. In the tropics, the seasonal pattern is variable with a less pronounced peak of activity.

The last reported indigenous case of poliomyelitis in the United States occurred in 1979, and the only identified imported case of paralytic poliomyelitis since 1986 occurred in a child transported to the United States for medical care in 1993. Since 1979, all other cases of polio, an average of eight per year between 1980 and 1996, have been oral poliovirus vaccine (OPV)-associated. With the elimination of OPV use in 2000, no cases of polio currently occur in the United States.

C. Rationale for vaccine use. Because of widespread vaccination, worldwide eradication of polio is now on the horizon. In the United States, the annual number of cases fell from more than 18,000 to essentially zero in two decades. Worldwide, there has been an 80% reduction in cases since the mid-1980s. Three WHO regions have eliminated or are close to eliminating poliovirus—the Region of the Americas has been polio-free since 1991, polio has not been detected in the Western Pacific Region since March of 1997, and transmission in the European Region is confined to southeastern Turkey. Reaching the goal of global eradication by 2005 will require accelerated activities in the remaining major foci of southern Asia and Africa.

These astonishing accomplishments have occurred primarily through the use of OPV. This was the vaccine of choice for children in the United States since the early 1960s because it induced optimal intestinal immunity, was painless to administer, and contributed to immunity at the population level through fecal-oral spread. For these same reasons, OPV continues to be used in many parts of the world. However, the continued use of OPV, with the attendant five to ten cases of vaccine-associated paralytic poliomyelitis (VAPP) per year, was felt to be unjustified in the United States in the absence of wild-type disease. Inactivated poliovirus vaccine (IPV) was known to be highly effective, was incapable of causing VAPP, and was used routinely in several countries that controlled or eliminated polio, including Finland, France, and the Netherlands. Accordingly, expanded use of IPV was recommended beginning in 1997, and as of January of 2000, the recommendation was made to substitute IPV for OPV in the United States. This marks one of the few times in history when the recommendation for a routine vaccine was withdrawn.

In 2000 to 2001, there was an outbreak of paralytic poliomyelitis in the Caribbean caused by a strain of OPV that had reverted to virulence. This occurred in areas of very low vaccine coverage, highlighting the need for vigilance in maintaining high immunization levels. After global eradication, it will be difficult to decide whether polio immunization should be discontinued. Theoretically, reserves of virus could still exist (e.g., in laboratories that have frozen stool specimens from the polio era), and infectious virus that can be used in bioterrorism can be reconstructed from the genetic material of the virus.

D. Vaccines. OPV is no longer manufactured and routinely available in the United States. The current IPV has enhanced potency compared to earlier versions. Two products are licensed in the United States, Poliovax (IPV; human diploid cell) and IPOL (IPV; monkey kidney cell), both manufactured by Aventis Pasteur (only IPOL is distributed). A third IPV is licensed only as part of the combination vaccine Pediarix (DTaP3/Hep-B/IPV) [see Chapter 6(V)]. IPOL (IPV) contains formaldehyde-inactivated poliovirus types 1, 2, and 3 and 2-phenoxyethanol as preservative. Potential contaminants may include formaldehyde, calf serum protein, neomycin, streptomycin, and polymyxin B. It is available as a liquid in prefilled syringes (one or ten) or in ten-dose vials. IPOL (IPV) is indicated for active immunization of individuals 6 weeks of age or older. The OPV produced and distributed in the United States by Wyeth (ORIMUNE) was discontinued in October 1999.

E. Storage, handling, and administration
- Maintain temperature at 35° to 46°F (2° to 8°C)
- Freezing can cause the vaccine to lose potency
- Each dose is 0.5 mL given intramuscularly [see Chapter 3(III)]

F. Schedule. A primary series of inactivated polio vaccine consists of three doses. The first dose may be given as early as 6 weeks of age, but is usually given at 2 months, with a second dose at 4 months of age. The third dose should be given at 6 to 18 months of age. The preferred interval between the second and third doses is 2 to 8 months. However, if accelerated protection is needed, such as before travel to an endemic area, the interval between doses can be shortened to 4 weeks. Children who receive three doses of IPV before the fourth birthday should receive a fourth dose before or at school entry. If the third dose is given on or after the fourth birthday, another dose is not needed.

G. Efficacy. Ninety percent or more of vaccinees develop protective antibody to all three serotypes after two doses, and 99% or more are immune after three doses. Protection against paralytic disease correlates with the presence of serum antibody. IPV appears to induce less mucosal immunity than does OPV, so persons who receive IPV are more readily infected in the gastrointestinal tract with wild poliovirus. Thus, a person immunized with IPV could become infected in an endemic area and shed virus on return to the United States. The infected person would be protected from paralytic polio, but the wild virus shed in the stool could be transmitted to a contact. The duration of immunity from IPV is not known with certainty but is probably many years after a complete series.

H. Official recommendations. All children should receive four doses of IPV according to the above schedule. The vaccine may be given concomitantly with any other vaccines as long as separate sites are used. Routine immunization of adults 18 years of age or older in the United States is not recommended. However, a three-dose series of IPV (0, 1 to 2, and 6 to 12 months) *is* recommended for *previously unvaccinated adults in the following circumstances* (an accelerated schedule can be used if necessary):

- Travel to countries where poliomyelitis is epidemic or endemic
- Community experiencing wild-type poliovirus disease
- Health care workers who will come into close contact with patients potentially excreting wild-type poliovirus
- Laboratory workers who will come in contact with specimens that may contain wild-type poliovirus

Adults who have received a primary series who are traveling to countries where poliomyelitis is still endemic should receive a single supplemental dose of IPV (this does not need to be repeated for subsequent travel). Those who are incompletely immunized should complete the primary series with IPV, regardless of which vaccine was given in the past.

The ACIP and AAP continue to support the global eradication initiative and use of OPV where polio is endemic. The Expanded Programme on Immunization of the WHO uses OPV at birth, 6 weeks, 10 weeks, and 14 weeks of age, and supplementary doses are often given during mass community programs. Breast-feeding does not interfere with successful immunization with OPV.

I. Safety. As with any vaccine, minor local reactions such as pain and redness may occur after IPV. No serious adverse events have been associated with use of the currently available vaccine.

J. Contraindications. Anaphylactic reaction to a previous dose or anaphylactic reaction to one of the antibiotics in the vaccine.

K. Precautions
- Moderate or severe acute illness
- The ACIP and AAP list pregnancy as a precaution for IPV because of the theoretic risk of harm to the fetus, even though this is an inactivated vaccine. No deleterious effects from IPV administered during pregnancy have been demonstrated, and the ACIP and AAP agree that if immediate protection against poliomyelitis is needed, IPV may be given.

KEY CONCEPTS: POLIO

- Last known indigenous case in the United States occurred in 1979
- Last case in the western hemisphere occurred in 1991
- Only IPV is used in the United States because of risk of poliomyelitis from OPV
- Global eradication of poliovirus expected by 2005

V. Measles, mumps, and rubella

Measles (rubeola) virus and mumps virus are enveloped, single-stranded RNA viruses in the *Paramyxoviridae* family. Rubella virus is an enveloped, single-stranded RNA virus in the Togavirus family. All three have only one known antigenic type.

A. Disease
- *Measles*

  Measles is characterized by a several-day prodrome of malaise, fever, anorexia, coryza, cough, and conjunctivitis. Temperature usually increases for 5 or 6 days and can be as high as 104°F (40°C). In uncomplicated cases, the temperature drops 2 to 3 days after the onset of exanthem. At some point between the second and fourth days after onset of symptoms, but before the rash appears, characteristic Koplik's spots appear on the buccal mucosa. The rash generally appears around the ears and hairline 3 to 5 days into the illness and spreads downward and outward to cover the face, trunk, and extremities over the next 3 to 4 days. It is initially erythematous and maculopapular and tends to become confluent as it spreads, especially on the face and neck. The rash usually lasts approximately 5 days and resolves in the order of appearance.
- *Mumps*

  Mumps usually presents as bilateral or, less commonly, unilateral parotitis that may be preceded by fever, headache, malaise, myalgia, and anorexia. Only

30% to 40% of mumps infections produce typical acute parotitis; 15% to 20% are asymptomatic, and up to 50% are associated with respiratory or nonspecific symptoms. Parotitis occurs more commonly among children aged 2 to 9 years, and inapparent infection may be more common among adults. Serious complications can occur without evidence of parotitis.

• *Rubella*
Rubella is characterized by nonspecific signs and symptoms, including transient, erythematous, and sometimes pruritic rash; postauricular or suboccipital lymphadenopathy; arthralgia; and low-grade fever. Twenty-five percent to 50% of infections are subclinical. The disease is generally considered benign and self-limited.

B. Epidemiology and transmission

• *Measles*
In temperate areas, measles occurs primarily in late winter and spring. There is no known animal reservoir, and asymptomatic human carriers have not been documented. Transmission is primarily person to person via large respiratory droplets. Airborne transmission has been documented in closed areas, such as office examination rooms, for up to 2 hours after the presence of an infected person. Measles is highly contagious, with secondary household attack rates exceeding 90%. It is estimated that before the introduction of the first vaccine in 1963, there were 3 to 4 million cases of measles each year in the United States. That number had fallen to approximately 1,500 by 1983. However, between 1989 and 1991, there were almost 56,000 reported cases and 123 deaths. This resurgence was due to pockets of low vaccine coverage in the population. Renewed efforts to vaccinate young children and the institution of a second vaccination at school entry effectively reversed this resurgence. The second dose is not given because of waning immunity; rather, it is intended to capture those children who either missed initial vaccination or did not seroconvert after the first dose.

• *Mumps*
The incidence peaks in winter and spring, but disease has been reported throughout the year. Mumps is a human disease. Although persons with asymptomatic or nonclassic infection can transmit the virus, no carrier state exists. Transmission occurs through airborne droplet nuclei or direct contact with saliva. Contagiousness is similar to that of influenza and rubella but less than that for measles and chickenpox. The infectious period is considered to be from 3 days before to the fourth day of active disease. In 1964, there were 212,000 cases in the United States; by 1983, after the vaccine had been licensed for 16 years,

that number had fallen to 3,000. There was a resurgence of disease among teenagers in the late 1980s, probably because this cohort had missed the universal infant vaccination recommendation. The resurgence was reversed by institution of the second measles, mumps, and rubella (MMR) vaccine at school entry.

- *Rubella*

  In temperate climates, rubella occurs in late winter and early spring. There is no animal reservoir, and although infants with congenital rubella syndrome (CRS) may shed large quantities of virus for up to a year, no true carrier state has been described. Rubella is only moderately contagious and spreads from person to person via airborne droplet nuclei shed from the respiratory tract. Transmission by subclinical cases, which constitutes 20% to 50% of all infections, can occur. The disease is most contagious when the rash is erupting, but virus may be shed from 7 days before to 7 days after rash onset. Between 1964 and 1965, there were over 12 million cases of rubella in the United States, and 20,000 babies were born with CRS. After vaccination was initiated in 1969, the number of cases of rubella and CRS declined dramatically, although disease is still seen, especially in immigrants from Latin America.

C. Rationale for vaccine use

- *Measles*

  Measles can be severe and is most frequently complicated by diarrhea, middle ear infection, or bronchopneumonia. Encephalitis occurs in approximately 1 out of every 1,000 cases, and survivors often have permanent brain damage. Death, usually from pneumonia or acute encephalitis, occurs in 1 to 2 out of every 1,000 cases; the risk is greater for infants, young children, and adults than it is for older children and adolescents. These two complications, encephalitis and death, constitute the main rationale for universal immunization. Subacute sclerosing panencephalitis can also be prevented by vaccination. This is a rare, fatal degenerative disease of the central nervous system that appears years after measles infection (5 to 10 per million cases) and is associated with persistent infection with a mutant form of the virus.

  In developing countries, measles is often more severe, with case-fatality rates as high as 25%. Measles can be severe and prolonged among immunocompromised persons, particularly those who have leukemia, lymphoma, or HIV infection. In these patients, the typical rash may be absent, and the patient may shed virus for several weeks.

- *Mumps*

  Mumps is usually self-limited, but complications do occur. Aseptic meningitis is common, occurring asymptomatically in 50% to 60% of patients and associated with headache and stiff neck in up to 15%. Adults are at greater risk for this complication than children, and boys are more often affected than girls. Encephalitis is rare, occurring in less than 2 per 100,000 cases. Orchitis is the most common complication in postpubertal males, occurring in up to 50% of cases. Approximately 50% of patients are left with some degree of testicular atrophy, but sterility is rare. Mumps was a leading cause of acquired sensorineural deafness in the prevaccine era, with an estimated incidence of 1 per 20,000 cases.

- *Rubella*
  The most severe effects of rubella occur in the fetuses of pregnant women who contract the infection during the first trimester of pregnancy. Infants born with CRS may have deafness, cataracts, microophthalmia, cardiac defects, and central nervous system abnormalities. The primary objective of rubella vaccination is to prevent CRS.

D. Vaccines. MMR vaccine contains the Moraten strain (derived from the Edmonston B strain) of measles virus, the Jeryl Lynn strain of mumps virus (which actually consists of two distinct strains), and the RA 27/3 strain of rubella virus (the original MMR, licensed in 1971, contained a duck-embryo–passaged rubella virus). All three are live-attenuated viruses; the measles and mumps viruses are grown in chick embryo cell culture, and the rubella virus is grown in human diploid cell culture. The MMR vaccine used in the United States, M-M-R$_{II}$, as well as the monovalent vaccines and other combinations, are all manufactured by Merck. Other iterations of these vaccines include ATTENUVAX (monovalent measles), MUMPSVAX (monovalent mumps), MERUVAX$_{II}$ (rubella), M-R-VAX$_{II}$ (also known as BIAVAX$_{II}$; measles and rubella), and M-M-VAX (measles and mumps, not currently available). The labeled indications are for prevention of measles, mumps, and/or rubella in susceptible persons 12 months of age or older. M-M-R$_{II}$ is supplied lyophilized as one-dose vials (one or ten per package) along with separate vials of diluent. Ten-dose vials are available to government agencies only. Potential contaminants and excipients include sorbitol, sucrose, gelatin, human albumin, fetal bovine serum, buffer and media ingredients, and neomycin.

E. Storage, handling, and administration
- Maintain temperature at 50°F (10°C) or less during shipping
- Freezing during shipment does not affect potency
- Store lyophilized vaccine before reconstitution at 35° to 46°F (2° to 8°C) or colder
- Vials must be protected from light at all times
- Store diluent in refrigerator or at room temperature (do not freeze)
- Reconstitute just before use and *only* with diluent supplied

- Use reconstituted vaccine immediately or stored in a dark place for up to 8 hours at 35° to 46°F (2° to 8°C)
- Each dose is 0.5 mL given subcutaneously [see Chapter 3(III)]

F. Schedule. Two doses of MMR separated by at least 1 month and administered on or after the first birthday are recommended for all children and for certain high-risk groups of adolescents and adults. The first dose is recommended at 12 to 15 months of age, and the second is routinely given at 4 to 6 years of age (and no later than 11 to 12 years of age). However, a second dose given any time 1 month or more after the first dose is valid, and no further doses are needed.

G. Efficacy. Measles immunization produces a mild or inapparent, noncommunicable infection. Antibodies develop in approximately 95% of children vaccinated at 12 months of age and 98% of children vaccinated at 15 months of age. Studies indicate that more than 99% of persons who receive two doses of vaccine, separated by at least 1 month on or after their first birthday, develop serologic evidence of measles immunity. Although vaccine-induced antibody titers are lower than those after natural disease, persistence of protective titers for as long as 16 years after vaccination has been demonstrated. Most vaccinated persons who appear to lose antibody have an anamnestic response on revaccination, indicating that they are most likely still protected. A small percentage of vaccinated individuals may lose protection after several years.

Mumps vaccine induces an asymptomatic, noncommunicable infection as well. More than 97% of susceptible recipients develop protective antibody titers, albeit lower than those after natural infection. Reported clinical efficacy ranges from 75% to 95%. The duration of vaccine immunity is unknown, but serologic data indicate the persistence of antibody for more than 30 years.

At least 98% of rubella-susceptible vaccinees 12 months of age or older develop protective antibody titers. Vaccine-induced rubella antibodies have persisted in more than 90% of vaccinees at least 16 years after receiving the RA 27/3 vaccine. Lifelong protection against clinical reinfection, asymptomatic viremia, or both usually results from a single dose of vaccine early in childhood. In some cases, vaccinees exposed to natural rubella develop an asymptomatic increase in antibody titer (reinfection with wild-type rubella virus has been observed in individuals with previous natural rubella). Reinfection of vaccinees is rarely associated with viremia or pharyngeal shedding, and person-to-person transmission has not been reported. The risk of CRS from rubella reinfection during pregnancy is extremely low.

Since vaccines containing measles, mumps, and rubella viruses were licensed, the number of reported cases of measles, mumps, rubella, and CRS has decreased by more than 99%. Since 1995, fewer cases of measles, mumps, and rubella have been reported than at any time since nationwide disease reporting began, and elimination of indigenous transmission appears feasible.

H. Official recommendations. MMR is the preferred vaccine, and there are very few, if any, indications to give the monovalent vaccines separately. Adults born before 1957, except for women who might become pregnant and health care workers, may be considered immune to measles because of previous natural infection, even if this is not documented. Those born in or after 1957 who have not been vaccinated and have no evidence of immunity (e.g., positive serology) should receive at least one dose of MMR; those in high-risk situations, such as health care workers or college students, should receive two doses. Women who do not have documentation of at least one dose of rubella vaccine or the presence of rubella antibody should receive one dose of the vaccine, preferably given as MMR, before becoming pregnant (pregnancy should be deferred for at least 28 days after vaccination). A clinical history of rubella is *not* proof of immunity, because other rash illnesses can mimic this disease.

During measles outbreaks, when the likelihood of exposure is high, measles vaccine can be given to infants as young as 6 months of age. Doses given before the first birthday, however, *do not count* in the series, and these children should receive two subsequent doses according to the usual schedule. Although measles vaccination is not a requirement for entry into any country, measles and mumps are still endemic in many parts of the world. Susceptible people who are traveling to these areas should be offered MMR before leaving. This includes infants 6 months of age or older, who should be revaccinated according to the schedule when they reach 12 months of age (vaccination of infants less than 6 months of age is not necessary, because most are protected by maternal antibodies).

Emphasis for rubella immunization should be placed on college students, women of childbearing age, foreign-born adults, and military personnel. Settings such as premarital screening, routine gynecologic examinations, postpartum visits, appointments for newborn infants, and well-child care provide opportunities for immunization. Rubella vaccine may be given after anti-Rho(D) immune globulin administration, but testing for seroconversion should be performed 6 to 8 weeks later. Although screening for rubella immunity before vaccination is acceptable, a more practical approach may be to immunize individuals without a documented history of immunization (there is no harm in vaccinating a person who is already immune).

Measles vaccine given within 72 hours of exposure to measles may prevent infection, but this is not true for mumps and rubella vaccines. Nevertheless, if exposure does not result in infection, the benefit of MMR vaccination is protection against future infection. MMR can be given simultaneously with any other childhood vaccine using separate syringes and separate sites. If not given simultaneously, other live virus vaccines should be deferred at least 1 month.

Guidelines for the use of MMR (and other live vaccines) in immunocompromised individuals, including those on steroids and those with HIV infection, are contained in Chapter 12(I).

I. **Safety.** Five percent to 15% of vaccinees develop fever of 103°F (39.4°C) or higher, and approximately 5% develop a mild morbilliform rash, usually within 7 to 12 days. Febrile seizures, seen 8 to 14 days after vaccination, are estimated to occur in 25 to 34 per 100,000 vaccinees and are not associated with subsequent seizures or neurodevelopmental disabilities. One case of thrombocytopenia occurs for every 30,000 to 40,000 doses distributed and is presumably due to the measles component. Although usually asymptomatic, thrombocytopenic purpura has been reported. Transient lymphadenopathy sometimes occurs after MMR, and parotitis has been reported rarely. Arthralgia is reported in up to 25% of susceptible adult women given MMR and is attributed to the rubella component; persistent or recurrent joint symptoms have been reported but are rare. It should be mentioned that the incidence of joint problems after immunization is lower than that after natural infection at the same age.

Most allergic reactions are minor and consist of a wheal and flare or urticaria at the injection site. Anaphylactic reactions are extremely rare. The vaccine does not contain significant amounts of egg protein and can safely be given to patients with allergies to eggs, chickens, and feathers without prior skin testing and without incremental dosing.

The viruses in MMR are not transmitted from person to person after vaccination and, therefore, the vaccine can be given to contacts of immunosuppressed and pregnant individuals.

J. **Contraindications**
   - Anaphylactic reaction to a prior dose of the vaccine or any of its components
   - Immunodeficiency or immunosuppression [except HIV-infected persons without severe immunosuppression; see Chapter 12(I)]
   - Pregnancy
   - Untreated active tuberculosis or positive skin test

K. **Precautions**
   - Moderate or severe acute illness
   - Recent administration of antibody-containing blood products [see Chapter 1(I)]
   - Thrombocytopenia or thrombocytopenic purpura, either active or by history

L. **Comments.** A vaccine that combines measles, mumps, rubella, and varicella vaccines into a single injection (MMRV) would be the most effective way to achieve universal immunization against these pathogens. Early studies indicated that interference between the viruses in MMRV combinations resulted in lower concentrations of antibody to varicella when compared to separate administration. Newer formulations have overcome this problem, and a licensed MMRV combination is expected in a few years.

KEY CONCEPTS: MEASLES, MUMPS, AND RUBELLA

- Main justifications for measles vaccine: encephalitis, pneumonia, death
- Main justifications for mumps vaccine: parotitis, orchitis, meningoencephalitis, hearing loss
- Main justification for rubella vaccine: congenital rubella syndrome
- Consists of three live-attenuated viruses
- Two doses necessary to ensure protection
- Can be given to people with egg allergy
- Horizontal transmission of the vaccine viruses does not occur

---

VI. Pneumococcal conjugate

Streptococcus pneumoniae is a facultatively anaerobic, catalase-negative, gram-positive coccus that produces an antiphagocytic, serotype-specific polysaccharide capsule.

A. **Disease.** Bacteremia without focal infection accounts for 70% of invasive disease among children younger than 2 years of age, and bacteremic pneumonia accounts for another 12% to 16%. With the disappearance of invasive Hib disease from the United States in the 1990s, pneumococcus became the leading cause of bacterial meningitis among children younger than 5 years of age. The highest incidence is in children younger than 1 year of age, with approximately 10 cases per 100,000 population. Pneumococcus is also a common cause of acute otitis media (AOM), accounting for 28% to 55% of cases. By age 12 months, 62% of children have had at least one episode of AOM, making this one of the most common reasons for sick pediatric office visits. Complications of otitis media include mastoiditis and suppurative intracranial infection.

B. **Epidemiology and transmission.** The reservoir for pneumococcus is the nasopharynx, and transmission occurs by direct person-to-person contact with droplets; autoinoculation from the upper respiratory tract also occurs. Spread within a household is influenced by such factors as crowding, season, and viral upper respiratory infection. The spread of pneumococcal disease is usually associated with increased carriage rates. However, high carriage rates do not always correlate with disease transmission in households. Pneumococcal infections are more common during the winter and early spring when viral respiratory diseases are most prevalent.

The incidence of invasive pneumococcal disease in the United States is approximately 21 per 100,000 population but varies greatly by age. The highest rates occur in young children, especially those younger than 2 years of age, and the lowest rates are in persons 5 to 17 years of age. Children with functional or anatomic asplenia, particularly those with sickle cell disease, and children with HIV infection are at very high risk, with rates in some studies more than 50 times those of age-equivalent children without these conditions. Alaskan Native, American Indian, and African American children are also at increased risk. The reason for this is not known, but the same racial and ethnic predilection was seen for invasive Hib disease. Day care attendance increases the risk of invasive pneumococcal disease and AOM two- to threefold among children 59 months of age or younger.

Mortality is highest among patients with bacteremia or meningitis, in patients with underlying medical conditions, and in the very young or old. In some high-risk groups, mortality from bacteremia is as high as 40% despite antibiotic therapy.

C. **Rationale for vaccine use.** Among children younger than 5 years of age in the United States, there are an estimated 17,000 annual cases of invasive disease, including 13,000 cases of bacteremia without focal infection and 700 cases of meningitis. Approximately 200 children die from pneumococcal infection every year. Although not considered invasive disease, an estimated 5 million cases of AOM occur each year in this age group.

The need for vaccination against pneumococcus is intensified by the emergence of antibiotic-resistant strains, making treatment more difficult. Children younger than 2 years of age respond poorly to the polysaccharide capsule of the organism. In addition, children up to 5 years of age may not respond well to serotypes 6B, 14, 19F, and 23F, common causes of pediatric infection and the most prevalent penicillin-resistant serotypes.

D. **Vaccines.** The pneumococcal conjugate vaccine contains the capsular polysaccharide of seven serotypes (4, 6B, 9V, 14, 18C, 19F, and 23F) linked to CRM_{197} (cross-reactive material, a mutant diphtheria toxin) and formulated with alum. These serotypes account for 80% of invasive infections in children. As with the Hib vaccine, conjugation converts T-cell–independent polysaccharide responses to T-cell–dependent ones, which are robust in infants and result in memory. The vaccine, called Prevnar (PCV-7), was licensed by Wyeth in 2000 and is indicated for immunization of infants and toddlers against invasive disease caused by the covered serotypes. In late 2002, the vaccine also received an indication for prevention of otitis media caused by vaccine serotypes, but it was specified that the degree of protection was expected to be substantially lower than that against invasive disease. It is supplied as a liquid in one-dose vials (five per package) without preservatives.

E. Storage, handling, and administration
- Maintain temperature at 35° to 46°F (2° to 8°C)
- Freezing can cause the vaccine to lose potency
- Shake well before use
- Each dose is 0.5 mL given intramuscularly [see Chapter 3(III)]

F. Schedule. The primary series beginning in infancy consists of three doses given at 2, 4, and 6 months of age. A booster dose is recommended at 12 to 15 months of age. For children vaccinated at less than 12 months of age, the minimum interval between doses is 4 weeks. Doses given at greater than 12 months of age should be separated by at least 8 weeks. The number of doses a child needs depends on the age and the presence of any high-risk conditions, as shown in Table 5.6.

G. Efficacy. After four doses of PCV-7, virtually all healthy infants develop antibody to all seven serotypes. PCV-7 is also immunogenic in infants and children with sickle cell disease and HIV infection. In a controlled clinical trial involving nearly 40,000 children, the vaccine reduced invasive disease caused by vaccine serotypes by 97%; there was also an 89% reduction in invasive disease caused by all serotypes, including those not in the vaccine. Efficacy against pneumonia varied depending on the specificity of the diagnosis. The vaccine also reduced x-ray–confirmed pneumonia with consolidation of greater than 2.5 cm by 73%. Children who received PCV-7 had 7% fewer episodes of AOM and underwent 20% fewer tympanostomy tube placements than unvaccinated children. Efficacy against AOM caused by vaccine-related pneumococcal serotypes in a Finnish study was 57%, but there was an increase of 33% in the rate of AOM episodes caused by nonvaccine serotypes. Despite this fact, the net effect on AOM caused by pneumococcus was a reduction of 34%. The duration of protection after PCV-7 is currently unknown. The effect of PCV-7 on nasopharyngeal carriage of pneumococci is also not clear at this time. One might expect a decrease in carriage, as was seen with the Hib conjugate vaccines, but the possibility of serotype replacement must be considered.

H. Official recommendations. Universal use of PCV-7 in children 23 months of age or younger is recommended as per the above schedule. Two doses of PCV-7, followed by one dose of Pne-PS, are recommended for children 24 to 59 months of age who are at high risk of invasive disease and have not previously been immunized. Routine

Table 5.6. Schedule for pneumococcal vaccination

Condition	Age at initiation (mo)	Total doses	Primary PCV-7 series	Booster
Healthy	2–6	4	3 doses (usually 2, 4, 6 mo)	12–15 mo
	7–11	3	2 doses 6–8 wk apart	12–15 mo
	12–23	2	2 doses 6–8 wk apart	None
	24–59[a]	1	—	None
High risk[b]	2–6	4	3 doses (usually 2, 4, 6 mo)	12–15 mo Pne-PS at 24 mo[c]
	7–11	3	2 doses 6–8 wk apart	12–15 mo Pne-PS at 24 mo[c]
	12–23	2	2 doses 6–8 wk apart	Pne-PS at 24 mo[c,d]
	24–59	2	2 doses 6–8 wk apart	Pne-PS[c,d]
	24–59 (previously immunized with Pne-PS but not PCV-7)	2	2 doses 6–8 wk apart	Pne-PS[e]

[a]Should be considered for all children but priority given to those aged 24 to 35 months, Alaskan Natives, American Indians, African Americans, those in group day care (4 hours per week or more with at least two unrelated children in the same center).
[b]Includes sickle cell disease; congenital or acquired asplenia or splenic dysfunction; HIV infection; congenital immune deficiency; chronic cardiac, pulmonary, or renal disease; cerebrospinal fluid leak; cochlear implants; diabetes; immunosuppressive therapy.
[c]A single repeat dose of Pne-PS can be considered 3 to 5 years later if high-risk condition persists.
[d]At least 8 weeks should elapse between the last dose of PCV-7 and Pne-PS.
[e]This dose should be given 3 to 5 years after the first dose of Pne-PS.
Adapted from AAP. Pneumococcal infections. In: Pickering LK, ed. *Red book: 2003 report of the Committee on Infectious Diseases*, 26th ed. Elk Grove Village, IL: American Academy of Pediatrics; 2003:490–500.

immunization of low- and moderate-risk children 24 to 59 months of age should be considered, with priority given to those aged 24 to 35 months, Alaskan Natives, American Indians, African Americans, and those who attend group day care centers.

High-risk children should be caught up according to Table 5.6. Revaccination after an age-appropriate primary series with PCV-7 is not recommended, and there is no indication for use of PCV-7 in older children or adults. PCV-7 can be administered at the same time as any other vaccine using a separate syringe and injection site.

I. Safety. Local reactions, which are more common with the fourth dose, occur in 10% to 20% of recipients. Fewer than 3% of local reactions are considered to be severe (e.g., tenderness that interferes with limb movement). In clinical trials, fever greater than 100.4°F (38°C) within 48 hours of any dose of the primary series was reported in 15% to 24% of children. However, in these studies, DTP was administered simultaneously with each dose and may have been responsible for the fever. In a study in which DTaP was given at the same visit as the booster dose of PCV-7, 11% of recipients developed a temperature greater than 102.2°F (39°C). No severe adverse events have been reported.

J. Contraindications. History of anaphylaxis to a previous dose or any of its components.

K. Precautions. Moderate to severe acute illness.

L. Comments. Because of the large number of serotypes that cause disease, development of conjugate pneumococcal vaccines has been more difficult than for Hib. Those under development differ in carrier protein, molecular size of the polysaccharide, and the method of conjugating the polysaccharide to the protein. To date, candidate carrier proteins have been the same as those used for Hib. Each antigen must be coupled to the protein in quantities large enough to induce an immune response without eliciting adverse reactions. Vaccines containing polysaccharides from serotypes 5, 7, 9, and 11 (in addition to the PCV-7 serotypes) conjugated to either tetanus toxoid, diphtheria toxoid, meningococcal outer membrane protein, or CRM_{197} are currently under study. Combinations that include polysaccharides from all three major pyogenic bacteria (i.e., pneumococcus, Hib, and meningococcus) are also under development.

KEY CONCEPTS: PNEUMOCOCCAL CONJUGATE

- Pneumococcus is leading cause of bacterial meningitis, bacteremia, and pneumonia in young children
- Antibiotic-resistant strains becoming common
- Overcomes poor antibody responses infants have to pure polysaccharide vaccines
- Contains serotypes 4, 6B, 9V, 14, 18C, 19F, and 23F, which account for 80% of invasive disease in children
- Universal immunization 23 months of age or younger recommended
- Selective immunization 24 to 59 months of age recommended
- Certain children should receive Pne-PS in addition to PCV-7

VII. Varicella

Varicella zoster virus is a large, enveloped, double-stranded DNA virus capable of establishing latency.

A. **Disease.** The incubation period ranges from 10 to 21 days but may be prolonged in immunocompromised patients and those who have received varicella zoster immune globulin (VZIG). In children, rash is often the first sign of disease, but adults may have a 1- to 2-day prodrome of fever and malaise. The rash is pruritic, usually beginning on the scalp or hairline, then moving to the trunk (where the highest concentration of lesions is) and extremities. Lesions are 1 to 4 mm in diameter and appear in successive crops over several days; at any given time, these crops are in different stages of development. Lesions characteristically evolve from macules to papules then to superficial, delicate vesicles containing clear fluid on an erythematous base ("dew drops on rose petals"). They rapidly become pustules that crust and fall off, leaving a shallow ulcer. Lesions can occur on mucous membranes and on the cornea. The average case consists of malaise and fever for 2 to 3 days and develops 200 to 500 lesions. Adults have more severe disease and higher complication rates. Immunocompromised individuals may develop *progressive varicella*, characterized by high fever, extensive vesicular eruption, and high complication rates. Mild hepatitis occurs in 20% to 50% of cases but is usually asymptomatic. Similarly, 5% to 16% of patients develop thrombocytopenia, but bleeding is rare. *Hemorrhagic varicella* is characterized by thrombocytopenia and extensive purpuric lesions.

Recovery from primary infection usually results in lifetime immunity. Periodic reexposure to natural varicella may lead to subclinical reinfection that boosts antibody titers. When immunity does wane (as, for example, with aging), reactivation of latent virus can result in *herpes zoster*, or *shingles*, characterized by a unilateral, vesicular eruption and pain in a dermatomal distribution. *Post-herpetic neuralgia*, characterized by persistent residual pain in the affected area, is a distressing complication with no adequate therapy. Herpes zoster is common in patients undergoing immunosuppressive therapy and in infants with intrauterine exposure to varicella or infection in infancy. In immunocompromised patients, herpes zoster may disseminate, causing generalized skin lesions, and central nervous system, pulmonary, and hepatic disease occurs. Although rare, *congenital varicella syndrome*, characterized by birth defects and neurologic devastation, occurs in 2% of pregnancies complicated by varicella in the first or second trimester.

B. **Epidemiology and transmission.** Varicella is less common in tropical than in temperate areas. In the United States, the incidence is highest between March and May and lowest between September and November. Transmission occurs through contact with respiratory tract secretions and airborne droplets or by direct contact with or inhalation of aerosols from vesicular fluid. Herpes zoster can cause chickenpox in susceptible individuals who come into contact with lesions or inhale aerosolized droplets.

Individuals with varicella are contagious from 1 to 2 days before onset of rash until the last lesion has crusted. Attack rates among susceptible individuals exposed in a household setting approach 90%. Attack rates in other settings such as day care, schools, and hospitals are not well established but are believed to be much lower than those observed in households.

C. **Rationale for vaccine use.** Varicella is now the most common classic childhood infectious disease in the United States. Before universal immunization, there were 4 million cases, 11,000 hospitalizations, and 100 deaths every year. Although the case-fatality rate in children is very low, the absolute number of childhood deaths is high (an average of 43 per year in the early 1990s) because there are so many cases. Ninety percent of children who die have no identifiable risk factors for severe varicella.

Five to 10% of cases in otherwise-healthy children experience complications. One-half of these are secondary bacterial infections usually due to *Staphylococcus aureus* or group A beta-hemolytic *Streptococcus* (GABHS). Otitis media occurs in up to 5% of cases. Serious secondary infections such as bacteremia, osteomyelitis, septic arthritis, endocarditis, necrotizing fasciitis, and toxic shock syndrome occur much less frequently. However, varicella increases the risk of severe GABHS infection among previously healthy children by a factor of 40- to 60-fold, and it is estimated that the prevention of varicella could prevent at least 15% of cases of severe pediatric GABHS infection. Further justification for universal vaccination includes the occurrence of cerebellar ataxia (1 in 4,000 cases) and encephalitis (1 in 5,000 cases).

Slightly greater than 1% of all adults with varicella are admitted to the hospital, and the case-fatality rate is 10 to 30 times higher than in children. Although only 5% of all cases occur in adults, 55% of annual deaths occur in this age group. As with children, the majority have no identifiable risk factor for severe disease. For this reason, susceptible adults should be vaccinated.

D. **Vaccines.** The vaccine available in the United States is VARIVAX (Merck), a live-attenuated virus derived from the Oka strain of varicella zoster virus [a similar vaccine called Varilrix (GlaxoSmithKline) is available outside the United States]. The strain was first isolated in the early 1970s from vesicle fluid of a child (named Oka) with chickenpox. It was attenuated by sequential passage in human embryonic lung cells, embryonic guinea pig fibroblasts, and human diploid cell culture, and it is currently produced in the latter. The vaccine is supplied lyophilized in one-dose vials (one or ten per package) along with diluent for reconstitution. Each 0.5-mL dose contains a minimum of 1,350 plaque-forming units of the virus. Potential contaminants and excipients include sucrose, gelatin, monosodium L-glutamate, residual cellular components, ethylenediaminetetraacetic acid (EDTA), neomycin, and fetal bovine serum. Varicella vaccine is licensed for use in individuals 12 months of age or older who have not had varicella.

E. Storage, handling, and administration
- Keep frozen at or below 5°F (15°C)
- Freezer must have a separate sealed freezer door (frost-free models are acceptable)
- Dormitory-style refrigerators with internal freezer compartments should not be used
- If the vaccine must be transported to a distant site, it should be kept frozen in a suitable container with dry ice. There should be enough dry ice to last through the return trip so that unreconstituted vaccine can be returned to the freezer. The container must be monitored to ensure that the temperature stays at or below 5°F (15°C).
- Vaccine can be stored at refrigerator temperature [35° to 46°F (2° to 8°C)] for 72 continuous hours prior to reconstitution; if not used within this period, it should be discarded
- Protect vaccine from direct sunlight
- Store diluent in refrigerator or at room temperature
- Reconstitute with the supplied diluent immediately before administration, and discard reconstituted vaccine if not used within 30 minutes
- Do not refreeze lyophilized or reconstituted vaccine
- Each dose is 0.5 mL given subcutaneously [see Chapter 3(III)]

F. Schedule. A single dose is recommended for children up to 12 years of age. Two doses separated by a minimum of 4 to 8 weeks is needed for individuals 13 years of age or older. If the interval to the second dose exceeds 8 weeks, no further doses need to be given.

G. Efficacy. Seroconversion occurs in greater than 96% of children 12 months to 12 years of age after one dose of vaccine. By 12 months of age, any maternally derived antibody that may still be present does not substantially reduce immunogenicity. There is an age-related decrease in the ability to develop a primary response to the vaccine; in individuals 13 years of age or older, seroconversion rates are 78% to 82% after one dose and 99% after two doses. In prelicensure trials, efficacy against any disease was 70% to 90% and against severe disease was greater than 95%. Postlicensure studies show efficacy of 87% to 100% in preventing severe disease. In fact, severe varicella, characterized by greater than 500 lesions, hospitalization, and complications, is rare in vaccinees. In adults and adolescents who have seroconverted, efficacy against disease is approximately 70% after household exposure. As many as 3% of vaccinated children per year develop breakthrough varicella. This rate does not change with time, which is further evidence that protective immunity does not wane. However, the number of cases accumulates with time such that, by 5 or 6 years from vaccination, 10% to 15% of vaccinated children have had breakthrough disease. When disease *does* develop in vaccinees, it is almost always attenuated, with fewer than 50 lesions (lesions tend to be macular rather than vesicular), no fever, and no systemic toxicity. It is important to emphasize that this vaccine is primarily intended to prevent severe disease, complications, and death, and it does so very effectively.

Antibodies and cellular responses to varicella have been detected in the majority of vaccinees as long as 20 years from immunization. However, these studies have been done in the context of the continued circulation of wild-type virus, raising the possibility that subclinical wild-type infections provide periodic boosts in immunity. Some studies demonstrate rising antibody titers during the years after vaccination, especially in those who have low responses originally. This could be due to exogenous reexposure to wild-type virus or possibly subclinical reactivation of latent vaccine virus.

Varicella vaccine has affected the epidemiology of disease in the United States. Active surveillance in three counties from 1995 through 1999 shows a 70% to 90% decline in cases coincident with coverage rates among 1- to 2-year-old children reaching 70%. Although the decline is most evident among children 1 to 4 years of age, there have been declines in all other age groups (including infants less than 1 year of age and adults), suggesting herd immunity. Studies in day care centers support the finding that herd immunity is occurring. Concerns have been raised that, as circulation of wild-type virus decreases, individuals not covered under the recommendation for universal childhood immunization might reach adulthood without natural or vaccine-induced immunity and, therefore, be susceptible to more severe disease. At this time, there is no evidence of a shift in incidence to older individuals; however, this concern highlights the need for all susceptible individuals to be immunized.

H. **Official recommendations.** All children should receive one dose of varicella vaccine between 12 and 18 months of age. Children 19 months to 12 years of age without a reliable history of chickenpox or vaccination should also receive one dose without prior serologic testing. A reliable history means a believable story, such as typical lesions and progression of illness after known exposure; physician documentation is not necessary. However, keep in mind that other rash illnesses such as enterovirus infection and scabies can mimic chickenpox. All susceptible individuals 13 years of age or older, including adults, should receive two doses according to the above schedule. Prior serologic testing for these individuals may be cost effective, as approximately 80% are found to be seropositive, and the cost of two doses of vaccine and the accompanying visits can be avoided.

Varicella vaccine is recommended for postexposure prophylaxis of susceptible individuals, although the product is not labeled for this indication. It should be given within 3 to 5 days of exposure to varicella. There is no evidence that administration of vaccine during the presymptomatic or prodromal stage of illness increases the risk for adverse events, but there is evidence that vaccination in this setting can prevent or modify disease.

There is no harm in giving the vaccine to someone who has already had chickenpox. Although there are no official recommendations, infants who had chickenpox before 6 months of age, and possibly before 9 months, should probably be vaccinated once they reach 12 months of age. This is because the immunity imparted by natural disease that is mitigated by maternal antibodies may be suboptimal.

Although all susceptible individuals should be immunized, the following high-risk groups deserve special attention:

- Adolescents and adults living in households with children
- Persons who live or work in environments where transmission of varicella is likely (e.g., schools, day care, institutional settings)
- Persons who live or work in environments where transmission can occur (e.g., college, correctional facilities, military)
- Women of childbearing age (who are not currently pregnant)
- International travelers
- Health care workers

The ACIP strongly supports the establishment of school entry requirements for varicella vaccine (or proof of immunity). In addition, vaccine use is encouraged for outbreak control.

Guidelines for use of varicella vaccine (and other live vaccines) in immunocompromised individuals, including those on steroids and those with HIV infection, are contained in Chapter 12(I). In general, this vaccine should not be administered to persons with cellular immunodeficiencies, but persons with isolated humoral immune defects *can* receive the vaccine (despite this being listed as a contraindication by the manufacturer). The vaccine can also be given to asymptomatic or mildly symptomatic HIV-infected children whose age-specific CD4 percentages are 25% or greater. Eligible children should receive two doses, with a 3-month interval between doses. Because there is some increased risk for complications, vaccinees should be encouraged to return for evaluation if they experience rash or other symptoms. Varicella vaccine should not be given to patients with blood dyscrasias, leukemia, lymphoma, or other malignancies of bone marrow or the lymphatic system. However, vaccine is available from the manufacturer under a research protocol for certain patients with acute lymphoblastic leukemia. Varicella vaccine can protect immunocompromised individuals from exposure to natural infection if given to their household contacts. However, vaccinees who develop a rash should be removed from contact with the immunocompromised person until the lesions are crusted over to avoid horizontal transmission.

The vaccine may be given at the same time as any other vaccine except smallpox, using separate sites and separate syringes. If not given simultaneously with MMR, 30 days or more should elapse between doses of MMR and varicella vaccine.

I. Safety. Injection-site reactions are reported in approximately 20% of vaccinees, and 15% may have low-grade fever. Approximately 3% of children and 1% of adults get a few vesicles at the injection site, and up to 5% may experience a generalized varicella-like rash (median of five lesions, mostly maculopapular). Herpes zoster due to the vaccine virus can occur, but the frequency appears to be much less than that after natural infection. Transmission of the vaccine virus from healthy vaccinees to susceptible individuals is extremely rare and is only known to occur when the vaccinee gets a rash after vaccination. In the few instances in which transmission has occurred, mild disease has resulted, and there is no evidence of reversion to virulence. More than 30 million doses of varicella vaccine have been distributed since licensure, and there have been no serious adverse reactions definitively linked to the vaccine.

J. Contraindications
- Anaphylactic reaction to a prior dose of vaccine or any of its components
- Pregnancy
- Immunodeficiency or immunosuppression (exceptions noted above)
- Untreated, active tuberculosis

K. Precautions
- Moderate to severe acute illness
- Recent administration of antibody-containing blood products [see Chapter 1(I)]

- Salicylate therapy (There are no known cases of Reye syndrome related to vaccination of patients on salicylates. Nevertheless, because of the association seen with natural infection, the manufacturer recommends withholding salicylates at least 6 weeks after administration of vaccine. Other nonsteroidal antiinflammatory agents can be used.)

L. Comments. The use of varicella vaccine in boosting immunity and preventing herpes zoster in older individuals is being studied. In addition, clinical trials are under way with combination vaccines containing measles, mumps, rubella, and varicella [see Chapter 10(II)].

KEY CONCEPTS: VARICELLA

- Varicella is the leading cause of death preventable by a routinely recommended childhood vaccine
- Does not prevent chickenpox entirely but does prevent severe disease
- Marked declines in cases and evidence of herd immunity since licensure
- May be used for postexposure prophylaxis

Combination Vaccines

I. General considerations

A. Preference for combination vaccines.
Combination vaccines consist of two or more separate immunogens combined in a single product and administered through the same syringe. Some of the first vaccines licensed in the United States were combination products. For example, the influenza vaccine (first licensed in 1945) is a combination of three different strains of influenza virus. Likewise, the hexavalent pneumococcal polysaccharide vaccine (1947); diphtheria, tetanus, and whole-cell pertussis vaccine (DTP) (1948); and trivalent inactivated poliovirus vaccine (IPV) (1955) and oral poliovirus vaccine (OPV) (1963) were also combinations. The "modern era" of combinations, however, began in the 1990s, when combinations of routinely administered childhood vaccines such as DTP; diphtheria, tetanus, and acellular pertussis vaccine (DTaP); *Haemophilus influenzae* type b (Hib); and hepatitis B vaccine (Hep-B) were developed.

At the present time, up to 23 separate injections may be needed to comply with all vaccine recommendations through age 6 years; depending on how vaccine visits are scheduled, up to five injections may be needed during a single immunization encounter. This causes distress for patients, parents, and health care professionals, enough so that compliance with universal vaccine programs may be threatened. Moreover, the situation is likely to worsen as new much-needed vaccines are introduced into the routine schedule (see Chapter 10). Combination vaccines offer distinct advantages and some potential disadvantages, both of which are listed in Table 6.1.

In 1999, recognizing the potential advantages, the Advisory Committee on Immunization Practices (ACIP), American Academy of Pediatrics (AAP), and American Academy of Family Physicians (AAFP) expressed a clear preference for combination vaccines over separate injections of their components. In addition, the agencies stated that licensed combination vaccines may be used even when some of the antigens are not indicated, provided that the vaccine components are not contraindicated. Such use might be justified when the appropriate monovalent vaccines are not readily available or would require extra injections, or when the benefits outweigh any potential risks of adverse events associated with extra antigens [whereas extra doses of Hep-B; Hib; measles, mumps, and rubella (MMR); varicella; and polio vaccines are not harmful, increased adverse reac-

Table 6.1.   Combination vaccines

Potential advantages	Potential disadvantages
Decreased injections, injection risks, and sharps injuries	Decreased immunogenicity
Decreased pain and anxiety	Increased reactogenicity and difficulty attributing adverse events
Decreased visits	Decreased visits[a]
Simplified schedule and improved record keeping	Confusion over antigen content and errors in record keeping
Increased compliance	Extra immunization
Decreased preparation time and more efficient well-child visits	Decreased flexibility
Decreased administration costs, overhead, and billing inefficiency	Increased cost of vaccines and decreased reimbursement[b]
Easier storage and inventory management	
Easier introduction of new vaccines	

[a]Other aspects of well-child care are delivered during immunization visits.
[b]Fewer administration fees are collected when separate injections are combined into a single injection.

tions may occur with extra doses or shorter-than-recommended intervals of tetanus and pneumococcal polysaccharide vaccines]. The agencies went on to encourage reimbursement by health insurance providers and managed-care systems, even when extra (and therefore "unnecessary") antigens are given. Finally, caution was raised against combining vaccines into the same syringe unless the products are specifically labeled for this purpose.

  B. **Development, evaluation, and licensure.** Producing safe and effective combination vaccines is far more complex than simply mixing disparate antigens together in a single vial. Adjuvants, buffers, stabilizers, and excipients can have *physical or chemical interactions* with antigens that reduce immunogenicity, and many of these interactions cannot be predicted *a priori*. For example, the preservative thimerosal reduces the immunogenicity of the polio type 1 antigen in IPV without affecting polio types 2 and 3. *Antigenic competition* can occur as vaccine components vie for position in binding to major histocompatibility molecules on antigen-presenting cells at the site of injection. This may explain, in part, the decreased Hib responses that were seen in initial attempts to combine Hib vaccine with DTaP. Another phenomenon, *carrier-induced epitopic suppression*, may cause decreased antibody responses to protein-polysaccharide conjugates (e.g., Hib) when there has been prior or simultaneous immunization with free (homologous) carrier protein. A similar effect is seen when different conjugates containing the same carrier protein are given at the same time. These interactions may be relevant, for example, in the hypothetical situation in which a child receives *tetanus* toxoid, Hib-*tetanus* conjugate, and pneumococcal-*tetanus* conjugate at the same time. When live viral vaccines are given together, *viral interference* may limit responses as the replication of one virus is inhibited by the replication of the other. This occurs, for example, between the different viral serotypes in OPV and is also relevant to combinations of measles, mumps, rubella, and varicella. Although these interactions are important considerations, they must be differentiated from "immune overload," a popular concept that has no scientific basis [see Chapter 13(IV)].

Once the compatibility issues are worked out in laboratory and animal models, extensive clinical trials are required to prove that a new combination vaccine is safe and effective. U.S. Food and Drug Administration (FDA) guidelines require that such trials compare the combination to separately but simultaneously administered monovalent components. Reactogenicity is compared to the most reactogenic of the individual components. For antigens that have an established serologic correlate of protection (e.g., diphtheria, tetanus, Hib, hepatitis B, and polio), it may be enough to demonstrate that the combination induces protective antibody responses. However, the FDA generally requires that *noninferiority* with monovalent vaccines be demonstrated, defined as "no more than a 10% reduction in seroprotection." Although this rule is intended to ensure that protection is not compromised for the sake of convenience, it has been an obstacle in the development of some combination vaccines, particularly those containing DTaP and Hib. Whereas Hib responses to DTaP-Hib combinations may fail the noninferiority test, they may nevertheless be robust enough (particularly with anamnestic responses) to protect the patient from disease. Because of uncertainty surrounding these issues, no premixed DTaP-Hib combination vaccines have been licensed in the United States to date.

For antigens (like pertussis) without established serologic correlates of protection, combination vaccines should demonstrate antibody responses similar to those measured in previous studies showing efficacy of individual vaccines. To further complicate matters, it is important to point out that component vaccines from different manufacturers have unique properties. Therefore, just because one combination vaccine performs as well as its component antigens, there is no guarantee that a similar combination of different manufacturer's components will perform just as well.

II. Diphtheria, tetanus, pertussis, and *Haemophilus influenzae*. The diseases, epidemiology and transmission, and rationale for vaccine use are given in Chapters 5(I) and 5(II).

A. Vaccine. Early attempts to combine DTaP vaccines with Hib conjugates in the same syringe resulted in diminished antibody responses to the polyribosylribitol phosphate (PRP) component. TriHIBit (DTaP2/PRP-T), manufactured by Aventis Pasteur, is the only such combination to achieve licensure in the United States (1996). Rather than a true preformed combination vaccine, TriHIBit (DTaP2/PRP-T) is actually a mixture of ActHIB (PRP-T) and Tripedia (DTaP2) made by reconstituting the former with the latter immediately before administration [see Chapters 5(I) and 5(II) for the constitution of each vaccine; the list of excipients and potential contaminants is the same]. TriHIBit (DTaP2/PRP-T) is labeled for the prevention of invasive Hib disease in children 15 to 18 months of age (fourth dose only) who have been immunized previously with three doses of either DTP or Tripedia (DTaP2) and three or fewer doses of ActHIB (PRP-T) in the first year of life. The product is packaged with a single lot number as one-dose vials (five per package) of lyophilized ActHIB (PRP-T) and one-dose vials (five per package) of liquid Tripedia (DTaP2) for reconstitution; both vials are preservative free. *No other DTaP and Hib vaccine can be combined in this fashion* or substituted for any of the components of TriHIBit (e.g., Infanrix should not be substituted for Tripedia). However, it *is* acceptable to combine ActHIB (PRP-T) and Tripedia (DTaP2) that have been supplied separately (i.e., not packaged as TriHIBit). In this situation, the diluent supplied with the ActHIB (PRP-T) should be discarded, and the lot numbers of both vaccines should be recorded in the medical record.

B. Storage, handling, and administration
- Maintain temperature for both vaccines at 35° to 46°F (2° to 8°C)
- Freezing can cause the vaccine to lose potency
- Reconstitute the ActHIB (PRP-T) with the Tripedia (DTaP2) and shake well
- Administer within 30 minutes of reconstitution
- Each dose is 0.5 mL given intramuscularly [see Chapter 3(III)]

C. Schedule. TriHIBit (DTaP2/PRP-T) can be used for the fourth dose of the DTaP series at 15 to 18 months of age. Using this vaccine reduces the number of shots in the first 2 years of life by one.

D. Efficacy. In clinical studies, children aged 15 to 20 months who had previously received three doses of a Hib conjugate vaccine and DTP were administered either Tripedia (DTaP2) and ActHIB (PRP-T) vaccines at separate sites or combined as a single injection. All children in both groups had serologic evidence of long-term protection from invasive Hib disease, as well as comparable antibody titers to diphtheria, tetanus, and pertussis. The protective efficacy of TriHIBit (DTaP2/PRP-T) has not been evaluated in a clinical trial. The vaccine was licensed based on seroconversion and safety data.

E. Official recommendations. All children should receive five doses of DTaP before 7 years of age and three or four doses of Hib conjugate vaccine (depending on the product) before 2 years of age. TriHIBit (DTaP2/PRP-T) should be used for the *fourth dose only* at 15 to 18 months of age. If administered as one or more doses of the primary series, the Hib doses should be disregarded, and the child should be revaccinated for Hib at the appropriate age (the DTaP doses should be considered valid and do not need to be repeated). TriHIBit (DTaP2/PRP-T) can be used regardless of which Hib conjugate vaccine was given for the primary series [including whether single antigen or the combination COMVAX (PRP-OMP/Hep-B) was used]. It can be used if the child is 12 months of age or older *and* has received at least one prior dose of Hib vaccine at least 2 months earlier *and* this will be the last dose in the Hib series. TriHIBit (DTaP2/PRP-T) should not be used if the child has received no prior Hib doses. Remember that there is a preference to use the same DTaP product for the entire immunization series [see Chapter 5(I)]. This would imply a preference to use Tripedia (DTaP2) for the primary series in children who will get TriHIBit (DTaP2/PRP-T) for the fourth dose. However, vaccination should not be withheld if a different product was used in the primary series, because the risks of missing an opportunity to immunize are probably greater than the risks of mixing products in the series. Although data are limited, it is assumed that TriHIBit (DTaP2/PRP-T) can be given at the same time as other vaccines at separate sites.

F. Safety. The rates of local and systemic reactions and adverse events are similar to those seen after administration of the individual component vaccines.

G. Contraindications and precautions. These are the same as for the individual vaccines [see Chapters 5(I) and 5(II)].

KEY CONCEPTS: TRIHIBIT (DTAP2/PRP-T)

- Mixture of ActHIB (PRP-T) and Tripedia (DTaP2) made immediately before administration
- Only approved for the fourth dose of the DTaP and Hib series

---

III. *Haemophilus influenzae* type b and hepatitis B. The diseases, epidemiology and transmission, and rationale for vaccine use are given in Chapters 5(II) and 5(III).

A. Vaccine. COMVAX (PRP-OMP/Hep-B), licensed by Merck in 1996, is essentially a combination of PedvaxHIB [PRP-OMP; see Chapter 5(III)] and RECOMBIVAX HB [Hep-B; see Chapter 5(II)]. Each dose contains 7.5 mg of PRP conjugated to a *Neisseria meningitidis* outer membrane protein (PRP-OMP) and 5 mg of hepatitis B virus surface antigen (HBsAg), as well as alum. The product is preservative free and is supplied as a liquid in one-dose vials (ten per package). Potential contaminants and excipients include formaldehyde and yeast proteins. COMVAX (PRP-OMP/Hep-B) is labeled for vaccination against invasive Hib disease and all known subtypes of hepatitis B infection in infants 6 weeks to 15 months of age born to HBsAg-negative mothers (the ACIP accepts use of the vaccine for infants of HBsAg-positive and -unknown mothers; see Official recommendations).

B. Storage, handling, and administration
- Maintain temperature at 35° to 46°F (2° to 8°C)
- Freezing can cause the vaccine to lose potency
- Shake well before use
- Each dose is 0.5 mL given intramuscularly [see Chapter 3(III)]

C. Schedule. COMVAX (PRP-OMP/Hep-B) can be used for Hib and Hep-B immunization in the routine childhood immunization schedule. The usual schedule is a dose at 2, 4, and 12 to 15 months of age. If this schedule cannot be followed, the interval between the first two doses should be at least 6 weeks, and although the minimum interval between the second and last doses is 8 weeks, the last dose should be given at 12 months of age or older. Because most infants receive a birth dose of Hep-B, use of COMVAX (PRP-OMP/Hep-B) at 2, 4, and 12 to 15 months results in the child's receiving four doses of Hep-B—one more than usual. There is no evidence that this compromises immune responses or results in increased reactogenicity. Extraimmunization with Hep-B, however, can be avoided by substituting PedvaxHIB (PRP-OMP) at 4 months of age.

D. Efficacy. Prelicensure clinical trials indicated that the immunogenicity of COMVAX (PRP-OMP/Hep-B) is equivalent to that of the monovalent vaccines. After two doses, 95% of approximately 570 subjects had anti-PRP antibody levels higher than 0.15 μg/mL, the level predictive of short-term protection. After three doses, 93% had levels higher than 1.0 μg/mL, the level predictive of long-term protection. Ninety-eight percent had anti-HBsAg antibody levels 10 mIU/mL or higher, the established protective level. The efficacy of COMVAX (PRP-OMP/Hep-B) is expected to be comparable to that of existing monovalent vaccines.

E. Official recommendations. COMVAX (PRP-OMP/Hep-B) *should not be used for the birth dose of Hep-B or before 6 weeks of age* because of the possibility of inducing tolerance to future doses of Hib conjugate vaccine. The number of total Hib conjugate vaccine doses depends on which vaccine is used and when the series is initiated [see Chapter 5(II)]; complete immunization with Hep-B requires three doses, regardless of age at initiation [see Chapter 5(III)].

Use of COMVAX (PRP-OMP/Hep-B) has not been studied in infants born to women who are HBsAg positive or women of unknown HBsAg status, and the product is labeled only for use in infants of HBsAg-negative women. However, there is no evidence of diminished postexposure prophylaxis effectiveness in infants who have received hepatitis B immune globulin (HBIG) and Hep-B vaccine at birth followed by PedvaxHIB (PRP-OMP) and RECOMBIVAX HB vaccines at 6 to 10 weeks of age and subsequent completion of each vaccine series. The ACIP considers it acceptable to give COMVAX (PRP-OMP/Hep-B) to infants of HBsAg-positive or -unknown mothers at 2, 4, and 12 to 15 months of age, as long as a birth dose of monovalent vaccine has been given.

The immunogenicity of COMVAX (PRP-OMP/Hep-B) when used in a series with other Hep-B or Hib conjugate vaccines has not been studied. However, immunogenicity data from studies of monovalent vaccines indicate that any combination of Hib conjugate vaccines may be used to complete the primary series. When COMVAX (PRP-OMP/Hep-B) and a Hib conjugate vaccine other than PedvaxHIB (PRP-OMP) are used to complete the primary series, three doses should be administered at ages 2, 4, and 6 months. Hep-B vaccines are considered completely interchangeable.

COMVAX (PRP-OMP/Hep-B) can be administered at the same time as any other vaccines given at separate sites.

F. **Safety.** COMVAX (PRP-OMP/Hep-B) has a reactogenicity profile similar to that for the individual components. The list of excipients and contaminating substances is the same as that for the individual vaccines.

G. **Contraindications and precautions.** These are the same as those for the individual vaccines [see Chapters 5(II) and 5(III)].

KEY CONCEPTS: COMVAX (PRP-OMP/HEP-B)

- Combination of PedvaxHIB (PRP-OMP) and RECOMBIVAX HB (Hep-B)
- Indicated only for infants born to HBsAg-negative mothers
- The ACIP accepts use for infants born to HBsAg-positive and -unknown mothers
- Can be incorporated into the routine childhood schedule
- Overimmunization with Hep-B (four total doses) is not a problem
- Should not be used before 6 weeks of age

IV. **Hepatitis A and hepatitis B.** The diseases, epidemiology and transmission, and rationale for vaccine use are given in Chapters 8(IV) and 5(III).

A. **Vaccine.** Twinrix (Hep-A/Hep-B), licensed by Glaxo-SmithKline in 2001, is essentially a combination of

Havrix [Hep-A; see Chapter 8(IV)] and Engerix-B [Hep-B; see Chapter 5(II)]. Each dose contains at least 720 enzyme-linked immunosorbent assay units of inactivated hepatitis A virus (equivalent to the pediatric formulation of Havrix) and 20 μg of recombinant HBsAg (equivalent to the adult formulation of Engerix-B), with 0.45 mg of aluminum as adjuvant. The product contains 2-phenoxyethanol as preservative and is supplied as a liquid in one-dose vials (one or ten per package) or pre-filled Tip-Lok syringes (five per package) without needles. The list of potential contaminants and excipients is the same as that for the individual vaccines. Twinrix (Hep-A/Hep-B) is labeled for active immunization of persons 18 years of age or older against hepatitis A and all known subtypes of hepatitis B.

B. Storage, handling, and administration
- Maintain temperature at 35° to 46°F (2° to 8°C)
- Freezing can cause the vaccine to lose potency
- Shake well before use
- Each dose is 1.0 mL given intramuscularly [see Chapter 3(III)]

C. Schedule. The series consists of three doses given at 0, 1, and 6 months. Table 6.2 gives a proposed schedule for patients who have received or will receive monovalent Hep-A.

D. Efficacy. In 11 clinical trials involving 1,551 healthy volunteers 17 to 70 years of age, 99.9% seroconverted to hepatitis A and 98.5% developed protective antibody levels to hepatitis B 1 month after completion of the three-dose series. In open randomized trials, the combination given as a three-dose series was found to have comparable immunogenicity to the individual monovalent vaccines (even though the Hep-A component is equivalent to the pediatric formulation of Havrix). Two clinical trials involving a total of 129 subjects demonstrated that antibodies to both hepatitis A and hepatitis B persisted for 4 years or longer. Efficacy is also expected to be similar to that of the monovalent vaccines.

Table 6.2. Completing vaccine series with monovalent vaccines

Initial vaccination	To complete Hep-A series	To complete Hep-B series
1 dose of Twinrix	1 dose of adult formulation Hep-A[a] ≥6 mo later	2 doses of adult formulation Hep-B[a] (1 and 6 mo later)
2 doses of Twinrix (0, 1 mo)	1 dose of adult formulation Hep-A[a] ≥6 mo from first Twinrix dose	1 dose of adult formulation Hep-B[a] at ≥6 mo from first Twinrix dose

[a]Any product is probably acceptable.

E. Official recommendations. Twinrix (Hep-A/Hep-B) is useful for susceptible individuals 18 years of age or older who are or will be at risk of exposure to both hepatitis A and hepatitis B. The respective risk categories are given in Chapters 8(IV) and 5(III). People in whom these risks overlap include the following:

- People traveling or relocating to areas of high or intermediate endemicity for both hepatitis A and hepatitis B who are at increased risk of hepatitis B due to behavioral or occupational factors
- Patients with chronic liver disease, including alcoholic cirrhosis, chronic hepatitis C, autoimmune hepatitis, and primary biliary cirrhosis
- Persons at risk through their work, including laboratory workers who handle live hepatitis A and hepatitis B viruses, police, health care workers and other personnel who render first aid or emergency medical assistance, and employees of day care centers and correctional facilities (workers who come in contact with feces or sewage are not felt to be at increased risk)
- Residents of drug and alcohol treatment centers
- Men who have sex with men or other persons at increased risk of disease due to their sexual practices
- Injecting drug users
- Individuals who are at increased risk for hepatitis A and who are in close household contact with individuals with acute or chronic hepatitis B infection
- Patients frequently receiving blood products, such as those with clotting factor disorders
- Military personnel

Although there are no specific data on interchangeability, it is assumed that Hep-A and Hep-B products can be interchanged as long as the correct schedules (above) are used. Likewise, it is assumed that Twinrix (Hep-A/Hep-B) can be given concomitantly with any other vaccines. When concomitant administration of immunoglobulin products is indicated, they should be given with different syringes and at different injection sites.

F. Safety. Local and systemic reactogenicity and adverse events are similar to those seen with the monovalent components. The frequency of solicited adverse events does not increase with successive doses. No serious vaccine-related adverse events have been observed.

G. Contraindications and precautions. These are the same as for the individual vaccines [see Chapters 5(III) and 8(IV)].

KEY CONCEPTS: TWINRIX (HEP-A/HEP-B)

- Combination of Havrix (Hep-A) and Engerix-B (Hep-B)
- Indicated for individuals 18 years of age or older who are or will be exposed to both hepatitis A and B
- Three doses are necessary

V. Diphtheria, tetanus, pertussis, hepatitis B, and polio. The diseases, epidemiology and transmission, and rationale for vaccine use are given in Chapters 5(I), 5(III), and 5(IV).

 A. Vaccine. Pediarix (DTaP3/Hep-B/IPV), licensed by Glaxo-SmithKline in late 2002, is essentially a combination of Infanrix [DTaP3; see Chapter 5(I)], Engerix-B [Hep-B; see Chapter 5(III)], and an IPV that is not currently licensed in the United States as an individual vaccine but is included in combination vaccines licensed in other countries. Each dose contains 25 Lf (limit of flocculation) units of diphtheria toxoid, 10 Lf units of tetanus toxoid, 25 μg of pertussis toxin (PT), 25 μg of filamentous hemagglutinin (FHA), 8 μg of pertactin (PRN), and 10 μg of HBsAg (all adsorbed to alum), as well as formaldehyde-inactivated poliovirus types 1 (Mahoney), 2 (MEF-1), and 3 (Saukett). The product contains 2-phenoxyethanol as preservative and is supplied as a liquid in one-dose vials (ten per package) and prefilled Tip-Lok syringes (5 or 25 per package), without or with (25 per package only) needles. Potential contaminants and excipients include formaldehyde, polysorbate 80, neomycin sulfate, polymyxin B, and yeast protein. Pediarix (DTaP3/Hep-B/IPV) is indicated for primary immunization of infants at 2, 4, and 6 months of age. It should not to be used in infants younger than 6 weeks of age or in children 7 years of age or older. The product is labeled only for use in infants born to HBsAg-negative mothers (the ACIP accepts use of the vaccine for infants of HBsAg-positive and -unknown mothers; see Official recommendations).

 B. Storage, handling, and administration
  • Maintain temperature at 35° to 46°F (2° to 8°C)
  • Freezing can cause the vaccine to lose potency
  • Shake well before use
  • Each dose is 0.5 mL given intramuscularly [see Chapter 3(III)]

 C. Schedule. Pediarix (DTaP3/Hep-B/IPV) can be used for the primary immunization series to protect against diphtheria, tetanus, pertussis, Hib, and hepatitis B as part of the routine childhood schedule. Doses are given at 2, 4, and 6 months of age. The vaccine should not be used for the birth dose of Hep-B, and it should not be used for booster doses. As most infants receive a birth dose of Hep-B, use of Pediarix (DTaP3/Hep-B/IPV) at 2, 4, and 6 months of age results in the child's receiving four doses of Hep-B, one more than usual. There is no evidence that this compromises immune responses or results in increased reactogenicity.

 D. Efficacy. In clinical trials, antibody responses to each antigen contained in Pediarix (DTaP3/Hep-B/IPV) were shown to be similar to those when the individual vaccines were given separately. Protective antibody levels for each antigen were achieved in greater than 95% of vaccinees. Although a 2-, 4-, and 6-month schedule for Hep-B is technically in compliance with official recommendations, there was some concern that this short-interval schedule might be less immunogenic than the traditional birth, 1-, and 6-month schedule. In fact, geometric mean concentrations of antibody to HBsAg are significantly lower when Pediarix (DTaP3/Hep-B/IPV) given at 2, 4, and 6 months is the only hepatitis B immunization that an infant receives. However, protective levels of antibody are achieved in greater than 99% of infants. Moreover, when the birth dose is given before the 2-, 4-, and 6-month schedule of Pediarix (DTaP3/Hep-B/IPV), as it should be in almost all infants, the anti-HBsAg titers are much higher.

E. **Official recommendations.** Pediarix (DTaP3/Hep-B/IPV) should not be used for booster immunization after the primary series. For infants born to HBsAg-negative mothers and given a birth dose of Hep-B, three doses of Pediarix (DTaP3/Hep-B/IPV) may be used to complete the primary immunization series. The ACIP considers it acceptable to give Pediarix (DTaP3/Hep-B/IPV) to infants of HBsAg-positive or -unknown mothers at 2, 4, and 6 months of age, as long as a birth dose of monovalent vaccine has been given. Pediarix (DTaP3/Hep-B/IPV) can be used to complete the primary series in infants who have already received one or two doses of Infanrix (DTaP3), Hep-B (RECOMBIVAX HB or Engerix-B), or IPV (IPOL) and are scheduled to receive the other components of the vaccine. Because data supporting the interchangeability of DTaP vaccines are limited, practitioners are encouraged to use the same DTaP vaccine for the entire series. Although this might limit the use of Pediarix (DTaP3/Hep-B/IPV) in infants who have received Tripedia (DTaP2) in the past, one study demonstrated comparable immunogenicity and reactogenicity of mixed schedules. Furthermore, if Pediarix (DTaP3/Hep-B/IPV) is available and otherwise indicated, the risks of mixing DTaP products are probably outweighed by the benefits of avoiding missed opportunities for immunization.

The vaccine may be given concurrently with Hib and pneumococcal conjugate vaccines.

F. **Safety.** In studies of more than 7,000 infants given a primary series of Pediarix (DTaP3/Hep-B/IPV), the most common adverse reactions were redness, swelling, and pain at the injection site, as well as fever and fussiness. In a study in which Hib and pneumococcal conjugate vaccines were given concurrently, Pediarix (DTaP3/Hep-B/IPV) was associated with a higher rate of fever 100.4°F (38°C) or higher after the first dose compared with separately administered vaccines (27.9% versus 19.8%, respectively); there was no difference in other adverse reactions. When fever did occur, it was generally mild and lasted for 2 to 3 days. Eight (1.2%) of 667 infants sought medical attention because of fever, and one infant was hospitalized for a thorough evaluation.

G. Contraindications and precautions. These are the same as for the individual vaccines [see Chapters 5(I), 5(III), and 5(IV)].

KEY CONCEPTS: PEDIARIX (DTAP3/HEP-B/IPV)

- Combination of Infanrix (DTaP3), Engerix-B (Hep-B), and IPV
- Indicated only for infants born to HBsAg-negative mothers
- Can be incorporated into the routine childhood schedule
- Overimmunization with Hep-B (four total doses) is not a problem
- Should not be used before 6 weeks of age
- Should not be used for booster doses

Vaccines for Adults and Selected Children

I. Tetanus and diphtheria

Clostridium tetani is a nonencapsulated, gram-positive, obligately anaerobic bacillus that produces a potent neurotoxin. *Corynebacterium diphtheriae* is an aerobic, pleomorphic gram-positive bacillus that produces a potent exotoxin.

A. Diseases. See Chapter 5(I).

B. Epidemiology and transmission. See Chapter 5(I).

C. Rationale for vaccine use. See Chapter 5(I). In addition to routine booster dosing, diphtheria and tetanus vaccine for adult use (Td) is used for prophylaxis of tetanus-prone wounds. In this setting, the benefits of using Td [as opposed to tetanus toxoid (TT)] to incidentally boost diphtheria antibody levels outweigh any possible added risks.

D. Vaccines. In the United States, the diphtheria, tetanus, and acellular pertussis vaccine (DTaP) cannot be used for adults because the quantity of diphtheria antigen is too reactogenic and the acellular pertussis components have not yet been licensed for use beyond 6 years of age. Therefore, periodic boosting of immunity to diphtheria and tetanus must be accomplished using monovalent or bivalent vaccines. Table 7.1 gives the available products in the United States.

Td and TT are labeled for use in patients 7 years of age or older.

E. Storage, handling, and administration
- Maintain temperature at 35° to 46°F (2° to 8°C)
- Freezing can cause the vaccine to lose potency
- Shake well before use
- Each dose is 0.5 mL given intramuscularly [see Chapter 3(III)]

F. Schedule. A dose of Td should be given at 11 to 12 years of age, provided that at least 5 years have elapsed since the last diphtheria and tetanus toxoid–containing vaccine. Thereafter, a dose should be given every 10 years. If a dose of Td or TT is given for wound management, the clock is reset for another 10 years. For individuals 7 years of age or older who have never been immunized, a primary series consists of three doses, with minimum intervals of 4 weeks between doses one and two and 6 to 12 months between doses two and three.

Table 7.1. Diphtheria and tetanus vaccines for adolescents and adults

Product name	Manufacturer	Content per dose (LF units)	Adjuvants/ contaminants/ excipients	Preservative	Packaging
Tetanus and diphtheria toxoids adsorbed for adult use (Td)	Aventis Pasteur	Tetanus toxoid: 5 Diphtheria toxoid: 2	Alum	Thimerosal	Liquid 10-dose vial Prefilled syringe (10/pk)
Tetanus toxoid adsorbed USP (TT)	Aventis Pasteur	Tetanus toxoid: 5	Alum Formaldehyde	Thimerosal	Liquid 10-dose vial
Tetanus toxoid USP for booster dose only[a] (TT)	Aventis Pasteur	Tetanus toxoid: 4	Formaldehyde	Thimerosal	Liquid 15-dose vial
Tetanus and diphtheria toxoids adsorbed for adult use	Massachusetts Public Health Biologic Laboratories (distributed by General Injectables & Vaccines, Inc.)	Tetanus toxoid: 2 Diphtheria toxoid: 2	Alum Formaldehyde	Thimerosal	Liquid 10-dose vial 15-dose vial

Lf, limit of flocculation; pk, package.
[a]This product cannot be used for primary immunization (i.e., the series of five doses before age 7 years).

G. Efficacy. A protective level of diphtheria antitoxin (greater than 0.1 IU/mL) is reached in more than 95% of adult recipients of diphtheria toxoid after three properly spaced doses. Clinical efficacy is estimated at 97%. Protection is thought to last at least 10 years, but vaccination does not eliminate carriage of *C. diphtheriae*. A minimal protective level of tetanus antitoxin (greater than 0.01 IU/mL) is reached in nearly all recipients of tetanus toxoid 7 years of age or older after three properly spaced doses. Efficacy of tetanus toxoid has never been studied in a clinical trial, but antibody responses would suggest efficacy of virtually 100%, and cases of tetanus in fully immunized persons whose last dose was within 10 years are extremely rare.

Tetanus antibody levels fall over time. Although some persons may be protected for life, most people approach the minimal protective level of antibody 10 years after the last dose of vaccine. This is the basis for the recommended boosters every 10 years.

H. Official recommendations. Td is the preferred vaccine for any tetanus booster doses, as it provides immunity to both tetanus and diphtheria. In the rare situation in which tetanus and diphtheria immunization in the absence of pertussis immunization is necessary before 7 years of age, the diphtheria and tetanus vaccine for pediatric use (DT) (with the higher dose of diphtheria toxoid) should be used. Routine recall of adolescents and adults every 10 years, beginning at 11 to 12 years of age, is recommended for Td immunization.

In the case of injury, a thorough attempt should be made to determine whether the patient has completed a primary immunization series. Patients with unknown or uncertain immunization histories should be considered to have had no previous tetanus toxoid doses and may require active and passive immunization after wound cleaning and débridement. Persons in military service since 1941 can be considered to have received at least one dose (although most will have completed a primary series, this cannot be assumed for each individual).

Table 7.2 can be used to determine the need for booster immunization and tetanus immune globulin (TIG) in patients with wounds.

Pregnant women who have not received a primary series should do so before delivery. If there is not enough time to complete the series, two doses of Td should be given at least 4 weeks apart, and the last dose should be at least 2 weeks before delivery. The last dose of the series can be given postpartum. Pregnant women whose last tetanus immunization was more than 10 years ago should receive a booster dose of Td.

Close contacts of a case of diphtheria should receive a booster dose of DTaP, DT, or Td (depending on age) if they have not received a booster of diphtheria toxoid

Table 7.2. Tetanus prophylaxis in wound management

Primary series	Age (yr)	Time since last dose of TT (yr)	Clean, minor wounds		Other wounds[a]	
			Vaccine	TIG[b]	Vaccine	TIG[b]
Complete[c]	<7	<5	None	No	None	No
		>5	None	No	DTaP[d]	No
	≥7	<5	None	No	None	No
		5–10	None	No	Td[e]	No
		>10	Td[e]	No	Td[e]	No
Unknown or incomplete[f]	<7	—	DTaP[d]	No	DTaP[d]	Yes
	≥7	—	Td[e]	No	Td[e]	Yes

TIG, tetanus immune globulin.

[a]Includes puncture, avulsion, crush, necrotic, and burn wounds; frostbite; and wounds contaminated with dirt, feces, soil, or saliva.

[b]TIG [250 units given intramuscularly; see Chapter 12(VII)]; equine tetanus antitoxin can be used if TIG is not available (3,000 to 5,000 units intramuscularly) but is difficult to get in the United States; vaccine and TIG should be given at separate sites.

[c]The primary series is considered complete if the patient has received three or more doses of an adsorbed (not fluid) tetanus toxoid; HIV-infected individuals should be considered *unimmunized* even if they have received the vaccine series.

[d]Use DT if pertussis immunization is contraindicated.

[e]Td is preferred, but TT can be used; only adsorbed products are indicated.

[f]For inadequately vaccinated patients of all ages, completion of a primary series at the time of discharge or at follow-up should be ensured.

within 5 years. Children who have not yet received a fourth dose should be immunized.

Tetanus and diphtheria disease do not confer immunity, because the illness is produced by very small amounts of toxin. Persons should begin or complete active immunization with Td during convalescence. Tetanus and diphtheria vaccines from different manufacturers are considered interchangeable. These vaccines can be given at the same time as any other vaccines as long as separate sites are used. Td and TIG should also be given at separate sites.

I. **Safety.** Erythema, induration, and pain at the injection site are common but are usually self-limited. A nodule may be palpable at the injection site for several weeks, and abscess formation has been reported. Fever and other systemic symptoms are uncommon. Exaggerated local (Arthus-type) reactions are occasionally reported after receipt of tetanus-containing vaccines. These are characterized by painful swelling beginning 2 to 8 hours after injection and often extending from the shoulder to the elbow. They are most often reported in adults, particularly those who have received frequent doses of tetanus toxoid and have very high serum tetanus antibody levels. They should not receive further doses of Td more often than every 10 years. Less severe local hypersensitivity reactions can occur in persons who have had multiple prior boosters.

Severe systemic reactions such as generalized urticaria, anaphylaxis, or neurologic complications have been reported after receipt of tetanus toxoid. A few cases of peripheral neuropathy and Guillain-Barré syndrome have also been reported. The Institute of Medicine (IOM) recently concluded that there probably is a causal relationship between tetanus toxoid and both brachial neuritis and Guillain-Barré syndrome, although these reactions are very rare.

J. Contraindications. Anaphylactic or neurologic reaction to a prior dose of vaccine or any of its components.

K. Precautions
   - Moderate or severe acute illness
   - Guillain-Barré syndrome 6 weeks or less after previous dose of tetanus toxoid–containing vaccine

L. Comments. If DTaP vaccines are approved for use in adolescents and adults, these may represent attractive alternatives to Td for wound management or booster immunization.

KEY CONCEPTS: TETANUS AND DIPHTHERIA

- Td is the agent of choice for immunization at 7 years of age or older
- Routine boosters recommended every 10 years
- Wound management requires booster dose in some patients
- Wound management requires TIG in some patients without history of primary series

---

II. Pneumococcal polysaccharide

Streptococcus pneumoniae is a facultatively anaerobic, catalase-negative gram-positive coccus that produces an antiphagocytic polysaccharide capsule that confers serotype specificity.

A. Disease. See Chapter 5(VI). Pneumonia is the most common presentation of pneumococcal disease in adults. Classically, there is abrupt onset of fever and a single rigor; repeated shaking chills are uncommon. Other symptoms include pleuritic chest pain; productive cough yielding mucopurulent, rusty sputum; dyspnea; tachypnea; hypoxia; tachycardia; malaise; and weakness. Nausea, vomiting, and headaches occur less frequently. Complications include empyema, pericarditis, and abscess. Pneumococcal meningitis also occurs in adults. Symptoms include headache, lethargy, vomiting, irritability, fever, nuchal rigidity, cranial nerve signs, seizures, and coma. The spinal fluid profile and neurologic complications are similar to those in other forms of bacterial meningitis. One-fourth of patients with pneumococcal meningitis also have pneumonia.

B. Epidemiology and transmission. See Chapter 5(VI).

C. Rationale for vaccine use. Pneumococcus accounts for greater than one-third of community-acquired and one-half of hospital-acquired pneumonia in adults. More than 60,000 cases of invasive disease and more than 6,000 deaths from bacteremia and meningitis occur annually in the United States. More than half of these cases occur in adults who have indications for pneumococcal polysaccharide (Pne-PS) vaccine. Mortality is most associated with bacteremia and meningitis, and death can occur despite adequate antibiotic therapy. Fatality rates increase from 30% to 40% in those 50 to 69 years of age to 55% to 60% in persons 70 years of age or older.

D. Vaccines. Pne-PS vaccines consist of liquid preparations of purified capsular polysaccharide from 23 different serotypes (1, 2, 3, 4, 5, 6B, 7F, 8, 9N, 9V, 10A, 11A, 12F, 14, 15B, 17A or 17F, 18C, 19A, 19F, 20, 22F, 23F, 33F; 25 μg of each per dose). Until 2002, two products were available in the United States, PNEUMOVAX 23 (Merck) and Pnu-Imune 23 (Wyeth); In late 2002, Wyeth announced plans to cease production of Pnu-Imune 23. PNEUMOVAX 23 contains serotype 17F rather than 17A, uses phenol as preservative, and is packaged as a liquid in one-dose vials (ten per package), five-dose vials, and prefilled syringes (five per package). Pnu-Imune 23 contained serotype 17A rather than 17F, used thimerosal as preservative, and was packaged as a liquid in five-dose vials and prefilled LEDERJECT syringes (five per package). The serotypes represented by the vaccines account for 90% of blood isolates and 85% of all pneumococcal isolates from sterile sites in the United States. There is also evidence that cross-reactivity may allow for protection against additional serotypes. Both vaccines include the six invasive serotypes that are most frequently antibiotic resistant (6B, 9V, 14, 19A, 19F, 23F) and the seven serotypes that are found in Prevnar (PCV-7; serotypes 4, 6B, 9V, 14, 18C, 19F, and 23F). They are indicated for vaccination against pneumococcal disease caused by those pneumococcal types included in the vaccine. Pne-PS is not immunogenic in patients younger than 2 years of age and should not be used in that age group.

E. Storage, handling, and administration
- Maintain temperature at 35° to 46°F (2° to 8°C)
- Freezing can cause the vaccine to lose potency
- Shake well before use
- Each dose is 0.5 mL given intramuscularly or subcutaneously [see Chapter 3(III)]

F. Schedule. Most individuals who qualify for vaccination should receive only a single dose. Consideration should be given to one-time revaccination for certain high-risk individuals; those 10 years of age or younger can receive this dose in 3 years, and those older than 10 years of age can receive it 5 years or more from the first dose. Otherwise-healthy persons 65 years of age or older should receive a second dose only if they received the first dose of vaccine more than 5 years ago at a time when they were younger than 65 years of age.

G. Efficacy. More than 80% of healthy adults who receive Pne-PS develop antibodies against the serotypes contained in the vaccine, usually within 2 to 3 weeks. Older adults and persons with some chronic illnesses or immunodeficiency states may not respond as well, or at all. Elevated antibody levels persist for at least 5 years in healthy adults but fall more quickly in persons with certain underlying illnesses. Overall, the vaccine is 60% to 70% effective in preventing invasive disease. It appears to be less effective in preventing nonbacteremic pneumonia, and it does not reduce pneumococcal carriage. No change in the distribution of pneumococcal serotypes causing invasive disease has been observed as the result of vaccination.

After vaccination, antibody levels decline after 5 to 10 years and decrease more rapidly in some groups than in others. However, the relationship between antibody titer and protection from invasive disease is not certain, so the ability to define the need for revaccination based only on serology is limited. Pne-PS elicits a T-cell–independent response characterized predominantly by IgM antibody and no immunologic memory. Available data do not indicate a substantial increase in protection in the majority of revaccinated persons.

H. Official recommendations. Pne-PS should be given to all adults 65 years of age or older. The vaccine should also be given to individuals 2 years of age or older at high risk of invasive pneumococcal disease. For those between 24 and 59 months of age, regimens that use PCV-7 and Pne-PS in sequence are optimal [see Chapter 5(VI)]. Beyond 59 months, only Pne-PS is indicated.

High-risk conditions include the following:

- Chronic cardiovascular disease such as congestive heart failure or cardiomyopathy
- Chronic pulmonary disease such as cystic fibrosis (but not asthma)
- Chronic renal failure or nephrotic syndrome
- Functional or anatomic asplenia (including sickle cell disease)
- HIV infection (including asymptomatic without evidence of immunosuppression)
- Immunosuppressive conditions including Hodgkin's disease, lymphoma, multiple myeloma, organ transplantation, long-term high-dose corticosteroid therapy, and chemotherapy (vaccinate 2 weeks or more before initiation if possible)
- Diabetes
- Alcoholism

- Cirrhosis
- Cerebrospinal fluid leaks
- Cochlear implants
- Elective splenectomy (vaccinate 2 weeks or more before surgery if possible)
- Persons living in special environments or social settings with increased risk of pneumococcal disease or its complications (e.g., Alaskan Native and certain American Indian populations)

The safety of Pne-PS in pregnant women has not been studied, although no adverse consequences have been reported among newborns whose mothers were inadvertently vaccinated during pregnancy. Women who are at high risk of pneumococcal disease should be vaccinated before pregnancy. If this is not accomplished and the risk of disease is high, vaccination during pregnancy is indicated.

The patient's verbal history may be used to determine vaccination status; those with uncertain or unknown vaccination status should be vaccinated if indicated. Pne-PS can be given at the same time as influenza vaccine in separate arms and is probably safe to administer with other vaccines as well.

Pne-PS is also used to assess the adequacy of polysaccharide antibody responses in individuals older than 2 years of age who are suspected of having immune deficiency. A serum specimen is drawn, the vaccine is administered, and a second serum specimen is obtained 3 or 4 weeks later. The specimens are then tested in parallel for serotype-specific antibodies.

I. **Safety.** Thirty percent to 50% of vaccinees report pain, swelling, or erythema at the site of injection. These reactions usually persist for less than 48 hours. Local reactions are reported more frequently after a second dose. Moderate systemic reactions, such as fever and myalgia, are seen in less than 1% of vaccinees. Severe systemic reactions (e.g., anaphylaxis) have rarely been reported.

J. **Contraindications.** Anaphylactic reaction to a prior dose of vaccine or any of its components.

K. **Precautions.** Moderate or severe acute illness.

KEY CONCEPTS: PNEUMOCOCCAL POLYSACCHARIDE

- More than 60,000 annual cases and 6,000 deaths from invasive pneumococcal disease in the United States
- Contains capsular polysaccharide from 23 serotypes representing over 90% of blood isolates
- Single dose indicated for all individuals 65 years of age or older
- Single dose indicated for certain high-risk groups with one-time revaccination in some circumstances

III. Inactivated influenza vaccine

> Influenza viruses are enveloped, single-stranded RNA viruses with a segmented genome.

A. **Disease.** The incubation period is usually 2 days but can vary from 1 to 5 days. Approximately 50% of infected persons develop classic symptoms of influenza, which include abrupt onset of fever, myalgia, sore throat, and nonproductive cough. Fever is usually 101° to 102°F (38.3° to 38.9°C) and is accompanied by prostration. Additional symptoms may include rhinorrhea, headache, eye pain, and photosensitivity. Systemic symptoms and fever usually last from 2 to 3 days and rarely more than 5 days. Recovery is usually rapid, although some patients may have lingering fatigue for several weeks.

The most frequent complication of influenza is bacterial pneumonia. Primary influenza viral pneumonia is uncommon but has a high fatality rate. Other complications include myocarditis, worsening of chronic bronchitis and other chronic pulmonary diseases, and encephalitis. The overall death rate is 0.5 to 1.0 per 1,000 cases.

B. **Epidemiology and transmission.** The virus is transmitted by inhalation of small-particle aerosols or large droplets or contact with secretions from the respiratory tract of infected persons. Maximum communicability occurs from 1 to 2 days before onset of illness to 4 to 5 days thereafter. Disease activity peaks between December and March in temperate climates. During 1976 to 2001, peak influenza activity in the United States occurred most frequently in January (24% of seasons) and February (40% of seasons). However, peak activity occurred in March, April, or May in 20% of seasons. Influenza occurs throughout the year in tropical areas.

Influenza A virus infects all age groups and causes the most severe disease. Influenza B is milder and occurs more often in children. Influenza C is rarely seen and does not cause epidemic disease. Influenza A viruses are subtyped based on two surface molecules, hemagglutinin and neuraminidase. The molecules regularly undergo *antigenic drift*, minor changes that result in slight variation in antigenicity. These changes account for the fact that experience with influenza in the prior year does not prevent infection with this year's strain, although severity of illness might be mitigated depending on how much drift has occurred. Occasionally, a major change, or *antigenic shift*, in antigenicity occurs, resulting in pandemic strains to which few people have immunity. The antigenic changes in influenza viruses necessitate yearly surveillance for emergent strains and incorporation of those strains into the current year's vaccines.

C. **Rationale for vaccine use.** Regular increases in mortality accompany influenza epidemics. The mortality results not only from influenza and pneumonia, but also from cardiopulmonary and other chronic diseases that can be exacerbated by the disease. During the 1990s (years with only antigenic drift), the average annual number of deaths attributable to influenza was estimated at 51,203. Ninety percent of these deaths occurred among persons 65 years of age or older.

The risk of complications and hospitalization with influenza are highest among persons over 65 years of age, the very young, and persons with certain underlying medical conditions. An average of 114,000 annual hospitalizations are related to influenza, with more than 50% occurring in persons younger than 65 years of age. In nursing homes, attack rates may be as high as 60%, with fatality rates as high as 30%. The cost of a severe epidemic has been estimated at around $12 billion.

D. **Vaccines.** Inactivated influenza vaccine contains three virus strains that are inactivated by formaldehyde or beta-propiolactone and are disrupted by organic solvents or detergents (only these so-called split-virus or subvirion vaccines are available in the United States). Two type A viruses and one type B virus are included, and the exact composition changes from year to year. For example, the vaccine for the 2002 to 2003 season contained types A/Moscow/10/99 (H3N2)-like, A/New Caledonia/20/99 (H1N1)-like, and B/Hong Kong/330/2001-like. The World Health Organization (WHO) has recommended the same constituents for the 2003 to 2004 season. The viruses are grown in the allantoic sac of chick embryos, and as such may contain enough egg proteins to cause allergic reactions in sensitized people.

The inactivated vaccines available for use in the United States are shown in Table 7.3.

E. **Storage, handling, and administration**
- Maintain temperature at 35° to 46°F (2° to 8°C)
- Freezing can cause the vaccine to lose potency
- Shake well before use
- Each dose is 0.5 mL given intramuscularly [see Chapter 3(III)]

F. **Schedule.** Influenza vaccine is usually given in October and November of each year but should still be given throughout influenza season. To avoid missed opportunities, high-risk individuals can be vaccinated when seen for other reasons as early as September. The vaccine should not be used in infants younger than 6 months of age. Between 6 and 35 months of age, the dose is 0.25 mL, and at 36 months of age or older, the dose is 0.5 mL. Children 8 years of age or younger who are being vaccinated for the

Table 7.3.   Inactivated influenza vaccines available in the United States[a]

Product name	Manufacturer	Labeling	Contaminants/ excipients	Preservative	Packaging
Fluzone	Aventis Pasteur	≥6 mo of age	Egg protein Gelatin	None	Liquid 0.25-mL prefilled syringe with needle (10/pk)
				None	Liquid 0.5-mL prefilled syringe with needle (10/pk)
				Thimerosal	Liquid 0.5-mL prefilled syringe with needle (10/pk)
				Thimerosal	Liquid 10- to 20-dose (0.25- to 0.5-mL) vial
Fluvirin	Evans Vaccines	≥4 yr of age	Egg protein	Thimerosal	Liquid 10-dose (0.5-mL) vial

pk, package.
[a]Production of FluShield (Wyeth) was discontinued in 2003.

first time should receive two doses separated by 1 month (the second dose should be received before December). This is true for the first vaccination only, even if several years go by before the next immunization.

G. **Efficacy.** Nearly all vaccinated young adults develop hemagglutinin-inhibition antibody titers that are likely to be protective against strains antigenically similar to those present in the vaccine. Efficacy is variable and depends on the degree of similarity between vaccine strains and circulating strains of influenza virus. Under optimal conditions of timing and strain relatedness, the incidence of disease may be reduced by 70% in healthy younger adults. Protection is transient, and yearly immunization is necessary irrespective of whether significant antigenic changes in the prevailing strains have occurred. Adequate protection is generally achieved in immunologically primed healthy individuals who receive a single dose, and the vaccine is most effective when it precedes exposure by no more than 2 to 4 months.

Immunogenicity is variable among immunocompromised individuals. Successful immunologic responses in these populations are most likely to occur when immunized individuals have previously been primed by exposure to antigenically similar influenza strains.

H. **Official recommendations.** All persons 50 years of age or older, regardless of underlying conditions, should be vaccinated. The following high-risk groups should be recalled each year and vaccinated:

- Residents of long-term care facilities
- Pregnant women who will be in the 14th week or beyond during influenza season (pregnant women who have other high-risk conditions should be vaccinated before influenza season regardless of the stage of pregnancy)
- Persons 6 months of age or older with chronic illness, including pulmonary illnesses (e.g., emphysema, chronic bronchitis, and asthma), cardiovascular illnesses (e.g., congestive heart failure), metabolic diseases including diabetes mellitus, renal dysfunction, hemoglobinopathies such as sickle cell disease, and immunosuppression including HIV infection
- Persons 6 months to 18 years of age on long-term aspirin therapy (to reduce the risk of Reye syndrome)
- Groups who have contact with high-risk persons, including health care workers, employees of long-term care facilities, household contacts of high-risk individuals, and providers of home care to high-risk persons (e.g., visiting nurses and volunteers)
- Persons who provide essential community services
- Students or others in institutional settings (e.g., schools and colleges)
- Foreign travelers (disease peaks in April through September in the Southern Hemisphere, so persons pre-

paring for travel there should be vaccinated if not vaccinated the previous fall)

As of the 2002 to 2003 season, the Advisory Committee on Immunization Practices (ACIP) and American Academy of Pediatrics (AAP) "encourage" vaccination of all children 6 to 23 months of age based on data showing particular susceptibility to hospitalization in this age group. Although this falls short of an official "recommendation," physicians should discuss the issue with parents who present for other vaccinations or other visits and should advocate for influenza vaccination. In addition, household contacts and caregivers of all infants 23 months of age or younger should be vaccinated. It is likely that universal use of influenza vaccine in young infants will be recommended in the next few years.

Any person who falls outside of the above risk categories and wishes to reduce his or her chance of getting influenza should be vaccinated. Practically speaking, this means that physicians should give the vaccine to patients who request it, but they do not need to institute recall procedures or post reminder notices for these individuals. The truth of the matter is that there are very few reasons *not* to get the influenza vaccine.

Inactivated influenza vaccines are interchangeable in the sense that one product can be used one year and another product the next year. Although no data are available regarding two consecutive doses in the same year, it is assumed that products are interchangeable.

I. **Safety.** Influenza vaccine cannot cause influenza because it is inactivated. Less than one-third of vaccinees have been reported to develop local redness or induration for 1 to 2 days at the site of injection. Fever, chills, headache, and malaise, although infrequent, most often affect children who have had no previous exposure to the antigens contained in the vaccine. These reactions generally begin 6 to 12 hours after vaccination and persist for only 1 to 2 days. Immediate reactions, presumably allergic, may consist of hives, angioedema, allergic asthma, or systemic anaphylaxis. These are rare and probably result from hypersensitivity to a vaccine component, most likely residual egg protein. Influenza vaccines have been associated with a slightly increased frequency of Guillain-Barré syndrome in adults, on the order of one case per million immunized.

J. **Contraindications.** Anaphylactic reaction to a prior dose of vaccine or any of its components, including egg protein.

K. **Precautions.** Moderate or severe acute illness.

L. **Comments**

A live-attenuated intranasal vaccine was licensed in June 2003 [see Chapter 10(VIII)].

KEY CONCEPTS: INFLUENZA

- Causes approximately 20,000 deaths per year in the United States
- Inactivated, subvirion vaccines that are formulated with the prevailing strains are used in the United States
- Optimal time for vaccination is October and November but should continue throughout the season
- Vaccination of all adults 50 years of age or older recommended
- Vaccination of all children 6 to 23 months of age encouraged
- High-risk groups should be recalled for yearly vaccination
- First-time vaccinees 8 years of age or younger need two doses
- Influenza vaccine cannot cause the flu
- Live-attenuated vaccine approved in June 2003

Vaccines for Specialized Use

I. Adenovirus

> Adenoviruses are small, nonenveloped DNA viruses of multiple serotypes.

A. Disease. Adenoviruses are most commonly associated with respiratory and gastrointestinal infections but may also affect other organ systems. Adenoviruses types 1, 2, 3, 5, and 7 cause nasopharyngitis, pharyngitis, tonsillitis, acute laryngotracheitis, and bronchitis but only occasionally cause common cold symptoms in the absence of pharyngitis. *Pharyngitis* is the most common manifestation in children and is characterized by fever, sore throat, exudative tonsillitis, and cervical adenopathy, often accompanied by cough, headache, malaise, myalgia, and chills. Symptoms usually last 5 to 7 days. Types 4 and 7 cause *epidemic acute respiratory disease*, classically seen in military recruits and characterized by fever, pharyngitis, laryngitis, tracheitis, bronchitis, and nonproductive cough that may become paroxysmal. Rhinitis, conjunctivitis, cervical lymphadenopathy, malaise, myalgia, chills, headache, dizziness, and abdominal pain may be present, and progression to pneumonia is not unusual.

Adenovirus types 3, 4, 7, and 21 rank third behind respiratory syncytial virus (RSV) and parainfluenza virus as causes of *pneumonia* in young children. This may be severe or even fatal, especially in neonates and children younger than 18 months of age. Typical features include fever, severe cough, respiratory distress, tachypnea, wheezing, rales, conjunctivitis, pharyngitis, lethargy, vomiting, and diarrhea. Extrapulmonary manifestations may include rash (erythematous and maculopapular, often confused with measles or rubella), hepatitis, splenomegaly, nephritis, myocarditis, seizures, meningitis, and encephalitis. Permanent respiratory sequelae such as *bronchiolitis obliterans* can occur. Adenoviruses (particularly type 5) can also cause a *pertussis-like illness* in infants and young children with paroxysmal cough, whoop, posttussive vomiting, cyanosis, and lymphocytosis.

Other syndromes caused by adenoviruses include *pharyngoconjunctival fever* (types 3, 4, and 7), *epidemic keratoconjunctivitis* (types 8 and 37), *hemorrhagic conjunctivitis* (type 11), *hemorrhagic cystitis* (type 11), and *acute gastroenteritis* (types 31, 40, and 41). Mortality rates as high as 50% to 70% have been seen in immunocompromised individuals.

B. **Epidemiology and transmission.** Transplacental antibody appears to protect most infants during the first 6 months of life. Infection rates peak between 6 months and 5 years of age such that, by school age, most children have been infected with several serotypes. Overall, 10% of children hospitalized with respiratory disease have adenoviral infection, as do 15% of children with diarrhea. Epidemic respiratory disease is seen more often in winter and spring, but sporadic disease occurs throughout the year. Epidemics of pharyngoconjunctivitis typically occur during the summer and have been associated with camps and swimming pools. During epidemics of respiratory disease in military recruits, as many as 90% are infected in the first 8 weeks of training.

Transmission occurs by close physical contact with respiratory secretions, small droplet aerosols, and fomites; enteric adenoviruses are transmitted by the fecal-oral route. Inoculation takes place at mucosal surfaces such as the conjunctiva, nose, and throat, and fecal shedding may last as long as 3 months. Effective spread is associated with crowded or closed conditions including day care centers and military barracks. Epidemics of pharyngoconjunctival fever have been associated with swimming pools, and epidemics of keratoconjunctivitis have been associated with contaminated ophthalmic instruments. Nosocomial outbreaks of respiratory and gastrointestinal infections are well described.

C. **Rationale for vaccine use.** Despite the significance of adenoviral disease in children, there has never been a concerted effort to develop vaccines for generalized use in this population. In contrast, the burden of disease in the military provided adequate justification for the development of a vaccine. Studies in the 1960s showed that as many as 20% of infected recruits required hospitalization and as many as 40% became incapacitated; at large posts, this added up to hundreds of admissions, tremendous costs, and the need to restart training for many soldiers. Because 60% of cases were caused by types 4 and 7, these became the focus of vaccination efforts.

D. **Vaccines.** Beginning in 1971, vaccines for adenovirus types 4 and 7 were routinely administered to recruits at U.S. military training centers. The vaccines, manufactured by Wyeth, were licensed by the U.S. Food and Drug Administration (FDA) for military use and were not available to the general public. They consisted of live, lyophilized viruses (10^5 tissue culture infective doses) embedded in an enteric-coated tablet (the type 4 tablet was white, the type 7 was yellow). Oral administration in this form allowed the viruses to bypass the stomach, where they might be inactivated, and establish infection in the intestine. The strains were not intrinsically attenuated, but because they were given enterically rather than in the respiratory tract, they were capable of inducing immunity without inducing disease. Wyeth stopped producing the vaccines in 1996, and by 1999, existing stockpiles were exhausted. In 2001, the Department of Defense awarded a contract to Barr Laboratories to develop and remanufacture the vaccines, with cooperation from Wyeth.

E. Storage, handling, and administration. The vaccines were stable for 2 years at 35° to 46°F (2° to 8°C). The two tablets could be given simultaneously but had to be swallowed without being chewed.

F. Schedule. Only one dose of each vaccine was given, sometimes within hours of arrival at the training center. Programs varied from routine administration to all recruits during winter months to year-round administration or selective administration based on surveillance data.

G. Efficacy. Initial studies with the type 7 vaccine showed high serum neutralizing antibody titers 2 to 3 weeks after vaccination. Interestingly, intestinal secretory IgA was not induced. The vaccine was estimated to reduce acute respiratory disease due to the homologous serotype by 95%. Studies of the type 4 vaccine in more than 42,000 military recruits demonstrated a reduction of acute respiratory disease by 50% and a reduction of adenoviral respiratory disease by greater than 90%. The type 7 vaccine demonstrated similar efficacy, and interference between the two strains when given simultaneously was not demonstrated.

Use of the two vaccines at an Air Force base over a 9-year period eliminated acute respiratory adenoviral disease. In two military installations, the vaccines reduced overall rates of acute respiratory disease by 69% to 84% and adenoviral disease by 95%. During the years that these vaccines were used, except for a period when vaccine potency was compromised in the 1970s, there was never an outbreak of acute adenovirus type 4 or 7 respiratory disease in any vaccinated group. Since cessation of adenovirus immunization programs, disease rates at training centers have increased to pre-1970s levels.

The duration of protection for these vaccines was never established.

H. Official recommendations. There were never recommendations to use these vaccines in nonmilitary personnel. Military recruits received them along with many other vaccines, including influenza, measles, rubella, diphtheria and tetanus (Td), polio, and meningococcal vaccines, during the first week of training.

I. Safety. In clinical studies, vaccinees demonstrated no increase in respiratory, gastrointestinal, or other illnesses requiring hospitalization or outpatient visits. Vaccinees shed the viruses in the stool beginning 4 days after immunization and continuing for 7 to 8 days, so there was some risk of spread to close contacts. No serious adverse events were reported. Traces of gentamicin sulfate, neomycin sulfate, and amphotericin B were in the vaccines, and the type 7 tablet contained Food, Drug, and Cosmetic (FD&C) yellow number 5 (tartrazine).

J. Contraindications
- Immunocompromised individuals were not given these vaccines because of the risk of disseminated adenoviral infection; however, a study in recruits with early human immunodeficiency virus (HIV) infection did not demonstrate increased adverse effects
- Pregnancy (counsel to avoid pregnancy for 3 months after immunization)
- Anaphylactic reaction to a prior dose of vaccine or any of its components

K. Precautions
- Moderate or severe acute illness
- Vomiting or diarrhea potentially interfered with effectiveness

L. Comments. Adenoviruses have been genetically altered to carry genes from other pathogens. Such live vector recombinant vaccines could induce immunity to multiple other organisms as well as to adenoviruses. Adenovirus vectors have been engineered to express genes from viruses such as HIV, cytomegalovirus (CMV), Epstein-Barr virus (EBV), RSV, rotavirus, and parainfluenza virus. There has been some success with these vaccines in animal models, but further work is needed before they can be used in clinical trials.

KEY CONCEPTS: ADENOVIRUS

- Cause of serious, epidemic acute respiratory disease in military recruits
- Live oral types 4 and 7 vaccines used in the military from 1971 to 1999
- Vaccines licensed but not available to the general public
- Efficacy against homologous strain respiratory disease greater than 90%
- Production stopped in 1996, but new contract awarded in 2001

II. Bacille Calmette-Guérin

Mycobacterium tuberculosis is a slow-growing, acid-fast bacillus capable of intracellular infection. *Mycobacterium bovis* is closely related.

A. Disease. Classic *pulmonary tuberculosis* presents as fever, anorexia, weight loss, night sweats, chills, chest pain, productive cough, and hemoptysis, with cavitary upper lobe infiltrate, hilar and mediastinal adenopathy, and a positive tuberculin skin test (TST). Intrathoracic complications such as bronchopleural fistula, pyopneumothorax, and pericarditis can occur. However, most infected people never develop active disease; instead, they experience a minor, asymptomatic, self-limited parenchymal infection and regional adenopathy and are left with a positive TST. This *latent tuberculous infection* (LTBI) can later reactivate and cause pulmonary disease. The lifetime risk of reactivation is 5% to 15% for immunocompetent adults, and if this occurs, it is usually within 2 years of primary infection. The risk is greater among children and immunocompromised individuals with LTBI. Extrathoracic disease is less likely after reactivation because the anamnestic immune response can limit lymphohematogenous spread.

Older children and adolescents with primary pulmonary tuberculosis are usually asymptomatic, although initial infection is occasionally marked by fever, cough, and flulike symptoms that spontaneously resolve. Reactivation of LTBI in this age group resembles adult disease. Primary infection resulting in disease is most common in infants, developing in 40% to 50% of those infected. The subpleural space is usually involved, resulting in pleural reaction and parenchymal disease. A localized infiltrate may be seen, but the hallmark finding is enlargement of hilar or mediastinal lymph nodes. Some infants develop bronchial obstruction due to enlarged lymph nodes, resulting in air trapping and consequent tachypnea, localized wheezing, and decreased breath sounds. Erosion into a bronchus can cause luminal infection, leading to partial or complete obstruction of the bronchus and radiographic findings similar to those associated with foreign body aspiration. Calcification of caseous lesions and parenchymal scarring or contraction may lead to bronchiectasis. Rarely, *progressive primary pulmonary tuberculosis* occurs when a parenchymal focus develops a large caseous center leading to severe intrathoracic complications; without therapy, the mortality rate is 30% to 50%.

In young children with both asymptomatic and symptomatic primary infection, dissemination to distant anatomic sites is universal. If the burden of organisms is high enough, disease can result coincident with or, more commonly, months after pulmonary disease. *Miliary tuberculosis*, most common in infants, usually occurs early and affects the lungs, spleen, liver, and bone marrow. Features include fever, hepatosplenomegaly, generalized lymphadenopathy, malaise, fatigue, anorexia, and weight loss. The most common form of extrapulmonary disease is *scrofula*, an infection of the anterior cervical, submandibular, supraclavicular, or tonsillar lymph nodes. Central nervous system infection, especially *meningitis*, is most common in children 6 months to 4 years of age and can occur with minimal apparent pulmonary disease. Other extrapulmonary infections include osteomyelitis, arthritis, enteritis, peritonitis, mesenteric adenitis, renal tuberculosis, genital tract disease, otitis media, mastoiditis, and cutaneous infection.

B. Epidemiology and transmission. Transmission occurs through droplet nuclei that may remain airborne for hours; direct contact with infected body fluids or fomites is an infrequent mode of transmission. Children are rarely infectious because they do not develop cavitary disease, have a low burden of organisms in endobronchial secretions, and have mild cough. For this reason, a case in a child almost certainly means active disease in an adult in the immediate environment. The probability of contagion from adolescents and adults correlates with the presence of organisms in the sputum; those whose sputum is acid-fast smear negative are no longer considered infectious (this generally occurs within 2 weeks of starting therapy).

Worldwide, 2 to 3 billion individuals are infected, 8 to 10 million develop tuberculosis annually, and 3 to 5 million die from the disease. The highest prevalence is in Asia and Africa, but rates have increased in all regions of the world except Western Europe. The HIV pandemic has contributed greatly to the number of cases. In the United States, the overall risk of children acquiring tuberculosis is less than 1% but ranges from 2% to 10% in urban populations, especially where many foreign-born persons reside.

Between 1953 and 1984 in the United States, the rate of new infections declined an average of 6% per year. However, after 1985 the rate increased due in part to HIV, the immigration of persons from endemic countries, decreased case finding and treatment, and increased transmission in jails and medical facilities. Risk factors for tuberculosis in the United States include (a) immigration from high-prevalence countries; (b) exposure to prisons, homeless shelters, nursing homes, and other institutions; (c) lower socioeconomic status, crowding, and poor nutrition; (d) close contact with a case or high-risk individual; (e) work in a health care setting; (f) illicit drug use; (g) homelessness; and (h) chronic medical conditions. Infection rates are twice as high in men than in women. Almost two-thirds of cases in children younger than 5 years of age occur in seven states: California, Florida, Georgia, Illinois, New York, New Jersey, and Texas.

C. Rationale for vaccine use. The cornerstones of prevention and control of tuberculosis in the United States are (a) early detection and treatment of patients with active disease, (b) treatment of LTBI to prevent progression to active disease, and (c) prevention of transmission in health care facilities and other institutional settings. This is a feasible approach because, as in other developed, industrialized countries, tuberculosis is generally confined to specific high-risk groups, and resources for case-finding and treatment are available. In the rest of the world, however, infection is distributed widely throughout populations, and resources are limited. Thus, the possibility that vaccination might curtail the spread and morbidity from tuberculosis has spurred great interest. In fact, routine recommendations for vaccination have existed at some time in every country except the United States and the Netherlands.

D. Vaccines. Bacille Calmette-Guérin (BCG) originated as a strain of *M. bovis* isolated from a cow in 1908. The organism was subcultured 231 times over 13 years, resulting in gradual attenuation. The original BCG strain was disseminated from the Pasteur Institute to laboratories in many different countries, and as each laboratory passaged the bacterium under slightly different conditions, daughter strains arose that differed in virulence and immunogenicity. After the vaccine was declared to be safe and effective during the First International BCG Congress in 1948 (despite a lack of data to support this claim), use of the vaccine increased dramatically. Currently, 100 million children receive the vaccine each year, and more than 4 billion persons have been immunized altogether. The World Health Organization (WHO) maintains a system of quality control for BCG vaccines made in various countries and implements worldwide vaccination programs through the Expanded Programme on Immunization.

There are two products licensed in the United States for prevention of tuberculosis: BCG VACCINE USP (Organon) and Mycobax (Aventis Pasteur); only the former is available. BCG VACCINE USP is made from the TICE strain of BCG developed at the University of Illinois. It is labeled for prevention of tuberculosis in persons who are at high risk for exposure and who are not previously infected. The vaccine is supplied as a one-dose vial containing 50 mg [1 to 8×10^8 colony-forming units (CFU)] of lyophilized organisms along with a vial of sterile water diluent.

BCG vaccines have also found use in the therapy of carcinoma *in situ* of the bladder and prophylaxis against recurrence of carcinoma *in situ* and certain papillary tumors. The mechanism of action is unknown but presumably involves the induction of local granulomatous inflammation. Two products are licensed in the United States for treatment of bladder cancer: TICE BCG (Organon) and TheraCys BCG Live (Intravesical) (Aventis Pasteur). Neither of these is indicated for use in prevention of tuberculosis.

E. Storage, handling, and administration
- Maintain lyophilized vaccine at 35° to 46°F (2° to 8°C)
- Freezing is not recommended
- Store diluent at 39° to 77°F (4° to 25°C)

- Protect vaccine from direct sunlight
- Reconstituted vaccine can be stored at 35° to 46°F (2° to 8°C) but must be used within 2 hours
- Reconstitute with the supplied diluent (1.0 mL for all ages except infants younger than 2 months of age, in which case 2.0 mL is used)
- Swirl gently and avoid forceful agitation
- Dispose of all materials as infectious waste

The vaccine is administered percutaneously using a multiple-puncture device consisting of a waferlike stainless-steel disk with 36 protruding points. Between 0.2 and 0.3 mL of reconstituted vaccine is dropped onto a cleansed area of skin over the deltoid region, which is held horizontal and taut. The vaccine is spread out over a 1-in. to 2-in. area using the edge of the device, and the device is applied to the skin over the liquid with firm pressure (without rocking) to penetrate the skin. The disk is then removed, and the vaccine is spread again into the puncture sites and allowed to dry. The site is kept loosely covered and dry for 24 hours.

F. Schedule. Most individuals receive a single dose. If an infant's TST is negative 2 to 3 months after immunization and the need for vaccination persists, a second (full) dose can be given at 1 year of age or older.

G. Efficacy. The establishment of a primary infection is unaffected by vaccination. Rather, protection appears to result from prevention of hematogenous spread of tubercle bacilli from the primary pulmonary focus. Induction of cellular immunity is critical, although the specific antigens and cellular responses are not understood.

Studies of BCG vaccine are difficult to interpret because of the variety of strains used and differences in study design and location. More important, because there is no serologic measure of immunity, the incidence of disease (as opposed to infection) is relatively low, and the incubation period is long, large populations must be studied for extended periods of time to determine efficacy. Moreover, there is no gold standard for diagnosis of tuberculosis, especially in children from whom sputum specimens may not be available.

Of the eight field trials conducted, three well-conducted trials showed excellent overall efficacy against active tuberculosis: one in North American Indians (80% efficacy), one in British school children (76% efficacy), and one in Chicago (75% efficacy). Two other studies, one in Puerto Rico and one in southern India, demonstrated efficacy rates of 20% to 29%. Three other trials showed poor efficacy, including one of the largest ever conducted. These diverse results are potentially explained by (a) differences in methodology; (b) differences in vaccine strain, dose, administration, and potency; (c) the presence of nontuberculous mycobacteria in the environment; (d) variations in the prevalent strains of *M. tuberculosis*; and

(e) difficulties in distinguishing exogenous reinfection from endogenous reactivation.

Nonrandomized effectiveness studies have yielded similar results, with efficacy rates between 0% and greater than 80%. In a study of neonatal vaccination, protection in children younger than 15 years of age was 82%, but this decreased to 20% by young adulthood. Most case-control and cohort studies have demonstrated effectiveness in the range of 30% to 66%. In one metaanalysis, protection against meningitis and miliary disease was 86% in randomized trials (n = 10) and 75% in case-control studies (n = 8). In another metaanalysis involving 14 prospective and 12 case-control studies, overall protection against tuberculous disease was estimated at 50% and was highest in children.

In summary, it is generally agreed that BCG is effective in preventing serious forms of tuberculosis in children. However, it does not prevent infection and, because it has little effect on the incidence of active pulmonary disease in adults, it is unlikely to contribute to overall control efforts at the population level.

H. Official recommendations. The recent resurgence of tuberculosis in the United States, coupled with the advent of multidrug resistance and new data regarding vaccine efficacy, prompted the Advisory Committee on Immunization Practices (ACIP) to release new recommendations for use of BCG in 1996. The vaccine is recommended only in TST-negative individuals (except healthy infants younger than 2 months of age who can receive BCG without a TST being performed). For children, vaccination should be considered in the following situations:

- Continuous exposure to a person with untreated or ineffectively treated contagious pulmonary tuberculosis, where the child cannot be removed from exposure or cannot be given long-term antituberculous therapy
- Continuous exposure to a person with untreated or ineffectively treated contagious pulmonary tuberculosis caused by *M. tuberculosis* resistant to isoniazid and rifampin, where the child cannot be removed from the exposure

For health care workers in settings associated with a high risk of transmission of tuberculosis, vaccination should be considered if *all* of the following criteria are met:

- A high percentage of patients are infected with *M. tuberculosis* resistant to both isoniazid and rifampin
- Transmission of drug-resistant strains and subsequent infection are likely
- Comprehensive infection-control precautions have been implemented and have not been successful

BCG should not be the primary method of prevention of tuberculosis in any institution. Health care workers who are considered for vaccination should be counseled regarding the risks and benefits associated with vaccination and preventive therapy for tuberculosis.

Vaccination of HIV-infected individuals is not recommended.

BCG can be administered concomitantly with other childhood vaccines. Other live vaccines, if not given simultaneously, should be deferred at least 4 weeks. Receipt of BCG can result in a false-positive TST for several years. Because such cross-reactions cannot easily be differentiated from true positives, the TST should be interpreted without regard for BCG vaccination history.

I. **Safety.** Nearly all vaccinees develop puncture-site reactions characterized by erythema, small red papules, induration, and tenderness. A 1-cm indurated papule develops at the puncture site within 10 to 14 days. A pustule forms that 6 weeks later may ulcerate, forming a scab or crust that eventually falls off (usually within 2 to 10 weeks). A permanent scar 5 to 15 mm in diameter often develops at the site. Hypertrophic scars occur in 28% to 33% of vaccinees, and keloid scars occur in 2% to 4%. Muscle soreness occurs in 75% of vaccinees, and 70% develop local ulceration with drainage. Systemic reactions include fever, myalgia, and anorexia.

Complications include enlargement of ipsilateral axillary, cervical, and supraclavicular lymph nodes, occurring in less than 1% of vaccinees. Suppurative lymphadenitis is more common in neonates than in older infants and children. Treatment is controversial, and it is not clear whether antituberculous chemotherapy, surgical drainage, or observation alone is adequate. More serious complications, which are rare in immunocompetent individuals but more common in infants, include osteitis (0.06 to 0.89 cases per million) and nonfatal disseminated infection (0.31 to 0.39 cases per million). Antituberculous therapy is recommended in these cases, but pyrazinamide cannot be used, because BCG is resistant. Fatal disseminated disease occurs in 0.06 to 1.56 cases per million and is well described in immunocompromised individuals, such as those with HIV infection. Allergy to BCG has not been described.

J. **Contraindications**
   - Immunocompromised state, including HIV infection, leukemia, lymphoma, generalized malignancy, and congenital immunodeficiency
   - Immunosuppressive therapy, including high-dose corticosteroids, cytotoxic drugs, and radiation therapy
   - Pregnancy
   - Anaphylactic reaction to a prior dose of vaccine or any of its components
   - Positive TST

K. **Precautions**
   - Moderate or severe acute illness
   - BCG can decrease elimination of theophylline

L. **Comments.** The mainstay of tuberculosis control in the United States continues to be case-finding and treatment strategies, and it is unlikely that BCG will find more widespread use. To have a major impact on the epidemiology of tuberculosis, more effective vaccines must be produced. BCG vaccines have varying efficacy, and there is a lack of understanding as to which antigens of *M. tuberculosis* are important for protective immunity. New candidate vaccines are being developed that include recombinant and mutant BCG vaccines, attenuated *M. tuberculosis* vaccines (which lack genes essential for virulence), subunit protein vaccines, and plasmid DNA vaccines.

KEY CONCEPTS: BACILLE CALMETTE-GUÉRIN

- As many as 3 billion people worldwide have tuberculous infection
- As many as 10 million people worldwide develop disease each year, and 3 to 5 million die
- Mainstay of control in the United States is case finding and treatment
- Almost all other countries vaccinate infants routinely
- Vaccine prevents severe disease in children but does not control tuberculosis at the population level
- Used in United States in very selected circumstances
- Vaccine also used to treat bladder cancer

III. Cholera

Vibrio cholerae is a noninvasive, gram-negative bacterium that colonizes the gut and produces a potent enterotoxin.

   A. **Disease.** Most infected people are asymptomatic; 25% have mild to moderate diarrhea, and 2% to 5% experience severe gastrointestinal disease. Diarrhea begins acutely and may be accompanied by vomiting and rapid dehydration; profuse watery diarrhea and massive fluid and electrolyte losses can progress within hours to shock and death. Diarrhea is usually painless, with liquid stools that progress to a "rice water" consistency. Patients may have decreased skin turgor, dry mucous membranes, sunken eyes, rapid pulse, tachypnea, decreased urine output, weakness, and altered mental status. Complications include hypotension, hypoglycemia, hypokalemia, seizures, intestinal ileus, cardiac arrhythmias, renal failure, acidosis, aspiration, and pneumonia. Children are especially susceptible to hypoglycemia and resultant seizures.
   B. **Epidemiology and transmission.** Cholera persists endemically around the Indian subcontinent, and worldwide pandemics probably originate from there. The first recorded pandemic occurred in 1817, and five more followed in the nineteenth century. These pandemics were

caused by toxigenic *V. cholerae* serogroup O1, which is divided into three serotypes (Inaba, Ogawa, and Hikojima) and two biotypes (classical and El Tor). The current pandemic, which began in 1961 in Indonesia, is caused by the El Tor biotype. In 1991, this pandemic spread to Latin America, thus affecting all five continents of the world. In 1992, a new epidemic caused by toxigenic *V. cholerae* serogroup O139 Bengal began in India and spread rapidly throughout the Indian subcontinent and southeast Asia. Unfortunately, vaccines derived from serogroup O1 strains are not protective against serogroup O139. The actual number of worldwide cholera cases each year is unknown but probably exceeds 1 million. More than 100,000 annual deaths occur, mostly in Asia and Africa.

The organism is acquired through ingestion of water contaminated with feces, and a high inoculum (10^8 to 10^{10} organisms) is necessary. Brackish surface water may remain contaminated for long periods of time due to the persistence of *V. cholerae* in invertebrates. Secondary spread occurs by the fecal-oral route through ongoing contamination of water and food supplies and is exacerbated by poor sanitation conditions, where contaminated water may be used for drinking, cooking, bathing, and washing. Interestingly, direct person-to-person spread has not been demonstrated. Raw or undercooked shellfish are sources of infection because they are harvested from or washed with contaminated water and may be handled by infected individuals. Human carriers have been described, and their importance in the spread of disease has been confirmed in recent years. Persons with achlorhydria or blood group O are more likely to develop severe disease.

C. **Rationale for vaccine use.** Cholera control relies on adequate sanitation and hygiene, which is not achievable in many parts of the world. Natural infection confers long-term protection against disease (especially severe disease), suggesting that vaccines might be efficacious. In fact, the first attempts to produce a vaccine began shortly after Koch isolated the causative agent in the early 1880s. Antibodies to lipopolysaccharide that block colonization and antibodies that neutralize the enterotoxin are important in protection, as is mucosal immunity conferred by secretory IgA.

D. **Vaccines.** One vaccine, Cholera Vaccine, USP (Wyeth), is licensed in the United States, but manufacture and sale were terminated in 2000. The vaccine consisted of phenol-inactivated Ogawa and Inaba serotypes in equal parts (8 units/mL) suspended in buffered sodium chloride and preserved with 0.5% phenol. The vaccine was given parenterally and was supplied in 1.5-mL and 20-mL vials. The labeled indication was for immunization of persons traveling to or residing in countries where cholera is endemic or epidemic.

Two other vaccines are available outside the United States:

- Dukoral is an inactivated oral vaccine produced in Sweden by Active Biotech. Each dose consists of inactivated *V. cholerae* (a total of 10^{11} organisms) and 1.0 mg of recombinant B subunit of the cholera toxin (whole-cell/recombinant B subunit, or WC/rBS). Four strains are included: heat-inactivated Inaba (classic) and Ogawa (classic) serotypes and formalin-inactivated Inaba (El Tor) and Ogawa (classic) serotypes. The B subunit is derived from a genetically modified strain that elaborates the B subunit but not the whole toxin.
- Orachol (Switzerland) and Mutacol (Canada) are the trade names for a live, oral vaccine produced by Berna in Switzerland. Termed CVD 103-HgR, it was engineered from an Inaba (classic) strain by deleting the toxin genes except for the B subunit.

E. Storage, handling, and administration. Cholera Vaccine, USP was stored at 35° to 46°F (2° to 8°C) and kept from freezing. It was administered intradermally, subcutaneously, or intramuscularly.

Dukoral (WC/rBS) and Orachol (CVD 103-HgR) are stored at 35° to 46°F (2° to 8°C) in a dry place protected from light. They are given orally at least 1 hour before food or drink, and an antacid is included to prevent inactivation of the B subunit. Before administration, the contents of a sachet containing buffer and one containing vaccine are mixed into 100 mL of water. The suspension is swallowed as soon as possible.

F. Schedule. Primary immunization with Cholera Vaccine, USP consisted of two doses separated by 1 week to 1 month or longer. Booster doses were given every 6 months in areas where cholera was endemic or epidemic.

Dukoral (WC/rBS) is given in two doses separated by 10 to 14 days. Yearly booster doses may be needed. Orachol (CVD 103-HgR) is given as a single dose, and the manufacturer recommends giving a booster dose every 6 months if indicated.

G. Efficacy. Cholera Vaccine, USP was regularly immunogenic. However, field studies demonstrated only 50% efficacy for periods not exceeding 6 months.

In a field trial of three doses of Dukoral (WC/rBS) in Bangladesh, efficacy was 85% at 6 months and 50% at 3 years. Protection waned rapidly during the first year for children younger than 5 years and disappeared completely by 3 years. A more recent study in Peruvian military recruits demonstrated an initial protection rate of 86%. Overall efficacy is estimated at 50% to 60%. There appears to be some cross-protection against enterotoxigenic *Escherichia coli*.

In challenge studies, Orachol (CVD 103-HgR) induced protection rates higher than 90% against moderate to severe disease. However, in an Indonesian field trial, protection rates were 60% during the first 6 months and 24% during the first year.

None of these vaccines is active against the O139 serogroup.

H. Official recommendations. The WHO no longer recommends immunization against cholera for any travelers to or from endemic or epidemic areas, and no country requires vaccination for entry. In addition, the ACIP does not recommend vaccination for U.S. citizens traveling abroad or for contacts of patients with cholera. Appropriate precautions to avoid contaminated food and water are sufficient to prevent disease.

Use of the parenteral vaccine is no longer recommended by any advisory body. The oral vaccines should be considered for preemptive use in endemic areas rather than as a means of outbreak control.

No interchangeability data for cholera vaccines are available. Administration of cholera and yellow fever vaccines within 3 weeks of each other may result in decreased antibody responses to both vaccines. Therefore, a minimum of 3 weeks should elapse if the vaccines are not given simultaneously.

I. Safety. Approximately 50% of individuals receiving the parenteral vaccine experienced injection-site erythema, pain, tenderness, and/or swelling; 10% to 30% developed fever, malaise, and/or headache, and 1% to 5% had more severe systemic symptoms requiring bed rest. Mild gastrointestinal symptoms have been reported in people receiving Dukoral (WC/rBS), and approximately 2% of people receiving Orachol (CVD 103-HgR) developed diarrhea.

J. Contraindications
- Anaphylactic reaction to a prior dose of vaccine or any of its components
- Immune deficiency or immunosuppressed state (live oral)
- Age younger than 2 years (live oral)

K. Precautions
- Moderate or severe acute illness
- Data on use during pregnancy are not available
- Antibiotics may decrease immunogenicity of live oral vaccines

L. Comments. The oral cholera vaccines available in much of the rest of the world are significantly better than the parenteral vaccine. However, new generation vaccines with improved efficacy, particularly in young children, are needed. Since the current pandemic is caused by the El Tor strain, live oral vaccines against this strain are being tested. In addition, because vaccines produced from serogroup O1 cholera do not protect against O139 strains, a new vaccine is needed. An effective bivalent O1/O139 vaccine would be ideal for use in Asia.

KEY CONCEPTS: CHOLERA

- Severe disease characterized by diarrhea, vomiting, dehydration, shock, and death within hours
- Endemic in parts of Asia, but worldwide pandemics occur
- Oral vaccines available outside the United States have modest efficacy
- Inactivated parenteral vaccine licensed in the United States no longer produced
- No country requires vaccination for entry
- Vaccination not recommended for travel anywhere in the world
- Mainstay of prevention is good sanitation and hygiene

IV. Hepatitis A

Hepatitis A virus is a small, nonenveloped, single-stranded RNA virus that is tropic for the liver but does not establish chronic infection. Hepatitis A vaccine (Hep-A) is not yet recommended for all U.S. infants, but it is routinely given in regions with high disease incidence.

    A. Disease. Ninety percent of children younger than 5 years of age with hepatitis A virus infection are asymptomatic, whereas 90% of adults experience symptoms such as jaundice. The incubation period ranges from 15 to 50 days. Onset is usually abrupt with low-grade fever, myalgia, poor appetite, nausea, vomiting, malaise, and fatigue, followed by dark-colored urine, scleral icterus, pale stools, jaundice, and weight loss. Diarrhea is more common in children. Hepatomegaly and right upper quadrant tenderness, and occasionally splenomegaly or rash, may be present. Symptoms generally subside within 3 to 4 weeks, although 10% to 15% of patients experience prolonged or relapsing disease for as many as 6 months. There is no chronic form of hepatitis A. Extrahepatic manifestations include arthralgias, pruritus, cutaneous vasculitis, cryoglobulinemia, hemophagocytic syndrome, and Guillain-Barré syndrome. Fulminant hepatitis is rare.

    B. Epidemiology and transmission. Hepatitis A virus is spread from person to person by the fecal-oral route. Peak infectivity occurs during the 2-week period before the onset of jaundice, and infants and children can shed the virus for several months. As infants and young children often have clinically silent infection and exposure to their feces may unavoidable, they are often the source of infection for adults in households or day care centers. Contaminated water and undercooked food (especially shellfish) are also common sources of transmission; often a food handler somewhere down the line is infected. Transient viremia in the donor occasionally leads to transmission through blood products.

Hepatitis A is most prevalent in Southeast Asia, Africa, and Latin America. In countries with high endemicity, the infection is usually acquired in childhood, whereas in many developed countries, most adults have not yet been exposed. Childhood disease often correlates with overcrowding, poor sanitation, limited access to clean water, and inadequate sewage systems. Risk factors in the United States include household or sexual contact with an infected individual (12% to 26%), exposure at a day care center or workplace (11% to 16%), foreign travel (4% to 6%), contaminated food or waterborne outbreaks (2% to 3%), and homosexual activities or illicit drug use (as great as 10%). However, nearly one-half of persons with hepatitis A have no identified exposure. Incidence is highest among children 5 to 14 years of age and among American Indians, Alaskan Natives, and Hispanics. Disease rates are substantially higher in the western United States; between 1987 and 1997, half of all cases occurred in 11 states west of the Mississippi.

C. Rationale for vaccine use. Each year there are 180,000 infections, 90,000 symptomatic cases, and 100 deaths attributable to hepatitis A in the United States. Most deaths occur in persons older than 50 years of age and in individuals with chronic liver disease. As many as 22% of patients are hospitalized; the average work lost is 27 days, and the cost of contact tracing and prophylaxis is substantial. In 1997, the overall costs of hepatitis A in the United States exceeded $300 million.

For many years, immune globulin intramuscular (IGIM) has been used to protect persons with known or anticipated exposure to hepatitis A virus. However, IGIM is cumbersome and expensive to produce and provides only transient protection, necessitating repeated injections if exposure is expected for greater than 5 months. Hep-A can protect individuals for many years and has the potential to reduce the incidence of disease in a community through large-scale vaccination programs. The primary target of such programs should be children because of their high infection rate and critical role in transmission. Previous strategies targeting only persons in the highest-risk groups and those at high risk of severe disease had little impact on the overall incidence of infection. New strategies use universal immunization of children living in regions that exceed national incidence rates.

D. Vaccines. Two vaccines are available in the United States (Table 8.1). Both consist of chemically inactivated hepatitis A virus grown on MRC-5 (human diploid) cells and adsorbed to alum. Other components of the final preparation may include amino acids, polysorbate 20, residual cellular proteins and DNA, formalin or formaldehyde, bovine albumin, sodium borate, and sodium chloride. Both products are labeled for preexpo-

Table 8.1.   Hep-A vaccines available in the United States

Manufac-turer	Trade name	Strain	Formulation	Packaging
Glaxo-Smith-Kline	Havrix[a]	HM175	2-dose pediatric (0.5 mL)[b] 720 ELISA units[c] Preservative: 2-phenoxyethanol	Liquid 1-dose vial (1 or 10/pk) Prefilled Tip-Lok syringe (5 or 25/pk)[d]
			Adult (1.0 mL) 1,440 ELISA units Preservative: 2-phenoxyethanol	Liquid 1-dose vial Prefilled Tip-Lok syringe (1, 5, or 25/pk)
Merck	VAQTA	CR326F	Pediatric (0.5 mL) 25 units[c] Preservative: none	Liquid 1-dose vial (1, 5, or 10/pk) Prefilled syringe (1 or 5/pk)[e]
			Adult (1.0 mL) 50 units Preservative: none	Liquid 1-dose (1 or 5/pk) Prefilled syringe (1 or 5/pk)[e]

ELISA, enzyme-linked immunosorbent assay; pk, package.
[a]Also available in combination with Hep-B vaccine [Twinrix; see Chapter 6(IV)].
[b]A pediatric formulation containing 360 ELISA units/0.5 mL and requiring three doses is no longer available.
[c]The units used to measure antigen content for these vaccines cannot be compared directly.
[d]Packages of 25 available with or without BD SafetyGlide needles.
[e]Needles included.

sure prophylaxis against hepatitis A virus infection in persons 2 years of age or older.
  E. **Storage, handling, and administration**
   • Maintain temperature at 35° to 46°F (2° to 8°C)
   • Freezing can cause vaccine to lose potency
   • Shake well before use
   • Each dose is 0.5 mL (pediatric formulation) for children and adolescents and 1.0 mL (adult formulation) for adults given intramuscularly [see Chapter 3(III)]
  F. **Schedule.** The vaccination schedules are given in Table 8.2.

Table 8.2. Hepatitis A vaccination schedule

Product	Age (yr)	Formula-tion (units)	Volume (mL)	Total doses	Timing (mo)
Havrix	2–18	720 ELISA	0.5	2	0, 6–12
	≥ 19	1,440 ELISA	1.0	2	0, 6–12
VAQTA	2–18	25	0.5	2	0, 6–18
	≥ 19	50	1.0	2	0, 6–12

ELISA, enzyme-linked immunosorbent assay.

G. Efficacy. Nearly 100% of individuals fully immunized with either vaccine achieve protective levels of antibody to hepatitis A virus, and infection is rare after immunization. Based on kinetic models of antibody decay, protective antibody may persist for longer than 20 years.

The efficacy of Havrix was evaluated in a study of 40,119 school children aged 1 to 16 years in Thailand. Two doses of vaccine (360 ELISA units each, equivalent to the discontinued formulation) or placebo were administered 1 month apart. Two children in the vaccine group and 32 in the control group developed hepatitis A, indicating an efficacy of approximately 94%. The efficacy of VAQTA was evaluated in a study of 1,037 healthy seronegative children 2 to 16 years of age in Monroe County, New York. A single dose of vaccine (25 units) or placebo was administered. Beyond the immediate postvaccination period, there were no cases of hepatitis A in the vaccine group and 34 cases in the placebo group, for an efficacy of 100%.

Recent studies have demonstrated control of community and institutional outbreaks of hepatitis A with large vaccination campaigns. For example, in an ongoing outbreak in Alaska, the incidence of disease decreased dramatically in areas where vaccine uptake was high, but cases continued to occur in villages where vaccination rates were low. Outbreaks in several Native American Indian communities have been curtailed by early and rapid vaccination programs. In Butte County, California, a mass immunization campaign in children 2 to 12 years of age between 1995 and 2000 resulted in a 93.5% decline in cases in the entire county population.

H. Official recommendations. Universal vaccination of all children 2 years of age or older *is recommended* in states, counties, and communities in which the average annual reported incidence of hepatitis A is 20 cases or more per 100,000 population (at least twice the national average between 1987 and 1997). Currently, the states in this category are Arizona, Alaska, Oregon, New Mexico, Utah, Washington, Oklahoma, South Dakota, Idaho, Nevada, and California. In addition, routine immunization *should be considered* for children living in areas where the average annual reported incidence is ten or greater but fewer than 20 cases per 100,000 population. Currently, these states are Missouri, Texas, Colorado, Arkansas, Montana, and Wyoming. For areas with high rates of disease, routine vaccination of children beginning at 2 years of age, catch-up vaccination of preschool children and vaccination of older children (10 to 15 years of age) should be instituted. In other areas, vaccinating one or more single-age cohorts of children or adolescents or those in selected settings may be appropriate. The vaccine may also be used for outbreak control.

The following persons are at increased risk for hepatitis A and *should be routinely vaccinated*:

- Persons traveling to or working in countries with high or intermediate endemicity, including Africa, Asia (except Japan), the Mediterranean basin, Eastern Europe, the Middle East, Central and South America, Mexico, and parts of the Caribbean
- Men who have sex with men
- Injecting and noninjecting illegal drug users
- Persons who work with hepatitis A virus–infected primates or with hepatitis A virus in a research laboratory (workers exposed to raw sewage are not at increased risk)
- Persons who have clotting-factor disorders (outbreaks were reported in the early 1990s, presumably due to blood from donors who were viremic at the time of donation)
- Persons who have chronic liver disease, including those who are waiting for or have received liver transplants (these individuals are particularly susceptible to severe disease)

Vaccination may also be *considered* in the following:

- Military personnel
- Alaska Natives and Native Americans
- Persons engaging in high-risk sexual activity (where fecal-oral contact may occur)
- Residents of a community experiencing an outbreak of hepatitis A
- Caretakers in institutions for the developmentally challenged
- Employees of day care centers
- Food handlers
- Juveniles in correctional facilities

Hep-A should be protective 4 weeks after one dose. If travel to a high-risk area will occur before 4 weeks, IGIM should be administered simultaneously with a dose of vaccine at a separate site; children younger than 2 years of age should receive IGIM alone because the vaccine is not approved in this age group [see Chapter 11(III)].

Hep-A vaccines appear to be interchangeable and can be given simultaneously with other vaccines at separate sites.

I. **Safety.** Reactions are usually mild and subside within 24 hours. Mild injection-site reactions including erythema, swelling, pain, and tenderness occur in as many as 21% of children and 56% of adults. Systemic reactions, including low-grade fever, malaise, and fatigue, are reported in fewer than 10% of vaccinees. No serious adverse events have been reported.

J. **Contraindications.** Anaphylactic reaction to a prior dose of vaccine or any of its components.

K. **Precautions.** Moderate or severe acute illness.

L. **Comments.** With the continuing spread of hepatitis A in the United States, recommendations to immunize all children may be anticipated at some point in the future.

KEY CONCEPTS: HEPATITIS A

- 180,000 cases and 100 deaths each year in the United States
- Children usually asymptomatic but capable of spreading infection to adults
- One-half of infected persons have no known exposure
- Two vaccines licensed in United States with indications for individuals 2 years of age or older
- Universal vaccination if regional incidence 20 per 100,000 or higher
- Selective vaccination of high-risk groups, including some travelers
- IGIM also indicated in some situations

V. Japanese encephalitis

Japanese encephalitis virus (JEV) is a mosquito-borne flavivirus with a single-stranded RNA genome surrounded by a protein nucleocapsid and a lipid envelope.

A. **Disease.** Only 1 in 250 infections with JEV results in symptomatic illness. However, as many as 25% of those who do develop encephalitis may progress to coma and death. Others may have less severe disease characterized by aseptic meningitis. Illness begins abruptly with fever, lethargy, headache, abdominal pain, nausea, and vomiting. Mental status changes including disorientation, personality change, agitation, delirium, and abnormal movements (including tremor, ataxia, choreoathetosis, rigidity, and extrapyramidal signs) are common, with progression to confusion, delirium, and coma. Mutism is a presenting sign in some cases. As many as 75% of patients present with or develop seizures. One-third of patients develop cranial nerve palsies, and some develop generalized or asymmetric muscular weakness, flaccid or spastic paralysis, and clonus.

Analysis of the CSF shows moderate lymphocytic pleocytosis and normal or moderately elevated protein. Imaging of the brain may show diffuse white matter edema, abnormal signal in the thalamus, and hemorrhage. Hyponatremia due to inappropriate secretion of antidiuretic hormone is a frequent complication. After a week of illness there may be gradual improvement, but some patients experience a rapidly fatal course. Complete recovery may require months to years, but one-third of patients have chronic neurologic sequelae such as memory loss, motor and cranial nerve paresis, movement disorders, chronic seizures, cortical blindness, and behavioral disorders. JEV may cause intrauterine infection and miscarriage when it is acquired in the first or second trimester of pregnancy.

B. **Epidemiology and transmission.** JEV is endemic throughout China, Southeast Asia, the Indian subcontinent, Indonesia, the Philippines, and Australia. In temperate areas, transmission generally occurs from May through September with periodic seasonal epidemics. In subtropical Asia, transmission is hyperendemic and the season is longer, from March through October. In tropical Asia, transmission occurs year-round without noticeable seasonable epidemics. The virus is spread from ground pool–breeding *Culex* mosquitoes to domestic pigs and aquatic birds that remain asymptomatic. Pigs have sustained viremia and serve as host to many feeding mosquitoes. Humans, horses, and domestic animals are incidental hosts. The risk of transmission is highest in rural areas where rice paddies exist. Disease incidence correlates with abundance of mosquitoes, proximity of pigs and birds, rainy season, and irrigation of agricultural fields. Incidence is highest in children 2 to 10 years of age; by adulthood, 80% of individuals have protective levels of antibody. Persons who travel extensively in or move to endemic areas acquire symptomatic infection at a rate of 1 per 50,000 persons per month; the risk to short-term travelers may be less than 1 per million. The risk of infection correlates with travel during transmission season, exposure to rural areas, extended period of travel or residence, and outdoor activities (especially in the evenings when mosquitoes are active).

C. **Rationale for vaccine use.** Residence in air-conditioned or screened-in areas, avoidance of outdoor activities, and the use of permethrin-treated mosquito nets, insect repellents, and protective clothing can reduce the risk of infection. Societal changes such as urbanization, less agriculture, use of pesticides, centralized pig rearing, and improved standards of living may also contribute to lower disease rates. However, there are still 175,000 annual cases worldwide among children younger than 15 years of age, resulting in 45,000 deaths and 78,000 survivors with chronic disabilities. Since 1996, childhood immunization programs in China, Taiwan, Japan, and Korea have resulted in marked decreases in the number of reported cases.

D. **Vaccines.** The only licensed vaccine in the United States is JE-VAX, manufactured by The Research Foundation for Microbial Diseases of Osaka University (Biken; Suita, Osaka, Japan) and distributed by Aventis Pasteur. The vaccine consists of the Nakayama-NIH strain of JEV purified from infected mouse brains and inactivated with formaldehyde. It is supplied lyophilized with thimerosal as preservative in one-dose (three per package) or ten-dose vials with vials of sterile water for diluent. The vaccine may contain gelatin, formaldehyde, polysorbate 80, and mouse serum protein. It is indicated for prevention of Japanese encephalitis in persons 1 year of age or older.

E. **Storage, handling, and administration**
- Maintain lyophilized vaccine at 35° to 46°F (2° to 8°C)
- Freezing can cause the vaccine to lose potency
- Reconstitute only with 1.3 mL of the supplied diluent, and shake well before use
- Store reconstituted vaccine at 35° to 46°F (2° to 8°C) and use within 8 hours
- Each dose is 1.0 mL given subcutaneously [see Chapter 3(III)] for individuals older than 3 years of age and 0.5 mL given subcutaneously for children 1 to 3 years of age

F. **Schedule.** A primary series consists of three doses given on days 0, 7, and 30. An abbreviated regimen given on days 0, 7, and 14 can be used when time constraints make the longer schedule impractical. The last dose should be given at least 10 days before international travel to ensure an adequate immune response and access to medical care in the event of delayed adverse reactions. A booster dose (0.5 mL if 3 years of age, 1.0 mL if 4 years of age or older) may be given after 2 years, and the need for further boosters can be determined by serologic testing.

G. **Efficacy.** Children 1 to 14 years of age were given a monovalent Nakayama-NIH strain vaccine (n = 21,628), a bivalent vaccine that also contained the Beijing strain (n = 22,080), or tetanus toxoid as placebo (n = 21,516) in a clinical trial in Thailand. Subjects received two doses of vaccine 7 days apart. Efficacy of each vaccine was 91%. Based on this study, a two-dose primary series is used in many parts of Asia. However, fewer than 80% of vaccinees in U.S. trials developed protective antibody levels after two doses, and responses were short lived. In contrast, more than 99% of subjects demonstrated adequate responses to regimens consisting of three doses over a 30-day period. The duration of protection after primary immunization is not well defined. In the Thai field trial, efficacy was maintained through 2 years of surveillance, but further follow-up data were not available. All 21 U.S.

Army personnel followed for 2 years after vaccination retained seroprotective antibody levels. In a Japanese study, individuals maintained seroprotective levels for 3 years after the primary series.

H. Official recommendations. JE-VAX is not recommended for all persons traveling to or residing in Asia. Factors that should be considered in the decision to administer vaccine include the incidence of Japanese encephalitis in the location of intended stay, the conditions of housing, nature of activities, duration of stay, and the possibility of unexpected travel to high-risk areas. In general, vaccine *should be considered* for use in persons spending a month or longer in epidemic or endemic areas during the transmission season, especially if travel will include rural areas. Depending on the epidemic circumstances, vaccine should be considered for persons spending less than 30 days who are at particularly high risk, such as those engaging in extensive outdoor activities in rural areas. Travelers are advised to take personal precautions to reduce exposure to mosquito bites. Current Centers for Disease Control and Prevention (CDC) advisories should be consulted with regard to disease activity in specific locales. The decision to use JE-VAX should balance the risks of exposure, the risk of disease, the availability and acceptability of repellents and other protective measures, and the side effects of vaccination.

Laboratory workers with potential exposure to infectious JEV *should be* vaccinated. Limited data suggest that JE-VAX can be given simultaneously with other vaccines at separate sites.

I. Safety. Injection-site tenderness, redness, and swelling have been reported in approximately 20% of vaccinees. Systemic side effects such as fever, headache, malaise, rash, chills, dizziness, myalgia, nausea, vomiting, and abdominal pain have been reported in approximately 10%. Most reactions occur within 3 days of the first dose and within 2 weeks of the second dose. In one study, less than 5% of travelers immunized with the three-dose regimen reported systemic complaints; 0.2% reported hives, and 0.1% reported facial swelling. Vaccinees may rarely experience generalized urticaria and angioedema. For this reason, patients should be observed for 30 minutes after vaccination and warned about the possibility of delayed urticaria and angioedema of the extremities, face and oropharynx, airway, and especially the lips. Most such reactions occur within 10 days of vaccination, so travelers should remain in areas where they have access to medical care for that period of time. Persons with a history of idiopathic urticaria or urticaria after hymenoptera envenomation, drugs, or other provocations appear to be at increased risk.

Vaccinees should avoid alcohol intake during the 48 hours after vaccination because of a study showing increased risk of hypersensitivity reactions in persons who had unusual alcohol consumption during this time period. The same study showed an increased risk for hypersensitivity reactions in persons who received other vaccines within the 7 days before receipt of a JEV vaccine. Therefore, other vaccines that must be given should be given concurrently rather than before JE-VAX.

J. Contraindications. Anaphylactic reaction (including generalized urticaria and angioedema) to a prior dose of vaccine or any of its components (this would include proteins of rodent or neural origin which were present in experimental hantaviral vaccines produced in Korea and China and a French neurotropic yellow fever vaccine strain that was discontinued in 1982).

K. Precautions
- Moderate or severe acute illness
- Pregnant women can be immunized when the risks of immunization are outweighed by the risk of infection for the mother and developing fetus

L. Comments. Candidate recombinant vaccines have been evaluated in which JEV genes have been inserted into attenuated vaccinia or canarypox viruses. These recombinants express the viral proteins and are protective in animal models, but they are not consistently immunogenic in humans. Inactivated whole-virus vaccines have been produced in cell culture and are being evaluated in clinical trials. Other areas of research include the development of DNA vaccines (which express viral proteins when taken up by cells) and a chimeric vaccine using the yellow fever vaccine virus to carry JEV coat proteins.

In China, inactivated and live-attenuated JEV vaccines are produced in primary hamster kidney cells. The inactivated vaccine has been China's principal vaccine since 1968, and approximately 70 million doses are distributed annually. The primary series is given each spring and consists of two doses given 1 week apart to children 12 months of age; booster doses are given 1 year later and at 6 and 10 years of age. The live-attenuated vaccine was licensed in 1988, and 30 million doses are distributed annually. One dose is administered in the spring to children at age 1 year, again at age 2 years, and, in some areas, a booster dose is given at age 6 years.

KEY CONCEPTS: JAPANESE ENCEPHALITIS

- Most infections are asymptomatic
- Case-fatality rate 25% with severe encephalitis
- Endemic throughout Asia
- One inactivated whole-virus vaccine available in the United States
- Indicated for selected individuals 1 year of age or older
- Generalized urticaria and angioedema of extremities and face may occur

VI. Lyme disease

> *Borrelia burgdorferi* is a fastidious, microaerophilic spirochete that is transmitted by *Ixodes* ticks and infects small mammals.

A. **Disease.** *Early localized disease* presents days to weeks after tick exposure and consists of *erythema migrans* (EM), a circular rash that begins as a red macule or papule at the site of the tick bite and expands with a flat red border and partial central clearing (the average final diameter is 15 cm). There may be associated fever, headache, myalgia, fatigue, malaise, and arthralgia. *Early disseminated disease* occurs several weeks after the tick bite and is characterized by multiple EM lesions (smaller than the first lesion) that develop away from the primary site. Associated symptoms often include fever, fatigue, myalgia, headache, conjunctivitis, and lymphadenopathy. Approximately 1% of children have associated aseptic meningitis. Fewer than 1% of children but 5% of untreated adults develop carditis with fluctuating degrees of atrioventricular block. As many as 15% of untreated adults develop focal neurologic disease, most commonly facial nerve (Bell's) palsy or radiculoneuritis. During this stage, migratory musculoskeletal pains often develop in joints, tendons, bursae, muscle, or bones, usually without joint swelling.

   Late disease, which develops months to years later, presents with arthritis and, less commonly, with demyelinating encephalitis or polyneuritis. The most commonly affected joint is the knee; symptoms resolve spontaneously in 1 to 2 weeks but often recur in other joints. Five percent to 10% of patients still experience recurrences despite antibiotic treatment; association with HLA types DR-2 and DR-4 suggests an immunopathologic basis for this chronic arthritis.

B. **Epidemiology and transmission.** In the United States, most cases occur in southern New England, the upper Midwest, and along the upper Pacific coast. Cases in Europe are concentrated in Scandinavia and the central continent. The incidence can be as high as 1% per year in hyperendemic areas. From 1993 to 1997, a mean of 12,451 cases were reported each year to the CDC. The highest rates were in children younger than 15 years and in adults 30 to 59 years of age. Most cases occur in the spring and summer and are acquired near the individual's home during routine outdoor activities. Approximately 50% of infections are asymptomatic.

   In the United States, *B. burgdorferi* is transmitted by *Ixodes scapularis* (the black-legged or deer tick) and *Ixodes pacificus* (the Western black-legged tick). Larvae or nymphs become infected as they feed on small animals such as mice. Although proportionally more adult ticks are infected than nymphs, most cases of human transmission come from nymphs because they outnumber adult ticks, are active during the spring and summer when more individuals are outdoors, and are small enough not to be detected on the skin while feeding. The risk of transmission is thought to be low during the first 24 to 36 hours after attachment because the organism must multiply in the midgut of the tick before migrating to the salivary glands.

C. **Rationale for vaccine use.** Lyme disease is the most common tick-borne illness in the United States, with more than 10,000 new cases reported each summer (the actual number is probably much more given the degree of underreporting). In some areas of New England, as many as 16% of residents have evidence of previous infection, and affected regions of the country continue to expand. The costs of Lyme disease include those associated with diagnosis, treatment of proven or suspected disease, days lost from school or work, and decreased quality of life; late disease is especially costly because of persistent symptoms, permanent disability, and poor response to therapy. Although these factors would seem to make vaccination attractive, Lyme disease is largely preventable by effective control of tick exposure and almost universally treatable if recognized early.

D. **Vaccines.** LYMErix (rOspA, GlaxoSmithKline) was licensed in the United States in 1998 but withdrawn by the manufacturer in 2002 because of decreased demand. The vaccine contained a lipoprotein from *B. burgdorferi* called outer surface protein A (OspA), derived from recombinant *E. coli*. OspA is expressed by *B. burgdorferi* as it replicates in the tick. LYMErix (rOspA) worked by inducing antibodies to OspA in the vaccinee that entered the tick via the blood meal and inactivated the bacterium before it was able to enter the host. This mechanism of action (antibody-mediated inactivation in the vector rather than the host) was unprecedented for a vaccine.

Each dose contained 30 μg of rOspA adsorbed to alum; 2-phenoxyethanol was used as a preservative. The vaccine was labeled for prevention of Lyme disease in individuals 15 to 70 years of age.

E. **Storage, handling, and administration**
   - LYMErix (rOspA) was stored at 35° to 46°F (2° to 8°C) and kept from freezing
   - Each 0.5 mL dose was given intramuscularly [see Chapter 3(III)]

F. **Schedule.** The vaccine was administered at 0, 1, and 12 months. Doses were timed so that the second dose and the third dose were given several weeks before the beginning of Lyme season.

G. **Efficacy.** A study conducted in 10,936 persons aged 15 to 70 years living in highly endemic areas of the United States showed efficacy against definite Lyme disease (typical symptoms with laboratory confirmation) of 49% and 76% after two and three doses, respectively. Efficacy against asymptomatic disease was 83% after two doses and 100% after three doses. A similar study using a rOspA vaccine manufactured by Aventis Pasteur showed efficacy against definite disease of 68% after two doses and 92% after three doses.

The duration of protection afforded by vaccination was unknown. In the efficacy trial of LYMErix (rOspA), antibody concentrations of 1,200 ELISA units/mL 1 month after the third dose correlated with protection for 1 year. Because antibody levels declined over time and sufficient levels were required to enter the tick during feeding, it was expected that booster doses would be required.

H. Official recommendations. There was never an official recommendation to routinely administer LYMErix (rOspA) to any individuals. Rather, it was recommended to *consider* the vaccine for high-risk individuals, but it was emphasized that vaccination was an adjunct to personal protective measures and that the cost–benefit ratio was not known. Vaccination was to be considered for individuals 15 to 70 years of age living in or traveling to endemic areas whose routine, occupational, or leisure activities would put them into frequent or prolonged contact with ticks. This included, for example, persons living in southern New England who worked in landscaping, brush clearing, forestry, or wildlife and parks management, as well as those participating in hiking, camping, fishing, or hunting. Individuals with a history of uncomplicated Lyme disease who were at continued risk were also considered, because previous infection does not necessarily confer protective immunity. However, those with chronic arthritis were excluded because of the possibility that this condition was immune mediated. Vaccination was *not* recommended for those living outside endemic areas or for those younger than 15 years of age.

Procedures to avoid tick bites continue to be emphasized, including the following:
- Avoiding tick-infested areas, especially in the spring and summer
- Clearing leaves, litter, brush, and woodpiles from around the house
- Wearing light-colored clothing so that ticks can be easily seen and removed
- Wearing long-sleeved shirts and long pants tucked into socks
- Applying DEET (n,n-diethyl-m-toluamide) insect repellant to clothing and exposed skin (permethrin can also be applied to clothing)
- Daily tick checks and prompt removal

There were no data regarding concomitant administration of LYMErix (rOspA) with other vaccines. When necessary, it was recommended to administer other vaccines at a separate site.

I. Safety. LYMErix (rOspA) was generally well tolerated, with mild local and systemic reactions that resolved in 72 hours or less. Injection-site pain was seen in 24% of vaccinees, with fever, chills, influenza-like symptoms, and myalgia in fewer than 5%. Headache, fatigue, and rash were common systemic complaints. In prelicensure trials, there was no significant difference between vaccinees and placebo recipients in the incidence of arthritis, aggravated arthritis, arthropathy, or arthrosis, although vaccinees did experience early arthralgia and myalgia more often. In subjects with positive Lyme serology before vaccination, there was no significant increase in adverse reactions. Subjects with a self-reported history of Lyme disease reported increased musculoskeletal symptoms within 30 days of vaccination compared to vaccinees with no history of Lyme disease (20% vs. 13%, p <.001).

Allergic reactions to LYMErix (rOspA) were rarely reported. The vaccine was capable of causing false-positive ELISA tests for antibody to *B. burgdorferi*, necessitating the use of Western blots for serologic diagnosis in vaccinated individuals.

J. Contraindications. Anaphylactic reaction to a prior dose of vaccine or any of its components.

K. Precautions
- Moderate or severe acute illness
- Antibiotic-resistant chronic Lyme arthritis
- Pregnancy (even though the vaccine was inactivated, it was not known whether fetal harm could result from vaccination)

L. Comments. New vaccines may be developed using OspC, another outer surface lipoprotein of *B. burgdorferi*. OspC is immunogenic and is upregulated during the blood meal when the organism migrates to the tick salivary gland. In animal models, immunization with OspC protects against challenge with the homologous strain of *B. burgdorferi*, but its usefulness is limited by strain heterogeneity. For that reason, a multivalent vaccine is under development. Other candidate components for a Lyme vaccine include OspB, OspF, decorin-binding lipoproteins (DbpA and DbpB), a 41-kd flagellar protein, a 110-kd fusion protein containing a portion of a *B. burgdorferi* heat-shock protein, the surface proteins P35 and P37, and a live-attenuated *B. burgdorferi* strain lacking flagella.

KEY CONCEPTS: LYME DISEASE

- Most common vector-borne infection in the United States
- Endemic to southern New England, upper Midwest, and Pacific Northwest
- LYMErix (rOspA) vaccine licensed in 1998 but withdrawn by manufacturer in 2002
- Considered for certain high-risk individuals in endemic areas
- Mainstay of prevention is physical measures to avoid tick attachment

VII. Meningococcus

> *Neisseria meningitidis* is a gram-negative coccus that produces an antiphagocytic, serotype-specific polysaccharide capsule as well as endotoxin that enhances pathogenicity.

A. **Disease.** *Meningococcemia* is characterized by the sudden onset of fever, lethargy, myalgia, rash, and vomiting, followed by altered mental status, high fever or hypothermia, tachypnea, and hypotension. Initially, the rash may be macular or maculopapular, but there is rapid transition to petechiae, purpura, or both. *Purpura fulminans* is characterized by rapid progression to disseminated intravascular coagulation, hypotension, shock, and possibly death within hours despite antimicrobial therapy and supportive measures. Case-fatality rates are as high as 40%. Survivors may lose extensive areas of skin or extremities due to ischemia. Interestingly, some individuals experience transient meningococcal bacteremia that resolves spontaneously without treatment. Differences in Fc-receptor function or polymorphisms in the genes that control coagulation may explain these differences in outcomes.

   Meningitis presents with fever, vomiting, headache, and photophobia. It is distinguished from other forms of pyogenic meningitis by the association with petechial or purpuric rash in two-thirds of patients. Neurologic sequelae include deafness, cranial nerve palsies, hydrocephalus, and developmental delay. Meningococcus also causes pneumonia, myocarditis, pericarditis, arthritis, conjunctivitis, endophthalmitis, urethritis, and pharyngitis. Immune-mediated arthritis, cutaneous vasculitis, or pericarditis can occur late in the course of infection after antibiotic therapy is instituted. *Chronic meningococcemia* occurs rarely and is characterized by recurrent episodes of fever, chills, rash, arthralgias, and headache over a 6- to 8-week period.

B. **Epidemiology and transmission.** Transmission is by close, direct contact with respiratory droplets. Whereas asymptomatic carriage of *N. meningitidis* in the general population is common, fewer than 5% of individuals carry pathogenic strains. In contrast, nasopharyngeal colonization with invasive strains approaches 50% in closed settings where a case has occurred. The secondary attack rate in households is approximately 5%.

   The highest incidence of invasive disease occurs in infants younger than 1 year of age, a time when maternal antibodies have waned. A second peak occurs in adolescence and young adulthood when intimate contact between people increases. The disease occurs predominately in the late winter and early spring, and outbreaks may parallel increases in influenza activity. Risk factors include overcrowding, low socioeconomic status, African-American race, chronic underlying illness, active and passive smoking, and preceding respiratory tract infection. Individuals with congenital or acquired immunodeficiency, especially complement deficiency (classically terminal components), asplenia, antibody deficiency, and HIV infection, are also at increased risk. During outbreaks, alcohol use and bar and nightclub attendance are implicated as risk factors.

Epidemics caused by serogroup A most commonly occur in the "meningitis belt" of sub-Saharan Africa, central Asia, the Indian subcontinent, and Saudi Arabia. Such epidemics are rare in developed countries. In the United States, 95% of cases are sporadic, but in recent years localized outbreaks have increased. Most U.S. cases are due to serogroups B, C, and Y. Cases due to serogroup Y have increased significantly in recent years.

C. **Rationale for vaccine use.** Approximately 3,000 cases of invasive meningococcal disease occur each year in the United States, with an overall case-fatality rate of 10%. Half of these patients have meningitis, making meningococcus the most common cause of bacterial meningitis in persons 2 to 18 years of age. The currently available polysaccharide vaccine (see Vaccines below) is not an attractive option for universal use because of the overall low incidence of disease in the general population, vaccine ineffectiveness in children younger than 2 years of age, the limited duration of protection, the fact that the vaccine does not cover serogroup B, the possibility of inducing immunological tolerance to future doses, and the availability of chemoprophylaxis for contacts. The vaccine does find use, however, in high-risk individuals and under outbreak conditions.

Recent studies demonstrate modestly increased risk among college freshmen living in dormitories, on the order of two- to fivefold higher than the general population or other students. Greater than 80% of these cases are caused by serotypes contained in the current polysaccharide vaccine, leading to interest in vaccinating college students. It has been estimated that vaccination of all college freshmen would prevent 37 to 69 cases of invasive disease, two to four deaths, and would cost $22,000,000 to $48,000,000 per death prevented; programs selective for freshmen living in dormitories would prevent 15 to 30 cases and one to three deaths and would cost $600,000 to $1,800,000 per death prevented.

D. **Vaccines.** The only vaccine licensed in the United States, Menomune–A/C/Y/W-135 (Men-PS, Aventis Pasteur), is composed of purified capsular polysaccharide from four serotypes, A, C, Y, and W-135. Type B polysaccharide is not included because it is not immunogenic, probably the result of antigenic relatedness to human neuronal tissue. As with other polysaccharide vaccines, responses are T-cell independent, resulting in short-term antibody production, poor immunogenicity in infants, and no memory. One dose of Menomune–A/C/Y/W-135 (Men-PS) contains 50 μg of each group-specific polysaccharide isolated directly from the organism. The vaccine is supplied lyophilized in one-dose vials (one or five per package) with 0.78 mL vials of preservative-free sterile water diluent. A ten-dose vial is also available along with a 6.0 mL vial of diluent that contains thimerosal as preservative. The reconstituted vaccine contains isotonic sodium chloride and lactose as stabilizer. It is labeled for active immunization against invasive meningococcal disease caused by serogroups A, C, Y, and W-135 in individuals 2 years of age or older (it may also be used at 3 months of age or older for control of outbreaks due to serogroup A).

E. **Storage, handling, and administration**
   • Maintain temperature of lyophilized vaccine at 35° to 46°F (2° to 8°C)
   • Multidose vial can be maintained at 35° to 46°F (2° to 8°C) for up to 35 days after reconstitution
   • Freezing can cause the vaccine to lose potency
   • Shake well before use
   • Use one-dose vial within 30 minutes of reconstitution
   • Each dose is 0.5 mL given subcutaneously [see Chapter 3(III)]

F. **Schedule.** Primary vaccination consists of one dose. *One-time* revaccination may be considered for some individuals (see Official recommendations), but there are no indications for *routine revaccination* and no indications for more than two doses (except for the rare instance of immunization of young infants during ongoing serogroup A outbreaks).

G. **Efficacy.** Serogroup A polysaccharide induces an antibody response in infants as young as 3 months of age, but responses are not comparable to adults and efficacy declines within 3 years. Serogroup C polysaccharide is poorly immunogenic in children younger than 18 months of age. In children younger than 5 years of age, antibodies to serogroups A and C wane by 3 years after receipt of a single dose. In healthy adults, antibody concentrations decrease with time but may be detectable for as long as 10 years after vaccination.

Serogroup C vaccine was tested in 20,000 U.S. Army troops between 1969 and 1970. Efficacy was 90%, even in the face of ongoing epidemics. During an epidemic of serogroup C disease in Sao Paulo, Brazil, in 1974, efficacy among 67,000 infants and young children was 67% in those aged 24 to 36 months of age. During an epidemic of serogroup A disease in Finland in 1975 and 1976, nearly 50,000 young children were given a serogroup A vaccine in a controlled trial, with demonstrated 100% efficacy. Efficacy of 100% against serogroup A was also observed in a New Zealand study in 1985 and 1986, in which two doses were given to children 3 to 23 months of age and one dose was given to those over 2 years. In children 3 to 23 months of age who failed to return for their second dose, the efficacy was only 52% and fell to 16% after 1 year. In the infants, however, antibody declined by 50% after 2 years and by 90% after 3 years.

Administration of serogroup C vaccine to all U.S. troops since 1972 resulted in the elimination of serogroup C disease in this population. During a mass immunization campaign among individuals 6 months to 20 years of age in Quebec in 1992 and 1993, 1.6 million doses of vaccine were distributed; 24% of these contained serogroups A, C, Y, and W-135, and 76% contained groups A and C only. Protection against serogroup C was 65% in the first 2 years but 0% in the next 3 years. Efficacy was strongly related to age, ranging from 83% for ages 15 through 20 years to 41% for ages 2 through 9 years. In Rwanda, a serogroup A epidemic was halted with the use of a serogroup A and C vaccine, although the carrier rate remained unchanged.

H. Official recommendations. Immunization *is recommended* for the following individuals or situations:

- Individuals 2 years of age or older in high-risk groups, including functional or anatomic asplenia, terminal complement component deficiency, and properdin deficiency
- Travelers to, and U.S. citizens residing in, countries recognized to have hyperendemic or epidemic disease caused by vaccine-preventable serogroups
- All U.S. military recruits

Immunization *should be considered* for the following individuals or situations:

- Control of outbreaks, defined as three or more confirmed or probable cases during a period of 3 months or less (population-based attack rate of 10 or higher per 100,000)
  - Serogroups C, Y, W-135: Individuals 6 months of age or older receive one dose; a booster dose is given 1 year later for children younger than 2 years of age and 3 to 5 years later for older children and adults (if outbreak continues or is recurrent)
  - Serogroup A: Infants 3 to 23 months of age receive two doses given 2 to 3 months apart and a booster dose 6 to 12 months after the second dose (if outbreak continues or is recurrent); individuals 2 years of age or older receive one dose and a booster dose 3 to 5 years later (if outbreak continues or is recurrent)
- Routine laboratory or industrial exposure to *N. meningitidis*
- College students, particularly those who live in dormitories or residence halls, should be *informed* about meningococcal disease and the benefits of vaccina-

tion; those who want to reduce their risk should be vaccinated

Children who were first vaccinated at younger than 4 years of age should be considered for revaccination after 2 to 3 years if they remain at high risk. Revaccination for older children and adults 3 to 5 years after their first dose *should be considered* if indications still exist for protection. College students should *not* routinely be revaccinated.

Menomune–A/C/Y/W-135 (Men-PS) can be given at the same time as other vaccines at separate sites. The only exception is concurrent administration with whole-cell pertussis or whole-cell typhoid vaccines, a situation in which the combined amount of endotoxin could potentially cause reactions.

Because the risk of disease in close contacts is 300 times that in the general population, chemoprophylaxis with rifampin, ciprofloxacin, or ceftriaxone should be given.

I. **Safety.** Reactions are generally mild and consist primarily of pain and erythema at the injection site. Fever is unusual and severe reactions are uncommon. Systemic allergic reactions and anaphylaxis occur at less than one case per million doses. The vial stopper does contain dry natural latex rubber and could be a cause of allergic reactions. Neurologic reactions, including Guillain-Barré syndrome, are rarely reported.

J. **Contraindications.** Anaphylactic reaction to a prior dose of vaccine or any of its components.

K. **Precautions.** Moderate or severe acute illness.

L. **Comments.** As with *Haemophilus influenzae* type b (Hib) [see Chapter 5(II)] and pneumococcal vaccines [see Chapter 5(VI)], efforts to improve immunogenicity in infants and engender memory responses have focused on the development of meningococcal polysaccharide–protein conjugates. Clinical trials of several candidate vaccines have demonstrated superiority over polysaccharide vaccines in infants and children. In fact, serogroup C conjugate vaccine was added to the routine childhood schedule in the United Kingdom in 1999, resulting in decreases in disease rates. Ultimately, combination vaccines may include meningococcal conjugates along with Hib and pneumococcal conjugates.

Approaches to immunization against serogroup B have focused on outer membrane proteins of the organism. One such vaccine licensed in Cuba demonstrated efficacy of 57% to 83% in large field trials. However, strain coverage with this vaccine is narrow. Other candidate vaccines have used outer membrane vesicles or the porin A protein of the organism. Clinical trials with a porin A vaccine using the six most prevalent serosubtypes have provided promising results.

KEY CONCEPTS: MENINGOCOCCUS

- 3,000 annual cases of invasive disease in the United States
- Highest incidence at younger than 1 year of age
- Risk in college freshmen living in dormitories is two to five times that in the general population
- Licensed vaccine consists of polysaccharides from serogroups A, C, Y, and W-135
- Not immunogenic in children younger than 2 years of age
- Indicated for high-risk individuals
- College students living in dormitories should be aware of disease and be offered vaccine
- Consider revaccination one time only for certain individuals
- Chemoprophylaxis indicated for close contacts of cases

VIII. Rabies

Rabies virus is a bullet-shaped, enveloped, single-stranded RNA virus in the Rhabdoviridae family that infects animals and is neurotropic.

A. **Disease.** Rabies presents in four sequential stages: the incubation period, prodrome, acute neurologic phase, and coma/death. Two-thirds of patients present with a *furious form*, characterized by fluctuating consciousness, phobic spasms, dilated pupils, and hypersalivation. The other one-third present with a *paralytic form*, which is differentiated from Guillain-Barré syndrome by the presence of fever, intact sensation, and urinary incontinence. The incubation period is typically a few weeks to 2 months but may be many years. Animal bites to the head usually result in shorter incubation periods than bites to the extremities.

There are no symptoms during the *incubation phase*, but the *prodrome*, which lasts 2 to 10 days, is characterized by fever, headache, malaise, fatigue, anorexia, anxiety, agitation, irritability, insomnia, and depression, as well as pain, pruritus, or paresthesia at the site of the bite. The *neurologic phase*, which lasts 2 to 12 days, is characterized by hyperactivity, disorientation, hallucinations, bizarre behavior, aggressiveness, seizures, paralysis, hydrophobia, aerophobia, hyperventilation, and cholinergic manifestations, including hypersalivation, lacrimation, mydriasis, and hyperpyrexia. Paralysis occurs in 20% of cases. Agitation may be precipitated by tactile, auditory, and visual or other stimuli; hydrophobia, characterized by painful spasms of the pharynx and larynx, may be precipitated by eating or drinking or even the sight of liquids. At the end of the neurologic phase, the patient may become comatose. Death from respiratory or cardiac arrest usually occurs within 7 days, although with supportive care, coma may last for months. There are only a handful of reported survivors, most of whom have neurologic sequelae.

B. Epidemiology and transmission. Transmission from animals to humans occurs by exposure to saliva, usually through an animal bite, scratch, or contact with mucous membranes. Infection by aerosol has been reported in laboratories that handle the virus and in caves inhabited by bats. Rabies can also be transmitted by allografts. In nature, dogs, wolves, foxes, coyotes, jackals, raccoons, skunks, weasels, bats, and mongooses are most commonly infected. However, in some areas of the world, dogs and cats account for the majority of animal rabies and the greatest number of exposures to humans. In the United States, where domestic animal rabies is well-controlled through vaccination of animals, most human exposures come from contact with wild animals such as skunks, raccoons, and bats. In recent years, silver-haired bats have become a particular problem because the strains they carry may infect human skin more easily and their bites may be too small to see. Small rodents (e.g., squirrels, rats, and mice) and lagomorphs (e.g., rabbits and hares) rarely carry rabies.

Most exposures in the United States occur in males 5 to 14 years of age who live in rural areas, and, not surprisingly, these exposures occur in the summer months. As illustrated in Table 8.3, most animal exposures in the United States involve dogs, cats, and rodents, and many such visits result in postexposure prophylaxis even though it is not appropriate (see Official recommendations below). Between 1980 and 1996 in the United States, bat exposure was the most common source of human rabies cases. In one-half of cases there was no known bite, suggesting that the bite may have occurred during sleep.

C. Rationale for vaccine use. There are an estimated 50,000 rabies cases each year worldwide; only one or two of these occur in the United States. The long incubation period makes rabies uniquely suited to postexposure prophylaxis through both active and passive immunization; in this respect, it is similar to hepatitis B. Although human disease in the United States is rare, animal exposures are common; for example, an estimated 1 million dog bites occur each year. This fact, combined with near certainty of death if rabies occurs, leads to frequent consideration of vaccination and administration of rabies immune globulin [RIG; see Chapter 11(V)]. Preexposure vaccination for individuals likely to encounter the virus can simplify treatment if exposure occurs and protect persons with inapparent exposure or in whom postexposure therapy is delayed.

D. Vaccines. Two rabies vaccines, IMOVAX RABIES (HDCV; Aventis Pasteur) and RabAvert (PCEC; Chiron), are available in the United States (Table 8.4).

Table 8.3. Animal exposure visits to emergency departments, 1996 to 1998[a]

Animal	Exposures (% of total)	Postexposure prophylaxis			
		Given		Not given	
		Number (% of category)	Inappropriate (% of number given)	Number (% of category)	Inappropriate (% of number not given)
Dog or cat	1,903 (93.7)	116 (6.1)	46 (39.7)	1,787 (93.9)	118 (6.6)
Rodent[b]	85 (4.2)	1 (1.2)	1 (100)	84 (98.8)	0 (0)
Raccoon	10 (0.5)	8 (80)	5 (62.5)	2 (20)	1 (50)
Bat	5 (0.2)	4 (80)	0 (0)	1 (20)	0 (0)
Other[c]	27 (1.4)	7 (25.9)	2 (28.6)	20 (74.1)	0 (0)
All	2,030 (100)	136 (6.7)	54 (39.7)	1,894 (93.3)	119 (6.3)

[a] 2,030 visits for mammalian exposures related to bites, body fluids, handling, and proximity were studied in 11 urban emergency departments.
[b] Rat, mouse, squirrel, gerbil, or gopher.
[c] Monkey, livestock, bear, rabbit, skunk, fox, bobcat, coyote, shrew, or opossum.
Adapted from Moran GJ, Talan DA, Mower W, et al. Appropriateness of rabies postexposure prophylaxis treatment for animal exposures. *JAMA* 2000;284:1001–1007.

Table 8.4.   Rabies vaccines available in the United States

Manufac-turer	Trade name	Virus strain	Cell line	Packaging
Aventis Pasteur	IMOVAX RABIES (HDCV)	PM-1503-3M	Human diploid cell	Lyophilized 1-dose vial, syringe containing diluent, and needles
Chiron	RabAvert (PCEC)	Flury Low Egg Pas-sage (LEP)	Purified chick embryo cell	Lyophilized 1-dose vial, vial of dilu-ent, syringe, and needles

Each consists of a different virus strain grown on a cell line, purified, and inactivated with beta-propiolactone. They are supplied as lyophilized preparations that require reconstitution and are preservative free. A third vaccine, Rabies Vaccine Adsorbed (RAV; BioPort), which was grown on fetal rhesus lung diploid cells, adsorbed to alum, and supplied as a liquid, is no longer available. In addition, a vaccine that was available from Aventis Pasteur for intradermal administration (IMOVAX RABIES I.D.) was discontinued in 2001.

IMOVAX RABIES (HDCV) may contain albumin, neomycin sulfate, and phenol red, and RabAvert (PCEC) may contain processed bovine gelatin, potassium glutamate, ethylenediaminetetraacetic acid (EDTA), ovalbumin, bovine serum, neomycin, chlortetracycline, and amphotericin. Both products are labeled for pre- and postexposure prophylaxis.

Persons exposed to rabies abroad might receive rabies biologics that are not used in the United States, and additional therapy may be indicated when they return to the country. State or local health departments should be consulted in this situation.

E. **Storage, handling, and administration**
- Maintain temperature at 35° to 46°F (2° to 8°C)
- Freezing can cause the vaccine to lose potency
- Protect from light
- Mix gently to reconstitute
- Use immediately after reconstitution
- Each dose is 1.0 mL given intramuscularly [see Chapter 3(III)]

F. **Schedule.** *Preexposure prophylaxis* consists of three doses of either vaccine given on days 0, 7, and 21 or 28. Certain individuals may require booster doses at regular intervals (see below). The management of animal bites or scratches should always include immediate and thorough washing with soap and water and application of a virucidal agent such as povidone-iodine solution. Tetanus prophylaxis should be given as indicated [see Chapter 7(I)], and antibiotic prophylaxis may be appropriate. Decisions regarding suturing of large wounds depend on cosmetic issues and the risk of infection.

The schedule for *postexposure prophylaxis*, including the use of RIG, depends on whether the individual has been previously immunized:

- *Previously immunized* (complete pre- or postexposure immunization regimen using a cell culture vaccine or immunization with another vaccine *and* documented rabies antibody titers after vaccination)
    - Two doses of either vaccine given on days 0 and 3
    - RIG is not necessary
- *Not previously immunized*
    - Five doses of either vaccine given on days 0, 3, 7, 14, and 28
    - One dose of RIG, 20 IU/kg (0.133 mL/kg), given at the same time as the first dose of vaccine (simultaneous administration is preferred, but if this does not occur, RIG can be given up to 7 days after vaccination is instituted); as much of the dose as possible should be thoroughly infiltrated into the wound and the surrounding tissues, and any remaining RIG should be given intramuscularly at a separate site from the vaccine

G. Efficacy. Essentially all persons given pre- or postexposure prophylaxis using the regimens above achieve seroprotective concentrations of antibody. In multiple studies, postexposure prophylaxis provided 100% protection against the development of disease. In rare situations in which postexposure prophylaxis has failed, deviations from standard protocols have occurred, including insufficient cleansing of wounds, late start of prophylaxis, passive immunization not given at all or not infiltrated into all wounds, and vaccine given in the gluteal region.

H. Official recommendations. Guidelines for administration of vaccine preexposure are given in Table 8.5.

The decision on whether to initiate postexposure prophylaxis must take into account the local and regional epidemiology of animal rabies. Each potential exposure must be individually evaluated, and local or state public health officials should be consulted. An unprovoked attack is more likely than a provoked attack to indicate a risk of rabies exposure (a bite incurred while attempting to feed or handle an apparently healthy animal should generally be regarded as provoked).

Exposures can be classified as follows:

- *Bite*: Penetration of the skin by teeth
    - Bites to the face and hands carry the highest risk, but the site of the bite should not influence the decision to begin treatment

Table 8.5.   Preexposure rabies prophylaxis

Intensity of exposure	Nature of exposure	Examples	Recommendation
Continuous	Continuous May go unrecognized Bite, nonbite, aerosol	Rabies research laboratory workers[a] Rabies biologics production workers	3-dose vaccine series Serology every 6 mo Booster dose if titer[b] falls below 1:5
Frequent	Episodic May go unrecognized Bite, nonbite, aerosol	Rabies diagnostic laboratory workers[a] Spelunkers Veterinarians and staff Animal control and wildlife workers in enzootic areas	3-dose vaccine series Serology every 2 yr Booster dose if titer[b] falls below 1:5
Infrequent	Episodic Bite or nonbite	Veterinarians and animal control and wildlife workers in nonenzootic areas Veterinary students Travelers to enzootic areas where access to immediate medical care is limited	3-dose vaccine series
Rare	Episodic Bite or nonbite	General U.S. population (including epizootic areas)	No preexposure vaccination

[a]Judgment of relative risk and monitoring of immunization status is the responsibility of the laboratory supervisor [see CDC and NIH. *Biosafety in microbiological and biomedical laboratories*, 3rd ed. Washington, DC: HHS Publication No. (CDC) 93-8395, U.S. Department of Health and Human Services, 1993].

[b]Rapid fluorescent focus inhibition assay.

Adapted from CDC. Human rabies prevention—United States, 1999: Recommendations of the Advisory Committee on Immunization Practices (ACIP). *MMWR* 1999;48(RR-1):1–21.

- Transmission can occur from minor or unrecognized bat bites. Postexposure prophylaxis should be considered for persons who were in the same room as a bat and who might be unaware that a bite or direct contact had occurred, especially if the bat is not available for testing. Examples would include a sleeping person who awakens to find a bat in the room or finding a bat in a room with an unattended child, mentally disabled person, or intoxicated person.
- *Nonbite*: This includes scratches, abrasions, open wounds, or mucous membranes contaminated with saliva or other potentially infectious material (e.g., brain tissue). Casual contact such as petting does not constitute an exposure.
- *Airborne*: Rare cases have occurred from airborne exposure in laboratories and in caves infested with millions of bats
- *Human-to-human transmission*: The only documented cases occurred in patients who received corneal transplants from persons who died of rabies that was undiagnosed at the time of death

Table 8.6 provides guidelines for instituting postexposure prophylaxis.

The vaccine from a single manufacturer should be used for the complete series whenever possible. If vaccines from more than one manufacturer are administered, an adequate antibody response should be confirmed by serologic testing. RabAvert (PCEC) was shown to elicit satisfactory responses when given as a booster in 41 persons who received a primary series with HDCV. Rabies vaccine is safe to administer simultaneously with other vaccines at separate sites.

I. **Safety.** Cell culture–derived vaccines are less reactogenic than previously available vaccines. Reactions are experienced more commonly in adults than in children. Pain, induration, swelling, or erythema occur at the injection site in 30% to 74% of vaccinees. Systemic reactions, reported in 5% to 40% of vaccinees, are usually mild or moderate and include headache, nausea, abdominal pain, malaise, myalgia, and dizziness. Fever is less common, and rarely, patients experience sweating, chills, circulatory reactions, monoarthritis, and transient paresthesias.

Approximately 6% of persons given booster doses of HDCV after preexposure immunization develop an immune complex–like illness 2 to 21 days later characterized by generalized urticaria and, in some cases, arthralgia, arthritis, angioedema, nausea, vomiting, fever, and malaise. This may be due to sensitization to human albumin that has been altered by beta-propiolactone. Persons who experience this type of reaction should receive no further doses of HDCV unless no

Table 8.6.   Postexposure prophylaxis guidelines

Animal	Animal evaluation and disposition	Recommendations
Dog, cat, ferret	Healthy and available for 10-d observation period[a]	Institute prophylaxis at first sign of rabies in animal
	Rabid or suspected rabid	Institute prophylaxis immediately
	Unknown (not available for observation)	Consult public health officials
Skunk, raccoon, fox, coyote, bobcat, wild animal crossbred to domestic dog or cat, other carnivores, bat	Regard as rabid[b]	Institute prophylaxis immediately
Livestock, rodents (including woodchuck and beaver), lagomorphs (rabbit and hare), other mammals	Consider individually	Consult public health officials
		Bites of squirrels, hamsters, guinea pigs, gerbils, chipmunks, rats, mice, other small rodents, rabbits, and hares almost never require prophylaxis

[a]The animal should be quarantined and observed for 10 days. This usually takes place under the supervision of the local health department, which specifies approved facilities (private or government) and monitors the animal's behavior. If signs of rabies develop (e.g., aggressive or combative behavior, irritability, hyperreaction to stimuli, paralysis), the animal should be euthanized and the brain sent for detection of rabies virus antigens by immunofluorescence (usually done at the state lab).
[b]Unless proved negative by euthanizing animal and testing brain for rabies antigens by immunofluorescence (usually done at the state lab); quarantine for observation is *not* recommended.
Adapted from CDC. Human rabies prevention—United States, 1999: Recommendations of the Advisory Committee on Immunization Practices (ACIP). *MMWR* 1999;48(RR-1):1–21. Postexposure prophylaxis regimens are given in the text.

other vaccine is available, they are exposed or are likely to be exposed to rabies, and they have unsatisfactory antibody titers. Once initiated, rabies prophylaxis should not be interrupted or discontinued because of local or mild systemic adverse reactions. Usually such reactions can be successfully managed with antiinflammatory and antipyretic agents.

Serious systemic anaphylactic reactions have been reported.

J. Contraindications
- Given the nearly uniform lethality of rabies, there are no absolute contraindications to postexposure prophylaxis
- For preexposure prophylaxis, anaphylactic reaction to a prior dose of vaccine or any of its components might be considered a contraindication; egg-allergic individuals should receive IMOVAX RABIES (HDCV) rather than RabAvert (PCEC)

K. Precautions
- Anaphylactic reaction to a prior dose of vaccine or any of its components
- Immunosuppressive agents should not be administered during postexposure therapy unless essential for the treatment of other conditions; in such situations, the patient's serum should be tested for rabies antibody

L. Comments. Oral vaccination of wildlife has proven effective in preventing spread of enzootic disease. Traditional approaches have used bait seeded with live-attenuated rabies strains. A more recent approach uses a vaccinia recombinant expressing the G protein of rabies virus.

KEY CONCEPTS: RABIES

- Disease in humans nearly always fatal
- Transmitted by exposure to animal saliva
- Most exposures in United States come from wild animals such as skunks, raccoons, and bats
- Long incubation period allows for postexposure vaccination
- RIG given postexposure along with vaccine unless individual is previously immunized
- Postexposure prophylaxis nearly 100% effective if done properly
- Certain high-risk individuals qualify for preexposure immunization
- Two cell culture–derived, inactivated vaccines available in United States

---

IX. Typhoid

Salmonella typhi is a motile, nonlactose-fermenting, gram-negative bacillus that produces a cholera-like toxin and easily invades the bloodstream from the intestinal lumen.

A. Disease. *Typhoid fever* refers to enteric fever caused by *S. typhi*, although other *Salmonella* species can cause a less severe form of enteric fever. The incubation period is 5 to 21 days depending on inoculum size and health of the host. The onset is insidious, with fever and abdominal pain accompanied by malaise and anorexia. Fever climbs to higher peaks each day, reaching 104°F (40°C) by the end of the first week; interestingly, adults display relative bradycardia for the level of fever. Early on, as many as 50% of patients have constipation and 30% diarrhea. Diarrhea is more common in infants and is typically small in volume and pea soup–like, containing red blood cells and leukocytes but not gross blood. During the first week of illness, children complain of headache and often are irritable, drowsy, or delirious. Adults may display psychosis or delirium, and arthralgia and back pain are common. Patients may appear toxic, have meningismus, a coated tongue with musty odor, and a tender doughy abdomen with slight guarding. During the second week of illness, a rash may appear on the abdomen or chest consisting of crops of 10 to 15 salmon-colored, blanching, slightly raised lesions measuring 2 to 4 mm, referred to as *rose spots*. The spleen may be palpable and tender and respiratory symptoms may develop. Untreated, the illness lasts 4 to 6 weeks.

Complications generally occur during the third or fourth week and include intestinal hemorrhage or perforation, which occurs in approximately 3% of patients. The patient's mental status may progress to coma. Additional complications include hepatitis, cholecystitis, arthritis, osteomyelitis, parotitis, endocarditis, myocarditis, pericarditis, pneumonia, meningitis, pyelonephritis, pancreatitis, and orchitis. Laboratory abnormalities include anemia, leukopenia or leukocytosis, thrombocytopenia, and elevated hepatic and muscle enzymes. Relapses occur in 5% to 20% of cases even after appropriate therapy, although they are usually milder than the initial illness. Infants are more likely than adults to develop massive hepatosplenomegaly and thrombocytopenia, and they have a higher mortality rate. However, young children may have *S. typhi* bacteremia with mild disease manifestations. Typhoid fever during pregnancy increases the risk of premature labor and spontaneous abortion. As many as 4% of patients who recover from typhoid fever become chronic carriers of *S. typhi* and are potential sources of infection for others.

S. typhi can also cause nontyphoidal gastroenteritis, bacteremia, and extraintestinal focal infection.

B. Epidemiology and transmission. There are an estimated 12 to 33 million cases of typhoid fever each year in the world, with the highest incidence in Asia (especially the Indian subcontinent), Central and South America, and Africa. In endemic areas, the annual incidence is as high as 500 to 900 cases per 100,000 people, and the peak is in school-aged children. In developed countries the incidence is only 0.2 to 3.7 cases per 100,000. Four hundred cases are reported in the United States each year, with the highest risk among international travelers.

Humans are the only reservoir of *S. typhi* and transmission is by the fecal-oral route; the infectious dose is approximately 10^7 organisms. Patients with cholecystitis or gallstones are especially vulnerable to chronic carriage and may excrete as much as 10^9 organisms per gram of stool. Direct person-to-person transmission is unusual; rather, disease spreads through feces-contaminated food or water. For this reason, countries with inadequate sanitation systems, overcrowded living conditions, and limited potable water have the highest rates of disease. Laboratory workers have acquired infection through accidents, and health care workers have acquired infection from patients because of poor handwashing. Occasionally, transplacental transmission occurs from a bacteremic mother to the fetus, and infants may be infected at the time of birth through exposure to bacteria shed in the mother's stool.

C. **Rationale for vaccine use.** Worldwide, approximately 500,000 people die each year from typhoid fever. In endemic areas, aside from the human costs, the direct medical and indirect societal costs are high. Interest in vaccination is highest in areas where antibiotic treatment is not readily available and where antibiotic-resistant strains have increased in prevalence. Outbreaks of multidrug-resistant *S. typhi* infection have occurred in the Indian subcontinent, Southeast Asia, and Africa and have been associated with high rates of complications and death. Vaccination might be beneficial for persons at high risk of disease, including children, international travelers, and military personnel. Persons who travel from low-risk to high-risk areas are particularly susceptible because they have not developed immunity through repeated exposure to low doses of *S. typhi* over time.

D. **Vaccines.** Two vaccines are available in the United States:

• Vivotif Berna (Ty21a; Berna Products, a subsidiary of Swiss Serum and Vaccine Institute Berne) is a live-attenuated strain of *S. typhi* (called Ty21a) that is orally administered. The bacterium was engineered by treatment of strain Ty2 with a mutagenic agent and selection for attenuation. It is formulated as lyophilized bacteria in gelatin capsules that are enteric coated and supplied as four capsules in a foil blister pack (a powdered formulation that is reconstituted in water and given in a three-dose regimen is available in other countries). Each capsule contains 2 to 6×10^9 CFUs of viable bacteria, as well as nonviable bacteria, sucrose, ascorbic acid, amino acids, lactose, and magnesium stearate. The preparation may also contain yeast proteins, casein, dextrose, and galactose. The vaccine is labeled for prevention of disease due to *S. typhi* in individuals 6 years of age or older.

• Typhim Vi (Ty-ViPS; Aventis Pasteur), consists of purified Vi capsular polysaccharide (25 μg per 0.5 mL dose) from the *S. typhi* Ty2 strain in isotonic phosphate buffered saline for parenteral administration.

The vaccine contains residual polydimethylsiloxane or fatty-acid ester-based antifoaming agents as well as phenol 0.25% as preservative. It is supplied in a prefilled syringe or, on special contract basis only, in 20- and 50-dose vials. The vaccine is labeled for prevention of disease due to *S. typhi* in individuals 2 years of age or older.

Typhoid Vaccine USP (Wyeth), a phenol-inactivated whole-cell vaccine for parenteral administration, is no longer produced.

E. **Storage, handling, and administration**
  • Both vaccines should be maintained at 35° to 46°F (2° to 8°C)
  • Freezing either vaccine can cause loss of potency
  • Each dose of Vivotif Berna (Ty21a) is one capsule given orally (the capsule should be swallowed whole 1 hour before a meal along with a cold or lukewarm drink [98.6°F (37°C) or cooler]; each dose of Typhim Vi (Ty-ViPS) is 0.5 mL given intramuscularly [see Chapter 3(III)]

F. **Schedule.** Table 8.7 gives the dosing schedule for each vaccine.

G. **Efficacy.** The efficacy of oral Ty21a was evaluated in a series of field trials. In Egypt, 16,486 children aged 6 to 7 years were given three doses of a liquid formulation on alternate days; 15,902 children were given placebo. Efficacy was 96% during a 3-year surveillance period. In Chile, school-aged children were given one (n = 27,618) or two doses separated by 1 week (n = 27,620) of an enteric-coated capsule; 27,305 children received a placebo. Efficacy during 24 months of surveillance was 29% and 59% for the one- and two-dose schedules, respectively, and protection was nearly absent 3 to 4 years out. Another Chilean study involving 109,594 school-aged children who received three doses of the capsules on alternate days or every 21 days showed efficacy of 67% and 49%, respectively. Efficacy with the shorter interval schedule was sustained 7 years out. Finally, another study in Chile involving nearly 190,000 school-aged children showed optimal efficacy using a four-dose, alternate-day regimen of the capsules. The results of this study were used to justify a four-dose schedule in the United States.

In a clinical trial of parenteral Ty-ViPS conducted in Nepal, subjects received the vaccine (n = 3,457) or a 23-valent pneumococcal vaccine as placebo (n = 3,450). Most subjects were 5 to 44 years of age. Efficacy against blood culture–confirmed typhoid fever was 74% during the 20-month follow-up period. In a second trial conducted in South Africa, the lyophilized formulation was evaluated in school children 5 to 15 years of age who received vaccine (n = 5,692) or a meningococcal polysaccharide vaccine as placebo (n = 5,692). Efficacy was 55% against blood culture–confirmed typhoid fever during a 3-year follow-up period.

Table 8.7. Administration of typhoid vaccines

Vaccine	Series	Age (yr)	Dose	Route	Number of doses	Interval between doses (d)	Boosting interval (yr)
Vivotif Berna (Ty21a)	Primary	≥6	1 capsule	PO	4	2[b]	—
	Booster[a]	≥6	1 capsule	PO	4	2	Every 5
Typhim Vi (Ty-ViPS)	Primary	≥2	0.5 mL	IM	1	—	—
	Booster[a]	≥2	0.5 mL	IM	1	—	Every 2

[a]Boosting is indicated for persons with repeated or continued exposure.
[b]If all four doses are not completed within 10 days (some sources say 21 days), the entire series should be repeated.
Adapted from CDC. Typhoid immunization. Recommendations of the Advisory Committee on Immunization Practices (ACIP). *MMWR* 1994;43(RR-14):1–7.

H. Official recommendations. Routine immunization is *not* recommended in the United States. This includes sewage sanitation workers, persons attending rural summer camps, and people living in areas where natural disasters such as floods have occurred. Further, there is no evidence that typhoid vaccine is useful in controlling common-source outbreaks.

Vaccination *is*, however, recommended for the following groups:

- Travelers to endemic areas (especially developing countries in Latin America, Asia, and Africa) who will have prolonged exposure to potentially contaminated food and water (individuals should be cautioned that vaccination is not a substitute for careful avoidance of contaminated food and drink); typhoid vaccine is not *required* for international travel, but it is *recommended*
- Persons with intimate exposure (e.g., household contact) to a documented carrier of *S. typhi* (the vaccine cannot be used to *treat* chronic carriers)
- Microbiology laboratory workers who are in frequent contact with *S. typhi*
- Persons living in endemic areas outside the United States

There are no data on interchangeability of typhoid vaccines. However, if a booster series is necessary in a person who previously received Typhoid Vaccine USP, it is reasonable to give four doses of Vivotif Berna (Ty21a) or one dose of Typhim Vi (Ty-ViPS). There is no evidence that concomitant administration of either vaccine with other live oral or live or inactivated parenteral vaccines impairs immune responses, although all permutations have not been tested.

I. Safety. Vivotif Berna (Ty21a) is the least reactogenic typhoid vaccine. Symptoms reported during clinical studies included abdominal pain (6%), nausea (6%), headache (5%), fever (3%), diarrhea (3%), vomiting (2%), and rash (1%), but only nausea occurred more frequently than in placebo groups. In field trials involving more than 500,000 school children, this vaccine did not cause serious adverse reactions. Postmarketing surveillance in the early 1990s, during which time 60 million doses were distributed, revealed only a handful of serious adverse events.

Typhim Vi (Ty-ViPS) causes injection-site induration and erythema in approximately 7% of vaccinees, but these resolve within 48 hours. Fever occurs in 1% and headache in as many as 3% of vaccinees. Reactions after booster doses are similar to those observed after primary immunization. Postmarketing surveillance in countries where over 14 million doses were distributed demonstrated some systemic reactions but very few serious adverse events.

Allergic reactions to either vaccine have rarely been reported, although it should be mentioned that the needle cover of Typhim Vi (Ty-ViPS) supplied in a syringe contains dry natural latex rubber.

J. Contraindications
- Both vaccines: anaphylactic reaction to a prior dose of vaccine or any of its components
- Vivotif Berna (Ty21a): immunodeficiency or immuno-suppressed state

K. Precautions
- Moderate or severe acute illness
- Pregnancy
- Vivotif Berna (Ty21a): acute gastrointestinal illness, concomitant antibiotics, mefloquine, or proguanil therapy (may inactivate the vaccine strain)

L. Comments. As with Hib and pneumococcal polysaccharides, the Vi capsular polysaccharide has been conjugated to protein carriers to improve immunogenicity. Carriers have included tetanus and diphtheria toxoid, cholera toxin, *E. coli* LT B subunit, and recombinant exotoxin A of *Pseudomonas aeruginosa* (Vi-rEPA). Most of these vaccines have been well tolerated and more immunogenic than the unconjugated Ty-ViPS. In a field trial involving 11,091 children aged 2 to 5 years in Vietnam, efficacy of Vi-rEPA for blood culture–proved typhoid fever was 92%. Another candidate vaccine consists of acetic anhydride–treated pectin, a polysaccharide of plants that resembles Vi, conjugated to a protein carrier. Recombinant strains of *S. typhi* are being developed with the goal of retaining the safety of Ty21a but improving immunogenicity. For example, derivatives of Ty21a have been developed in which genes encoding specific enzymes are inactivated, resulting in limited growth potential in mammalian tissues. Some of these have shown promise in animal and limited human studies.

KEY CONCEPTS: TYPHOID

- Prolonged systemic illness characterized by bacteremia, high fever, rash, splenomegaly, and pancytopenia
- Acquired from contaminated food or water
- Travelers to endemic areas at greatest risk
- One live oral and one inactivated parenteral vaccine licensed in the United States
- Vaccines indicated for some travelers and those in close contact with carriers or laboratory isolates

---

X. Yellow fever

Yellow fever virus (YFV) is a mosquito-borne flavivirus with a single-stranded RNA genome surrounded by a protein nucleo-capsid and a lipid envelope.

A. Disease. YFV infection may be asymptomatic or present as a viral syndrome of varying severity. The classic triad of jaundice, hemorrhage, and albuminuria occurs in 10% to 20% of patients, and the associated case-fatality rate is 20% to 50%. The onset of symptoms is abrupt with fever, headache, backache, malaise, myalgia, nausea, vomiting, prostration, photophobia, restlessness, irritability, and dizziness; epistaxis and bleeding from the gums may also occur. Children may experience febrile seizures. Examination reveals congestion of the skin, conjunctivae, and mucous membranes. Leukopenia, albuminuria, and elevated serum transaminase levels may be present. After approximately 3 days of illness, most patients experience a remission of symptoms, but this may be brief and relapse may occur with prostration, marked venous congestion, extreme bradycardia, severe nausea and vomiting, epigastric pain, jaundice, marked albuminuria and anuria, hematemesis, and melena. The hemorrhagic manifestations may be so severe as to cause hypotension, shock, acidosis, myocardial dysfunction, arrhythmias, and death, usually after 7 to 10 days. Central nervous system signs include delirium, agitation, seizures, stupor, and coma, and complications include pneumonia, parotitis, skin infections, and renal abscesses.

B. **Epidemiology and transmission.** Transmission of the *jungle* form of yellow fever involves tree hole–breeding mosquitoes and nonhuman primates in the rain forests of Africa and South America. Humans exposed to the mosquitoes in this environment, such as forestry workers, soldiers, and settlers, may acquire the infection and travel to urban areas where *Aedes aegypti* mosquitoes become infected after feeding on them. These mosquitoes may in turn infect other persons leading to epidemics of *urban* yellow fever (jungle and urban yellow fever are clinically indistinguishable). *A. aegypti* breeds in and around houses and thereby sustains interhuman transmission. YFV is also transmitted vertically from infected female mosquitoes to their offspring. This mode of transmission is important to survival of the virus during prolonged dry periods.

Yellow fever occurs throughout sub-Saharan Africa and tropical South America. Epidemics are common in Africa, where approximately 20,000 cases and 5,000 deaths were reported between 1986 and 1991. After accounting for underreporting, the true annual number of cases is thought to be approximately 200,000. Epidemics of yellow fever have reappeared in the urban centers of West Africa and may reappear in tropical urban centers in the Americas in the near future. In South America, approximately 100 cases are reported in forested areas annually. Mass vaccination campaigns and mosquito control programs have been instituted in South America in an attempt to prevent urban outbreaks. Yellow fever has never been reported in Asia.

C. **Rationale for vaccine use.** As with Japanese encephalitis, control of mosquitoes and mosquito exposures can reduce the risk of infection, but this is not always possible. Between 1986 and 1995, a total of 23,543 cases and 6,421 deaths were reported to the WHO, a dramatic increase compared with previous intervals. The case-fatality rate during this same period was 24% in Africa and 64% in South America. Perhaps the most important rationale for vaccination is the risk of reemergence of yellow fever carried by *A. aegypti* mosquitoes in urban areas of the Americas. This is a possibility because *A. aegypti* infests many areas that are currently free of yellow fever, including coastal regions of South America, the Caribbean, North America, the Middle East, coastal eastern Africa, the Indian subcontinent, Asia, and Australia. Travelers to and expatriates living in tropical Africa and America are candidates for vaccination as well.

D. **Vaccines.** The only licensed vaccine in the United States is YF-VAX, manufactured by Aventis Pasteur. This live-attenuated vaccine is made from serially passaged 17D strain of YFV that is cultured in chicken embryos. It is supplied lyophilized with sorbitol and gelatin stabilizers in one-dose (five per package), five-dose, and 20-dose vials along with sodium chloride diluent. The vaccine is provided only to WHO-designated Yellow Fever Vaccination Centers authorized to issue a valid Certificate of Yellow Fever Vaccination. Each 0.5-mL dose contains not less than 5.04 $\log_{10}$ plaque forming units of virus. The vaccine is labeled for active immunization of persons 9 months of age or older.

E. **Storage, handling, and administration**
   - Maintain lyophilized vaccine at 32° to 41°F (0° to 5°C) [the ACIP states that 35° to 46°F (2° to 8°C) is acceptable]
   - Reconstitute only with the supplied diluent, and swirl gently before use
   - Use reconstituted vaccine within 1 hour [multidose vials should be stored at 35° to 46°F (2° to 8°C) until they are discarded after 1 hour]
   - Each dose is 0.5 mL given subcutaneously [see Chapter 3(III)]

F. **Schedule.** One dose is given at least 10 days before anticipated exposure. International Health Regulations require revaccination at intervals of 10 years.

G. **Efficacy.** Although the efficacy of yellow fever vaccine has never been tested in a controlled clinical trial, numerous observations suggest efficacy. For example, neutralizing antibodies can be demonstrated in 95% or more of vaccinees. Infection of laboratory workers disappeared after vaccination became routine, and in Brazil and other South American countries, yellow fever only occurs in people who have not been immunized. Immunization during outbreaks results in rapid disappearance of cases, and high rates of coverage in endemic areas are followed by marked reduction in disease incidence. During an epidemic in Nigeria in 1986, vaccine efficacy was estimated at 85%, although there were important methodologic problems with the assessment. Immunity persists for at least 30 to 35 years and probably for life.

H. Official recommendations. Vaccination is *recommended* for the following individuals:

- Those traveling to or living in areas of South America and Africa where yellow fever is officially reported
- Those traveling outside of urban areas in countries that do not officially report the disease but that lie in yellow fever–endemic zones
- Travelers to countries that require a certificate of vaccination against yellow fever
- Laboratory personnel who might be exposed to virulent YFV or to concentrated preparations of the 17D vaccine strain

Up-to-date information regarding the risk of yellow fever in various regions and vaccination requirements for travelers can be found at the following sources:

- WHO International Travel and Health home page: www.who.int/ith (accessed 12/03/02)
- National Center for Infectious Diseases (CDC) Travelers' Health home page: www.cdc.gov/travel (accessed 12/03/02)

Vaccinees should receive an International Certificate of Vaccination that has been completed, signed, and validated with the center's stamp. Certain countries in Africa require evidence of vaccination from all entering travelers. Some countries waive the requirements for travelers who are staying less than 2 weeks from areas where no evidence of substantial risk exists. Certain countries require persons, even if only in transit, to have a valid certificate if they have been in countries either known or thought to have yellow fever, or even where yellow fever does not exist but where *A. aegypti* mosquitoes are found. The best advice is to check the above-referenced Web sites before travel.

The risk of vaccine-associated encephalitis is highest for young infants. For this reason, the ACIP recommends *against* immunizing infants younger than 6 months of age under any circumstances. The AAP and the manufacturer place the cutoff age at younger than 4 months. In any event, physicians considering immunization of infants between 4 and 9 months of age should contact the Division of Vector-Borne Diseases (970-221-6400) or the Division of Global Migration and Quarantine (404-498-1600) at the CDC. Vaccination of pregnant women may also be considered if travel cannot be postponed and if exposure is very likely, even though this is a live virus vaccine (only 1 of 81 infants born to mothers vaccinated during pregnancy had evidence of fetal infection and none had congenital anomalies). However, seroconversion may be markedly reduced, and the CDC should be contacted in these cases as well.

In general, immunosuppressed individuals should not be vaccinated, including those with congenital or acquired immunodeficiency, symptomatic HIV infection, leukemia, lymphoma, generalized malignancy or those taking corti-costeroids, alkylating medications, antimetabolites, or radiation. Patients with HIV infection who are not immu-nosuppressed can be offered the vaccine. Low-dose (20 mg or less prednisone or equivalent) or short-term (less than 2 weeks) corticosteroid therapy or intraarticular, bursal, or tendon injections with corticosteroids should not be immunosuppressive. In any circumstance, if international travel requirements are the *only* reason for vaccination of an individual at high risk for vaccine complications, con-sideration should be given to writing a waiver letter.

There is no evidence that concomitant administration of YF-VAX with vaccines other than cholera impairs immune responses, although all permutations have not been tested. In general, if other live vaccines are not given simultaneously, 4 weeks or more should elapse between them, unless time constraints do not allow. Neither IG nor chloroquine therapy adversely affect antibody responses.

I. **Safety.** Reactions to yellow fever vaccine are typically mild; 2% to 5% of vaccinees experience mild headaches, myalgia, low-grade fever, or other minor symptoms for 5 to 10 days. Approximately 1% of vaccinees need to cur-tail regular activities. Two important serious adverse events should be mentioned:

- *Vaccine-associated neurotropic disease*: Formerly known as *postvaccination encephalitis*, this has been reported in 23 persons since the 17D vaccine strain was introduced in 1945. Sixteen of these cases were in children 9 months of age or younger, and only three cases occurred in the United States. The overall risk is estimated at less than 1 per 8,000,000 vaccinees.

- *Vaccine-associated viscerotropic disease*: Formerly known as *febrile multiple organ system failure*, it typi-cally begins 2 to 5 days after vaccination and is charac-terized by fever, hypotension, respiratory failure, elevated hepatocellular enzymes, hyperbilirubinemia, lymphocytopenia, thrombocytopenia, and renal failure. There is probably a spectrum of disease ranging from moderate illness with focal organ dysfunction (as many as 4% of vaccinees experience mild, transient elevation of hepatic transaminases) to severe disease with multi-ple organ failure and death. Seven cases were reported to have occurred between 1996 and 2001, and six of these patients died; three additional suspected cases have recently been identified. Although the vaccine virus can be isolated from the blood in most cases, the syndrome appears to be due to an aberrant host response rather than reversion of the vaccine virus to virulence. The risk is estimated at 1 per 400,000 vac-cinees and is greatest after the first vaccination. Persons 65 years of age or older might be at increased risk.

Immediate hypersensitivity reactions are estimated to occur in 1 per 130,000 to 250,000 vaccinees and principally involve persons with a history of egg allergy. Less severe or localized manifestations of allergy to egg or to feathers are not contraindications to vaccination, and persons who are able to eat eggs or egg products can receive the vaccine. Egg-sensitive individuals can be tested with the vaccine with scratch, prick, puncture, or intradermal tests, and those with positive tests can be desensitized if vaccination is imperative (the procedure is described in the package insert). Allergic reactions can also occur to the dry natural latex rubber contained in the stopper and to gelatin that is used as a stabilizer.

J. Contraindications
- Anaphylactic reaction to a prior dose of vaccine or any of its components, including egg protein
- Age younger than 6 months
- Immune deficiency or immunosuppression

K. Precautions
- Moderate or severe acute illness
- Pregnancy
- Nursing mother

L. Comments. A method for developing new yellow fever vaccines based on the 17D strain uses a full-length cDNA clone of the virus that is modified by site-directed mutagenesis. The goal is to further attenuate the marginally acceptable neurovirulence profile of the current vaccine. In addition, the new vaccine would be genetically homogeneous as opposed to the heterogeneous mixtures currently used. In addition, investigators have produced a new seed stock in primary chick embryo cell culture rather than the embryonated eggs currently in use; cell culture–derived vaccine should reduce manufacturing costs. Finally, combination vaccines with measles, Hep-A, typhoid, and other travel vaccines are being investigated.

KEY CONCEPTS: YELLOW FEVER

- Classic triad of jaundice, hemorrhage, and albuminuria
- Case-fatality rate 20% to 50%
- Endemic in sub-Saharan Africa and tropical South America
- Potential to spread to Central and North America
- One live-attenuated vaccine available in the United States
- Indicated for certain travelers who are 9 months of age or older
- Infants younger than 6 months of age should not be immunized
- Individuals with egg hypersensitivity or immune deficiency should not be vaccinated
- Vaccine-associated neurotropic and viscerotropic disease can occur

Bioterrorism

Bioterrorism refers to the deliberate release of a harmful biologic agent to intimidate civilians and their government (*biowarfare* more accurately refers to the use of such agents by warring parties to inflict mass casualties). The discovery in the 1990s that the Soviet Union and Iraq had well-established bioweapons development programs and the occurrence of high-profile domestic and international terrorist events—the Murrah Building in Oklahoma City, the U.S. embassies in Nairobi and Dar es Salaam, the U.S.S. Cole, the World Trade Center, and the Pentagon—combined to raise alarm that governments, individuals, or small groups could mount effective biologic attacks. This fear was realized in the U.S. anthrax attacks of September and October 2001.

The following characteristics make certain biologic agents ideal for use as agents of terrorism:
- Ability to cause high morbidity and mortality
- Potential for person-to-person transmission
- Low infective dose
- Infectious by aerosol dissemination
- Effective vaccine unavailable or in short supply
- Absence of natural immunity
- Availability of the agent and feasibility of large-scale production
- Environmental stability
- Ability to induce panic based on historical fears of infectious diseases

Agents that are presently considered potential threats are listed in Table 9.1. Many of these agents have already been weaponized in several countries.

Vaccines (and passive immunoprophylactics) have a role in biodefense, but that role is complicated by a number of factors. First, until recently, there have been few incentives to develop vaccines against many of these agents. In addition, the development process is long and arduous, and great forethought is needed to anticipate which vaccines might become necessary. Second, there are few—if any—historical precedents for the use of vaccines in biodefense. Third, for many diseases, efficacy cannot be tested directly, and surrogate markers of protection are not known. Fourth, biologic agents can be genetically manipulated to change their antigenicity and render conventional vaccines less useful. Finally, the balance between the benefits of preexposure vaccination and safety concerns must be addressed, and the infrastructure for large-scale postexposure vaccination must be developed. However, for some agents with short incubation periods, postexposure vaccination would not be useful.

Table 9.1.   Potential agents of bioterrorism

Category	Characteristics	Disease/condition	Agent
A	Highest priority Easily disseminated or transmitted from person to person High mortality Potential for major public health impact Potential for public panic and social disruption Require special action for preparedness	Anthrax Botulism Plague Smallpox Tularemia Viral hemorrhagic fevers	*Bacillus anthracis* *Clostridium botulinum* toxin *Yersinia pestis* Variola virus *Francisella tularensis* Filoviruses, arenaviruses, bunyaviruses, flaviviruses
B	Second highest priority Moderately easy to disseminate Moderate morbidity and low mortality Require specific enhancements of diagnostic capacity and surveillance	Brucellosis Epsilon toxin Food safety threats Glanders Melioidosis Psittacosis Q fever Ricin toxin Enterotoxin B Typhus fever Viral encephalitis Water safety threats	*Brucella* species *Clostridium perfringens* *Salmonella* species, *E. coli* O157:H7, *Shigella* *Burkholderia mallei* *Burkholderia pseudomallei* *Chlamydophila psittaci* *Coxiella burnetii* Derived from castor beans (*Ricinus communis*) *Staphylococcus aureus* *Rickettsia prowazekii* Alphaviruses (e.g., Venezuelan equine encephalitis, eastern equine encephalitis, western equine encephalitis) *Vibrio cholerae, Cryptosporidium parvum*
C	Could be used in the future Available Easy to produce and disseminate High mortality and morbidity Major public health impact	Emerging infectious diseases	Nipah virus, hantavirus

Adapted from CDC. Biological diseases/agents. Public health emergency preparedness and response Web site. www.bt.cdc.gov/Agent/agentlist.asp (accessed 02/03/03).

I. Smallpox

Variola virus is a very large, brick-shaped, enveloped DNA virus in the genus *Orthopoxvirus* that replicates in the cytoplasm and is closely related to vaccinia, cowpox, and monkeypox.

A. **Disease.** Initial infection takes place at mucosal surfaces of the oropharynx or respiratory tract. Three to 4 days later, viremia leads to visceral dissemination, but the patient remains asymptomatic. Secondary viremia leads to a marked prodromal illness that begins 12 to 14 days after infection and is characterized by high fever, malaise, headache, backache, prostration, chills, vomiting, delirium, and/or abdominal pain. Rash begins 1 to 4 days into the prodrome and is coincident with a decrease in fever; maculopapular lesions initially appear in the mouth and on the face and forearms, spreading to the trunk and legs. The lesions evolve slowly into vesicles and pustules, which are characteristically deep seated, round, firm and discrete, although some may coalesce. Eventually, the lesions develop an umbilicated appearance with a central dimple. Fever usually continues until scabs form, approximately 2 weeks into the illness. Scars are evident after the scabs separate.

Variola major refers to the typical smallpox syndrome that is easily recognized and accounts for the vast majority of cases; mortality rates approximate 30%. *Hemorrhagic smallpox* follows a shorter incubation period and is characterized by an extreme prodrome, the development of dusky erythema, and the eruption of petechiae and hemorrhage into skin and mucous membranes. Pregnant women are disproportionately affected, and the syndrome is uniformly fatal. In *malignant (flat) smallpox*, the onset is equally abrupt, but the initial confluent lesions never evolve into pustules, remaining flat, soft, and velvety instead. Mortality in this form approaches 100% as well. *Modified smallpox* occurs in previously vaccinated individuals, and although the prodrome may be severe, the lesions are fewer in number, more superficial, and evolve more rapidly; death is rare. *Variola minor (alastrim)*, caused by a less pathogenic strain of the virus, is differentiated by fewer constitutional symptoms, sparse rash, and excellent prognosis. *Variola sine eruptione* is asymptomatic or self-limited with fever and flulike symptoms; it occurs in previously vaccinated individuals or infants with maternal antibodies.

Direct organ damage by viral infection is unusual, as is secondary bacterial infection. Instead, death results from toxemia associated with circulating immune complexes and viral antigens. Encephalitis can occur and is similar to the acute perivascular demyelination syndromes that may complicate measles and varicella infection, or vaccinia vaccination. There is no clinical experience with antiviral treatment, but cidofovir may have some activity and would be made available under an investigational protocol in the case of an outbreak.

Failure to diagnose the first wave of cases during a smallpox attack would have grave consequences. For this reason, and given the fact that most practicing physicians today have never seen a case, attention has focused on recognizing the clinical signs and symptoms and differentiating smallpox from other conditions that bear similarities, most notably chickenpox. Table 9.2 provides clues to accurate and timely diagnosis. Suspected cases should immediately be reported to state or local health departments; if laboratory diagnostics are indicated, the Centers for Disease Control and Prevention (CDC) Rash Illness Evaluation Team (770-488-7100) should be consulted.

B. Epidemiology and transmission. Some historians believe that smallpox has killed more people than all other infectious diseases combined. Although global eradication through vaccination was conceived by Jenner as early as 1801, this did not become a real possibility until 1967, when the following factors converged: (a) the World Health Assembly resolved to eradicate the disease and increased funding was secured; (b) large amounts of stable, lyophilized vaccine became available, and reference testing centers were established; (c) a highly effective bifurcated needle was adopted for administration; and (d) the strategy of ring vaccination was developed, wherein active cases were hunted and their contacts vaccinated. As a result, the last natural case of smallpox on the planet occurred in 1977 (the last case in the United States was in 1949), and on December 9, 1979, the World Health Organization (WHO) certified that smallpox had been eradicated. Because there is no reservoir of the virus in nature and there is no human carrier state, the elimination of natural disease was felt to be definitive. In the United States, routine vaccination of civilians ceased in 1972, health care workers in 1976, and military personnel in 1990. Until recently, the only individuals in the United States who continued to be vaccinated were laboratory and animal care workers with potential exposures to orthopox viruses and health care personnel conducting clinical trials with recombinant vaccinia virus vaccines. No country has routinely immunized civilians since 1984.

It was remarked that smallpox eradication was one of the few things that needed to be done only once in the history of the world. This sentiment preceded serious concerns about the use of smallpox as a weapon. Worldwide stocks of virus were intentionally consolidated at the CDC and the Institute of Virus Preparations in Moscow (now the Russian State Centre for Research on

Table 9.2. Diagnosis of smallpox

Clinical finding	Smallpox[a]	Chickenpox[b]
Major criteria		
Prodrome	Fever ≥101°F (38.3°C) beginning 1–4 d before rash and at least one of the following: prostration, headache, backache, chills, vomiting, severe abdominal pain	None or mild
Lesion morphology	Deep-seated, firm, round, well-circumscribed vesicles or pustules, may be umbilicated or confluent	Superficial vesicles ("dewdrops on a rose petal")
Lesion development	Same stage of development on any one part of the body	Appear in crops and are at different stages of development on any one part of the body
Minor criteria		
Distribution	Centrifugal (concentrated on face and distal extremities)	Centripetal (concentrated on trunk)
Initial lesions	Oral mucosa, palate, face, forearms	Face or trunk
General appearance	Toxic or moribund	Well appearing
Evolution	Slow (from macules to papues to pustules over days)	Rapid (from macules to papules to vesicles to pustules to crusts in <24 h)
Palms and soles	Involved	Spared

Note: If the patient has all three major criteria, the risk of smallpox is high, and authorities should be notified immediately. If the patient has a febrile prodrome and one other major criterion or four or more minor criteria, the risk is moderate and urgent evaluation is indicated. Pictures of smallpox lesions are available at www.bt.cdc.gov/agent/smallpox/smallpox-images (accessed 01/31/03).
[a]Other conditions to be considered in the differential diagnosis include disseminated herpes zoster or herpes simplex, impetigo, drug eruptions, erythema multiforme, Stevens-Johnson syndrome, enteroviral infection, scabies, secondary syphilis, bullous pemphigoid, and molluscum contagiosum. Cowpox and monkeypox resemble smallpox but are usually acquired directly from animals. The differential diagnosis of hemorrhagic smallpox includes meningococcemia, hemorrhagic varicella, Rocky Mountain spotted fever, ehrlichiosis, and gram-negative sepsis.
[b]Other clues to the diagnosis of chickenpox include absence of a personal history of varicella or varicella vaccination and exposure to chickenpox or shingles. Most cases occur in children, because most adults are immune. The lesions are typically intensely pruritic, and scarring is unusual.
Adapted from CDC. Poster: evaluating patients for smallpox. Public health emergency preparedness and response Web site. www.bt.cdc.gov/agent/smallpox/diagnosis/evalposter.asp (accessed 01/31/03).

Virology and Biotechnology, Koltsovo, Novosibirsk Region, Russian Federation), but it is possible that unauthorized vials were retained at other sites. More importantly, it is now known that the Soviet Union had an active program to weaponize the virus, and with the political unrest and economic hardship that ensued in Russia during the 1990s, it is feared that the virus and the technology to deliver it may have fallen into the hands of terrorists or rogue nations. Even a single case anywhere in the world would strongly hint at this possibility and would be considered an international medical and strategic emergency. In the 1990s, several dates that were set for destruction of the last known stocks of variola virus came and went. On December 20, 2001, the WHO issued a report recommending a stay of execution to facilitate continued research into molecular diagnosis, genetic analysis, serological assays, animal models, antiviral drugs, and vaccines.

Certain features of smallpox make it attractive as a weapon, including the small infectious dose, high mortality rate, absence of natural and vaccine-induced immunity at the population level, lack of established therapy, historical fear and panic related to the disease, and person-to-person spread, which would amplify the effect of a primary release by generating secondary and tertiary cases. Epidemic disease in developed countries today would have the potential for great devastation because of the high point prevalence of atopic skin disease and relative immunoincompetency resulting from immunosuppressive therapy, chronic conditions, human immunodeficiency virus (HIV) infection, and aging.

Fortunately, variola virus is labile, and less than 90% remains viable for 24 hours after aerosol release in the presence of ultraviolet light. Transmission occurs through direct contact with body fluids and inhalation of aerosols and droplet nuclei expelled from the oropharynx of infected persons. Close contact is usually required, and secondary attack rates vary from approximately 40% to 90% under these circumstances. Distant airborne transmission is rare, but fomites such as bedding or clothing can transmit the virus. Transmission does not occur through insects or animals. Patients are most infectious 7 to 10 days after the rash develops; as this occurs after a debilitating prodromal illness, patients are likely to be easily recognized and bedridden at the time they are most contagious. Transmission from subclinical cases is of little epidemiologic importance.

C. **Rationale for vaccine use.** Possible scenarios for a smallpox attack are given in Table 9.3. *Universal preevent vaccination* would constitute an absolute deterrent to a smallpox attack and could be conducted under controlled conditions. However, this approach is not favored because the overall risk of an attack is considered to be low, the population at risk cannot be determined, and the risks of vaccination are substantial. The strategy of *surveillance*

Table 9.3. Smallpox attack scenarios

Attack	Description
Laboratory release	Laboratory facility in a metropolitan area is sabotaged. Previously vaccinated laboratory workers develop modified illness but transmit to unvaccinated household contacts, who then infect others.
Human vectors	Distantly vaccinated terrorists infect themselves and develop moderate illness. They use the mass transit system of a metropolitan area and infect close contacts.
Building attack	Aerosolized virus is released into the ventilation system of a federal office building, exposing hundreds of workers and visitors.
Airport attack	Terrorists use portable nebulizers to distribute virus aerosols at domestic terminals of multiple airports during busy travel times. In the low-impact scenario, 5,000 people are infected; in the high-impact scenario, 100,000 people are infected.

Adapted from Bozzette SA, Boer R, Bhatnagar V, et al. A model for a smallpox-vaccination policy. *N Engl J Med* 2003;348:416–425.

and containment, or *ring vaccination*, involves the isolation of suspected and confirmed cases and the identification, vaccination, and monitoring of their contacts. Vaccination can be extended to household contacts of contacts as well and to other people with indirect exposure, and the strategy can be supplemented by local quarantine and travel restrictions. The strategy, which was highly successful during the global eradication campaign, is workable because postexposure vaccination is effective if given soon after exposure. Ring vaccination, however, might not work as well in a largely nonimmune, highly mobile population experiencing a multisite intentional aerosol release of virus. In addition, the logistical complexity of this approach is daunting, especially in the face of the potential for public panic. The CDC has developed large-scale vaccination clinic guidelines (available at www.bt.cdc.gov/agent/smallpox/response-plan/files/annex-3.pdf, accessed 02/22/03) to assist state and local health departments in expanding vaccination rings if this becomes necessary. *Universal postevent vaccination* would be logistically difficult and would provide little additional benefit to ring vaccination, although the CDC National Pharmaceutical Stockpile has protocols for simultaneous delivery of vaccine to every state and territory within 24 hours of an event. The current U.S. vaccination plan (see Official recommendations) combines limited preevent vaccination with ring vaccination.

  D. Vaccines. The origin of vaccinia virus is not clear, but it appears to be a hybrid between cowpox and smallpox that is not found in nature. On October 25, 2002, the U.S. Food and Drug Administration (FDA) relicensed Dryvax (smallpox vaccine, dried, calf-lymph type), a product manufactured by Wyeth until 1982 but in storage at the CDC since then, for active immunization against smallpox. Relicensure was intended to facilitate administration of the vaccine outside of investigational protocols, although the vaccine remains available to civilians only through the CDC. Dryvax is a lyophilized preparation of the New York City calf-lymph strain of vaccinia, derived from the New York City Board of Health strain. It was harvested from lymph contained in skin lesions that develop after scarification of calves. Reconstituted vaccine contains approximately 10^8 pock-forming units of vaccinia virus, not more than 200 contaminating bacterial organisms per mL, as well as small amounts of polymyxin B, streptomycin, chlortetracycline, and neomycin. The diluent contains 50% glycerin and 0.25% phenol. It is supplied as a package containing one vial of lyophilized vaccine, one 0.25 mL diluent syringe, one vented needle, and 100 individually wrapped bifurcated needles (enough to vaccinate 100 individuals).

As of December 16, 2002, two lots of Dryvax with a total of 2.7 million doses were approved for release under licensure, with more lots expected soon thereafter. Studies indicate that Dryvax may be diluted up to 1:5 without diminution in the response rate in naïve subjects; with this information, it is estimated that at least 75 million doses would be available in the event of an emergency. In 2002, approximately 85 million doses of a similar vaccine (in liquid formulation) that had been in cold storage since the 1950s were discovered by Aventis Pasteur and donated to the CDC. This product is now being studied under an investigational new drug protocol and appears to be potent. Finally, in 2001 the federal government contracted with Acambis (Cambridge, UK and Cambridge, MA) to manufacture at least 209 million doses of two new cell-culture derived vaccines, ACAM1000, grown in MRC-5 (human embryonic lung) cells and ACAM2000, grown in Vero (African green monkey kidney) cells. The safety and immunogenicity of these vaccines is currently under study, and soon there should be enough effective doses of vaccine to immunize the entire U.S. population, if that were necessary.

E. Storage, handling, and administration
- Unreconstituted Dryvax is stored at 35° to 46°F (2° to 8°C)
- Do not freeze
- Reconstituted vaccine may be used for 15 days if stored at 35° to 46°F (2° to 8°C)
- *Reconstitution*
  - Provider *should wear gloves* and use aseptic technique

- Lift up tab of aluminum seal on vaccine vial but do not break off or tear down
- Wipe off vial stopper with alcohol and allow to dry
- Place vaccine vial upright on a hard, flat surface. Insert sterile 21-gauge or smaller needle (not supplied) into rubber stopper to release the vacuum. Discard needle in a biohazard sharps waste container
- Warm diluent-cartridge in palm of hand for 1 minute
- Aseptically remove vented needle (provided) from package
- Remove rubber cover from end of diluent syringe
- Attach vented needle to hub of diluent syringe
- Remove protective cover from vented needle and expel air from the diluent syringe
- Insert needle through rubber stopper into vaccine vial up to the first hub
- Depress the plunger to ensure that entire volume of diluent is delivered into vial
- Withdraw diluent syringe and vented needle and discard in a biohazard sharps waste container
- Allow vaccine vial to stand undisturbed for 3 to 5 minutes. Afterward, if necessary, swirl vial gently to achieve complete reconstitution
- *Administration*
  - Provider s*hould wear gloves*
  - Preparation of the skin with alcohol is not required (this may inactivate the virus). Soap and water should be used if the site is grossly contaminated. If alcohol is used, the skin must be allowed to dry thoroughly before inoculation
  - Tear off aluminum seal completely, and remove rubber stopper (maintain under sterile conditions for later recapping)
  - Dip bifurcated needle into reconstituted vaccine and withdraw. A sufficient amount of liquid (approximately 0.0025 mL) is retained between the prongs by capillary action
  - The wrist of the vaccinator's hand should lay on the vaccinee's arm below the deltoid region. The vaccinator's other hand should be used to pull the skin taut from underneath
  - Using firm strokes from the wrist, make rhythmic perpendicular insertions into the skin of the deltoid region within a 5-mm area. A trace of blood should be visible after 15 to 30 seconds. For primary vaccination, two to three punctures are recommended. For revaccination, 15 punctures are recommended. If no blood is visible after vaccination, an additional three insertions should be made *without* reinserting the needle into the vial
  - Discard bifurcated needle immediately in a biohazard sharps waste container

- Absorb excess vaccine and blood with sterile gauze and discard in a biohazard container
- Cover site with gauze and a semipermeable dressing such as OpSite (Smith & Nephew) or Tegoderm (3M) (some of these products are supplied with attached gauze pads). Vaccinees should make sure that a layer of clothing covers the dressing and should exercise meticulous hand hygiene after touching the site. Gauze alone can be used by vaccinees who are not in the health care setting, but semipermeable dressings should not be used alone because they macerate the skin
- *Postvaccination care*
  - Change dressing every 3 to 5 days or more often if exudates accumulate (dressings can be discarded in the household trash if sealed in a plastic bag)
  - Avoid rubbing and scratching
  - Wash hands with soap and water or alcohol-based hand rub after contact with vaccination site or contaminated bandages
  - Keep site dry. Showering or bathing can continue. If the site is uncovered, it should not be touched. The site should be blotted dry with gauze which should then be discarded in a sealed plastic bag in the household trash. If a towel is used for drying the site, it should not be used on the rest of the body
  - Wash clothing or other material that comes into contact with the site

The subject should return for examination in 7 days. A red, pruritic papule should form 3 to 4 days after vaccination. By 5 to 6 days, there should be a vesicle with surrounding erythema, which by 7 to 11 days becomes umbilicated then pustular. This begins to dry, and the redness subsides. Two to 3 weeks out, the lesion becomes crusted, and by 21 days the scab detaches, leaving a pink scar that ultimately becomes flesh colored. Revaccination is considered successful if a pustule or area of induration surrounding a central scab or ulcer is present 1 week out. *Any reaction other than those described above is considered equivocal and means that vaccination was unsuccessful and should be repeated.* Images of normal and adverse reactions to smallpox vaccination can be viewed at www.bt.cdc.gov/training/smallpoxvaccine/reactions (accessed 02/01/03).

F. **Schedule.** Until 1972, smallpox vaccine was given in the United States one time to children at 1 year of age. For those who receive preevent vaccination today, a single dose is recommended with a booster every 10 years. Revaccination every 3 years should be considered for workers with occupational exposure to orthopox viruses. The vaccine completely prevents or significantly modifies smallpox if given 3 to 4 days postexposure; vaccination 4 to 7 days postexposure probably modifies the severity of the disease.

G. Efficacy. Protection against smallpox persists for at least 5 years after primary vaccination. Many U.S. citizens who were born before 1972 were probably vaccinated one time in childhood. It is known that antibody levels steadily decline 5 to 10 years after vaccination, and although detectable cellular responses may persist, it must be assumed that these individuals are not immune to smallpox. Revaccination even one time results in boosted antibody levels that may persist for 30 years. Recent studies of Dryvax show vigorous antibody, cytotoxic T-cell, and interferon-γ responses in subjects who develop vesicles at the inoculation site.

H. Official recommendations. On June 22, 2001, the Advisory Committee on Immunization Practices (ACIP) released a statement recommending against preevent vaccination of any group other than laboratory and health care workers involved in orthopox research. Certain groups were targeted for vaccination postevent, including people with primary exposure, close contacts of cases (face-to-face, household, or less than 2 m distance), medical personnel with potential patient contact, clinical laboratory personnel, and ancillary personnel with potential exposure to infectious waste. The earliest vaccinations would be targeted to persons who had been vaccinated in the past. These recommendations were reviewed in the wake of the anthrax attacks of September and October 2001, and supplemental recommendations to vaccinate the following groups were made on June 20, 2002:

- *Smallpox Response Teams*: At least one team would be maintained in each state and territory, to include a medical team leader, public health advisor, epidemiologists, disease investigators, diagnostic laboratory scientists, nurses, medical personnel, vaccinators, and security and law enforcement officials.
- *Smallpox Health Care Teams*: These are individuals who would care for initial cases at predesignated isolation and care facilities.

Under these recommendations, 10,000 to 20,000 individuals would have received preevent vaccination.

Recognizing the fact that smallpox patients would likely present to any hospital, the ACIP issued revised recommendations on October 21, 2002. Supplemental recommendations from ACIP and the Healthcare Infection Control Practices Advisory Committee (HICPAC) were issued on February 10, 2003 in draft form and were published on April 4, 2003. It is recommended that all acute care hospitals establish Smallpox Health Care Teams. These teams would provide hospital-based in-room evaluation and management for the first 7 to 10 days, using 8- to 12-hour shifts. Team members would include the following persons:

- Emergency department and intensive care unit staff, including physicians and nurses

- General medical and primary care staff
- House staff
- Medical subspecialists, including infectious disease specialists, experienced physicians, dermatologists, ophthalmologists, pathologists, surgeons, and anesthesiologists
- Infection control professionals
- Respiratory therapists
- Radiology technicians
- Security personnel
- Housekeeping staff

The following comments were also offered:

- Clinical laboratory workers were not included because clinical specimens were expected to contain low levels of virus, and standard precautions were considered to be protective
- Although emergency medical technicians (EMTs) would not be routinely vaccinated, hospital-based EMTs could be vaccinated if included on the teams
- Designated vaccinated staff would examine all vaccinated health care workers each day, assess vaccine take, and change the dressings if indicated
- Persons handling the vaccine would also be vaccinated
- Routine leave for vaccinated health care workers was not recommended. However, leave would be indicated for systemic illness, extensive lesions that cannot be covered, or inability to adhere to infection-control precautions.
- Institutions would take a phased-in, staggered approach to vaccination, beginning with groups of previously vaccinated individuals
- Rigorous screening for contraindications (see Contraindications below) was recommended, but routine pregnancy and HIV testing was not

The federal plan announced on December 13, 2002 called for compulsory vaccination of as many as 500,000 military personnel and voluntary vaccination of as many as 500,000 health and safety workers constituting local Smallpox Response Teams. Although vaccination of the general public was not immediately recommended, plans were formulated to offer unlicensed vaccine on a voluntary basis to adults without medical contraindications sometime in 2003 and with a licensed vaccine in 2004. Under all circumstances, preevent vaccination of civilians is voluntary.

- Monkeypox

  In May and June of 2003, an outbreak of monkeypox occurred in the United States related to contact with prairie dogs. The virus was introduced by Gambian giant rats imported from Ghana and housed with other animals. The disease is characterized by a prodrome of fever, headache, backache, and fatigue, followed by a rash that is similar to that associated with smallpox. Lymphadenopathy is prominent. historical case-fatality rates are 1% to 10%, and person-to-person transmission is considered a possibility.

Smallpox vaccine is highly effective against monkeypox. Therefore, on June 11, 2003, the CDC offered the following guidelines:

- Close (household or three or more hours of direct exposure within 6 ft) or intimate (exposure to body fluids or lesions) contact with animal or human cases in the past 4 days *should be* vaccinated. Vaccination *should be considered* for persons with close or intimate contact or exposure to contaminated surfaces in the past 2 weeks
- Persons investigating suspect human and animal cases should have been vaccinated in the past 1 to 3 years. If this is not feasible, individuals should be vaccinated immediately before deployment
- Health care workers caring for suspect or proven cases *should be* vaccinated. Ideally, previously vaccinated individuals should care for patients. If this is not feasible, workers can be vaccinated immediately before beginning clinical duties
- Vaccination is *not* recommended for unexposed veterinary workers

Smallpox vaccine may be administered simultaneously with all inactivated vaccines and live vaccines except for varicella, in which case 4 weeks or more should separate the two inoculations. Tuberculin skin tests should be deferred at least 1 month after smallpox vaccination to minimize the risk of false negatives. In December 2002, the FDA issued a guidance recommending deferral of blood donation by vaccinees (as well as individuals with contact vaccinia) until the scab spontaneously separates or 21 days postvaccination, whichever is later.

I. **Safety.** Smallpox vaccine is the most reactogenic and dangerous of all licensed vaccines. By definition, successfully vaccinated individuals develop a pustule at the inoculation site that lasts several weeks. Many experience additional local reactions and associated systemic complaints, listed in Table 9.4. In approximately one-third of patients, these symptoms may lead to missed work, school, or recreational activities, or trouble sleeping. Potential complications of vaccination and their frequency, based on historical data, are given in Table 9.5. Suggestions for management of these complications are included in the CDC's Guidance for Clinicians (see Chapter 15), including recommendations for use of vaccinia immune globulin (available only from CDC). CDC also has established a Smallpox Vaccine Adverse Events Monitoring and Response System. Clinicians can contact the CDC at 877-554-4625 at any time for assistance in evaluating adverse events. Adverse events should also be reported to the Vaccine Adverse Event Reporting System (VAERS) [see Chapter 13(III)].

In March 2003, the CDC reported ten cases of myopericarditis occurring shortly after vaccination among

Table 9.4.   Adverse reactions after primary smallpox vaccination

Reactogenicity	Days after vaccination[a]	Proportion of vaccinees (%)[b]
Local[c]		
Erythema >4 cm	10–12	50%
Moderate or severe pain	7–9	34%
Erythema >10 cm	10–12	10%
Local satellite lesions	13 and 14	6%
(Maximum induration, mean)	10–12	(5 cm)
Systemic		
Missed school, work, recreational activities, or had trouble sleeping	Anytime	36%
Any regional adenopathy	7–9	31%
Moderate or severe muscle aches	7–9	21%
Moderate or severe fatigue	7–9	20%
Moderate or severe headache	0–6	15%
Rash outside of vaccination site	Anytime	14%
Temperature ≥100°F (37.7°C)	7–9	9%
Moderate or severe chills	10–12	7%
Temperature ≥101°F (38.3°C)	7–9	3%

Note: Pictures of reactions to smallpox vaccination are available at
www.bt.cdc.gov/agent/smallpox/vaccineimages.asp (accessed 01/31/03).
[a]Time period with greatest proportion of reactions.
[b]Includes subjects who received both diluted and undiluted vaccine. Subjects receiving undiluted vaccine had larger areas of induration and a higher incidence of regional adenopathy; those receiving diluted vaccine had a higher incidence of local satellite lesions.
[c]Differentiating robust takes from bacterial cellulitis may be difficult. Clues: the latter include occurrence within 5 days or after 30 days of vaccination, progression in the absence of treatment, and the development of fluctuant regional lymph nodes.
Adapted from Frey SE, Couch RB, Tacket CO, et al. Clinical responses to undiluted and diluted smallpox vaccine. *N Engl J Med* 2002;346:1265–1274.

240,000 primary military vaccinees, as well as two similar cases in civilians. The incidence of myopericarditis was substantially higher than in unvaccinated historical cohorts, raising suspicion of a causal relationship. Five civilians with cardiac ischemic events were also reported. As a precaution, new guidelines were issued to exclude at-risk individuals from preevent vaccine programs (see the section Contraindications).

Section 304 of the Homeland Security Act of 2002 (P.L. 107-296) provides liability protection (with certain caveats) in the case of injury to a vaccinee or a contact for smallpox vaccine manufacturers, health care institutions and public health agencies that administer vaccine programs, and licensed providers and other individuals authorized to administer vaccine (see www.bt.cdc.gov/agent/smallpox/vaccination/section-304-qa.asp, accessed

Table 9.5. Complications of primary smallpox vaccination

Complication	Description	Risk factors or predisposition	Number per 1,000,000 vaccinated
Inadvertent inoculation	Transfer of virus from inoculation site to a second location, usually the face, eyelid, nose, mouth, lips, genitalia, or anus Includes keratitis and conjunctivitis	Manipulation of vaccination site Age <4 yr Disrupted skin integrity	529
Generalized vaccinia	Disseminated maculopapular or vesicular rash Occurs 6–9 d after vaccination Lesions follow same course as primary site Patients are nontoxic and condition is self-limited	Hematogenous spread More serious in immunocompromised persons	242
Erythema multiforme	Erythematous target lesions with central pallor Occurs 10 d after vaccination May be pruritic Can progress to Stevens–Johnson syndrome	Hypersensitivity reaction	165
Eczema vaccinatum	High fever Extensive vesiculopustular eruption Associated lymphadenopathy At risk for secondary bacterial infection High mortality rate	History of eczema or atopic dermatitis irrespective of disease activity or severity	39
Postvaccinal encephalitis or encephalomyelitis	Abrupt onset of fever, headache, malaise, lethargy, vomiting, meningeal signs, seizures, paralysis, drowsiness, altered mental status or coma Mortality 25% Neurologic sequelae 25%	Age <1 yr	12

(continued)

Table 9.5. *Continued*

Complication	Description	Risk factors or predisposition	Number per 1,000,000 vaccinated
Vaccinia necrosum (progressive vaccinia)	Painless progressive necrosis at vaccination site Possible spread to distant sites Poor prognosis	Immunodeficiency	2
Other	Severe local reactions Bacterial superinfection at the vaccination site Fetal vaccinia		266
Contact vaccinia	Predominantly eczema vaccinatum and inadvertent inoculation Occurs 5 to 19 d after exposure Aerosol transmission, if it occurs, is not epidemiologically important	Household contact with other predisposing condition	20–60
Any			1,254
Death			1–2

Note: Pictures of complications of smallpox vaccination are available at www.bt.cdc.gov/agent/smallpox/vaccineimages.asp (accessed 01/31/03).
Adapted from CDC. Smallpox vaccination and adverse reactions: guidance for clinicians. *MMWR* 2003;52(RR-4):1–28.

02/01/03). A declaration on January 24, 2003 by the Secretary of the Department of Health and Human Services stating the advisability of instituting voluntary smallpox countermeasures brought these protections into effect. Questions remain, however, about administrative leave for health care workers experiencing bad reactions or unable to adhere to infection-control measures, coverage by disability insurance, and workers' compensation.

J. Contraindications
- *In the event of known exposure to smallpox, there are no contraindications to vaccination*
- *For preevent vaccination, the following contraindications apply to both potential vaccinees and their household contacts (this includes sexual contacts):*
  - *Eczema, atopic dermatitis, other acute, chronic, or exfoliative skin conditions*: burns, impetigo, chickenpox, contact dermatitis, shingles, herpes, severe acne, psoriasis, Darier's disease (keratosis follicularis), even if currently inactive. Two screening questions have been suggested by the CDC:
    - Have you or a member of your household ever been diagnosed with eczema or atopic dermatitis?
    - Have you or a family member ever had an itchy, red, scaly rash that lasts for more than 2 weeks and often comes and goes?
  - *Immunodeficiency or immunosuppression*: solid organ or bone marrow transplantation; generalized malignancy; leukemia; lymphoma; agammaglobulinemia; autoimmune disease; treatment with radiation, antimetabolites, alkylating agents, corticosteroids [in similar doses to those outlined in Chapter 5(VII)], chemotherapy agents, or organ transplant medications; and HIV infection (routine testing is not recommended but should be done in individuals with risk factors, those who are unsure of their status, and those who are concerned that they could have HIV infection)
  - *Pregnancy*: currently pregnant or plans to become pregnant in the next 4 weeks (vaccinated women should be counseled not to become pregnant for 4 weeks)
    - For reassurance, women can perform a urine pregnancy test on the first morning void on the day of vaccination
    - Routine pregnancy testing is not recommended
    - Inadvertent vaccination during pregnancy is not ordinarily a reason to terminate the pregnancy, although the mother should be aware of the extremely rare occurrence of fetal vaccinia
  - *For preevent vaccination, the following contraindications apply only to vaccinees:*
    - Allergic reaction to smallpox vaccine or any vaccine components
    - Moderate or severe acute illness

- Infants younger than 12 months of age (ACIP advises against vaccination of individuals younger than 18 years of age)
- Breast-feeding
- Cardiac risk
  - Known underlying heart disease, with or without symptoms
  - Persons with three or more risk factors, including hypertension, diabetes, hypercholesterolemia, first-degree relative with heart disease under age 50 years, and smoking
  - Verbal screening for risk factors is recommended
  - Special follow-up for persons with risk factors who have already been vaccinated is not recommended
- *Monkeypox*: For individuals closely exposed within the past 2 weeks to a symptomatic human or animal with confirmed monkeypox, the risk of monkeypox disease is probably greater than the risk of vaccinia exposure
  - In this setting, neither age, pregnancy, nor history of eczema (including active disease) is an absolute contraindication to smallpox vaccination
  - Vaccination is still contraindicated for HIV-infected adults with CD4 counts less than 200 (or age-appropriate equivalent counts in children), transplant recipients, patients receiving high-dose immunosuppressive therapy, and persons with lymphosarcoma, hematologic malignancies, or primary T-cell immunodeficiencies

K. Precautions. The vial stopper contains dry natural rubber and may cause reactions if contacted by individuals with latex sensitivity.

II. Anthrax

> *Bacillus anthracis* is a large, aerobic, spore-forming, toxin-producing gram-positive rod with a "jointed bamboo-rod" appearance and "Medusa's head" colony morphology.

A. Disease. Table 9.6 lists five recognized clinical syndromes along with their distinguishing features and differential diagnoses. *Inhalational* and *cutaneous* anthrax would be the most likely consequences of a bioterrorism attack because they result from inhalation or contact with spores; meningitis can develop with either of these forms. The gastrointestinal and oropharyngeal forms result from ingestion of large numbers of vegetative bacilli (usually in poorly cooked meat) and would therefore be unlikely to result from an attack. After the spores are ingested by phagocytes, they are transported

Table 9.6. Clinical features of anthrax and differential diagnosis

Anthrax disease form/key features	Differential diagnosis/etiologic agents	Clues to differential diagnosis
Inhalational Biphasic Prodromal flulike illness lasting hours to days with fever, malaise, dyspnea, nonproductive cough, headache, vomiting, chills, weakness, abdominal pain, chest pain Fulminant second stage with fever, dyspnea, stridor, diaphoresis, cyanosis, shock Widened mediastinum, pulmonary infiltrates and pleural effusion Hemorrhagic thoracic lymphadenitis and mediastinitis Absence of typical bronchopneumonia Associated with hemorrhagic meningitis Mortality 50% with antibiotic therapy and supportive care	**Viral pneumonia** Influenza virus, adenovirus, RSV	Seasonal Rhinorrhea common Shortness of breath, nausea, vomiting uncommon
	Community-acquired bacterial pneumonia *Streptococcus pneumoniae, Haemophilus influenzae, Staphylococcus aureus, Moraxella catarrhalis,* group A streptococcus, *Klebsiella pneumoniae*	Rarely fulminant Predisposing medical condition Positive Gram stain
	Atypical pneumonia *Chlamydia pneumoniae, Mycoplasma pneumoniae*	Nontoxic Low-grade fever
	Legionnaires' disease *Legionella pneumophila*	Predisposing condition Exposure to cooling towers
	Psittacosis *Chlamydophila psittaci*	Exposure to caged birds
	Hantavirus pulmonary syndrome Sin Nombre virus	Exposure to mouse droppings Fulminant noncardiogenic pulmonary edema
	Pneumonic plague *Yersinia pestis*	Hemoptysis common *(continued)*

Table 9.6. Continued

Anthrax disease form/key features	Differential diagnosis/etiologic agents	Clues to differential diagnosis
	Pneumonic tularemia *Francisella tularensis*	Indolent Exposure to rabbits or outdoor yard work in endemic areas
	Q fever *Coxiella burnetii*	Rarely fulminant Exposure to parturient cats, cattle, sheep or goats
Cutaneous May occur at break in skin Initial pruritic macule or papule enlarges into a round ulcer surrounded by vesicles Painless, depressed, ulcer with extensive, non-pitting, gelatinous surrounding edema Black eschar forms in 1–2 d and sloughs off within 2 wk Lymphangitis and painful lymphadenopathy Low-grade fever and malaise Mortality rare with antibiotic treatment	**Ecthyma gangrenosum** *Pseudomonas aeruginosa*	Neutropenia Bacteremia Edema uncommon
	Ulceroglandular tularemia *Francisella tularensis*	Indolent Nontoxic Exposure to ticks or rabbits
	Bubonic plague *Yersinia pestis*	Extremely tender regional lymphadenopathy Ulceration and eschar formation usually absent
	Bacterial cellulitis *Staphylococcus aureus*, group A streptococcus	Trauma No eschar Painful
	Necrotizing cellulitis and fasciitis Group A streptococcus, *Clostridium* species	Severe systemic toxicity Disproportionately painful

	Necrotizing viral infection Herpes simplex virus	Immunocompromised
	Brown recluse spider bite Venom of *Loxosceles reclusa*	Southeastern United States Exposure to barns or woodpiles Painful
	Rickettsialpox *Rickettsia akari*	Generalized maculopapular rash
	Scrub typhus *Orientia tsutsugamushi*	Travel to Asia and Western Pacific Generalized maculopapular rash
	Orf Orf virus	Farm worker No eschar Edema absent
Gastrointestinal Severe bloody diarrhea, vomiting, and signs of acute abdomen Ulcerative lesions in terminal ileum and cecum Hemorrhagic mesenteric lymphadenitis with ascites Mortality 25–60%	**Typhoid fever** *Salmonella typhi*	No ascites
	Gastrointestinal tularemia *Francisella tularensis*	Less severe No ascites Nonacute abdomen Fever less prominent
	Bacillary dysentery *Shigella dysenteriae*	No ascites
	Bacterial gastroenteritis *Campylobacter jejuni*, toxigenic *Escherichia coli*, *Yersinia enterocolitica*	Less severe No ascites Nonacute abdomen Fever less prominent

(continued)

Table 9.6. *Continued*

Anthrax disease form/key features	Differential diagnosis/etiologic agents	Clues to differential diagnosis
		Association with hemolytic uremic syndrome
	Bacterial peritonitis Gram-negative organisms, *Streptococcus pneumoniae*	Gastrointestinal symptoms not prominent Predisposing condition
Oropharyngeal Oral or esophageal ulcer leading to regional lymphadenopathy, edema, and sepsis Fever, severe sore throat, neck swelling, dysphagia, respiratory distress Occasional pseudomembranes Mortality up to 50%	**Diphtheria** *Corynebacterium diphtheriae*	No history of vaccination Prominent membranes No ulcerative or necrotic lesions Bleeding after removal of membrane
	Oropharyngeal tularemia *Francisella tularensis*	No neck edema Exudative pharyngitis Exposure to rabbits
	Bacterial pharyngitis Group A streptococcus	Exudative pharyngitis No ulcerative or necrotic lesions No neck edema, but may have cervical lymphadenopathy Positive rapid test
	Infectious mononucleosis Epstein-Barr virus	Splenomegaly No neck edema, but may have cervical lymphadenopathy
	Herpangina Coxsackievirus	Painful vesicular lesions No neck edema

	Condition / Etiology	Distinguishing features
	Herpetic pharyngitis Herpes simplex virus	May have shallow ulcers No neck edema, but may have cervical lymphadenopathy
	Vincent's angina Polymicrobial Anaerobes	Severe gingivitis Tonsillar abscesses No neck edema
	Ludwig's angina Polymicrobial Anaerobes	Dental source or trauma Predisposition Brawny edema of submandibular spaces Bull neck appearance Elevated floor of mouth No pharyngitis
Meningitis Often complicates other forms of disease Fever, nuchal rigidity, headache, nausea, vomiting, change in mental status, seizures Bloody cerebrospinal fluid Usually fatal	**Bacterial meningitis** *Neisseria meningitidis, Streptococcus pneumoniae, Haemophilus influenzae, Listeria monocytogenes,* group B streptococcus	No hemorrhage Suggestive Gram stain
	Aseptic meningitis Enteroviruses	No hemorrhage Negative Gram stain Monocytic pleocytosis
	Subarachnoid hemorrhage Trauma	No fever Findings on noncontrasted computed tomographic scan

Adapted from Bioterrorism information and resources. Infectious Diseases Society of America Web site. www.idsociety.org/bt/biotemplate.cfm?template=an_summary.htm (accessed 02/02/03).

to regional lymph nodes, where they germinate into vegetative cells after variable (and potentially extended) periods of time. Replicating cells then elaborate toxins that lead to massive hemorrhage, edema, necrosis, and cytokine release. Early antibiotic therapy for symptomatic disease is essential, but the effects of local tissue damage and systemic toxinosis may be irreversible.

B. **Epidemiology and transmission.** Anthrax spores are found in soil worldwide and may remain viable for years. Infection occurs in grazing animals who ingest the spores, and natural human infection occurs almost exclusively after contact with infected animals and animal products (one classic example is *woolsorter's disease*, inhalational anthrax linked to the processing of hides and wool in enclosed spaces). As many as 20,000 annual cases of anthrax are estimated to occur worldwide, but disease in the United States was extremely rare until the fall of 2001. Only 18 cases of inhalational anthrax were reported between 1900 and 1976, and no cases were reported after 1976. Between 1944 and 1994, only 224 cases of cutaneous anthrax were reported, with one case occurring in 2000.

Anthrax is an attractive agent of bioterrorism because the infection can be lethal, natural immunity does not exist, the organism can be engineered into antibiotic resistance, and the infectious dose of spores is very low. It is easily grown in the laboratory, and the spores can be *"weaponized"* into a highly concentrated powder with uniform small particle size and low electrostatic charge, features that reduce clumping and facilitate aerosol dispersal. Such aerosols are odorless and invisible, can spread over large areas, and would probably not be detected until cases occurred. The lethality of aerosolized weapons-grade anthrax was demonstrated after the accidental release of anthrax spores (possibly as little as 1 g) on April 2, 1979 from a Soviet bioweapons facility in Sverdlovsk (now called Ekaterinburg). As many as 250 cases and 100 deaths occurred downwind (away from the city of over 1,000,000 people) of the release, mostly from inhalational disease. Most cases occurred within 10 days, but some occurred 6 weeks later. Although the majority of victims were exposed in a narrow 4-km band extending from the military facility to the southern city limit, cases did occur many miles away, and livestock in several towns downwind of the release were affected.

In September and October of 2001, at least five letters containing high-grade Ames strain anthrax spores were mailed through the U.S. postal service from Trenton, New Jersey to sites in Florida, New York City, and Washington, DC. One letter was known to contain 2 g of powder and between 100 billion and 1 trillion spores. A total of 22 anthrax cases occurred in seven eastern states between September 22 and November 16; 11 were inhalational (five deaths) and 11 cutaneous (no deaths). Twelve victims were mail handlers, demonstrating the propensity for weaponized spores to disperse from relatively sealed containers. Cross-contamination was evidenced by the isolation of anthrax from more than 100 environmental samples along the path of the letters.

In 1970, the WHO estimated that a release of 50 kg of spores over an urban population of 5 million would result in 250,000 cases and 100,000 deaths. The recent U.S. experience indicates that this might have been an underestimate. Unlike smallpox, all cases occurring after an attack would result from primary exposure, because the infection is not transmitted from person to person. However, secondary aerosolization of particles that settle after a primary release could continue to cause disease for some time.

C. **Rationale for vaccine use.** Antibiotic therapy after exposure can prevent inhaled spores from germinating and causing disease. In fact, there were no cases of anthrax among more than 10,000 people who took antibiotics (primarily ciprofloxacin or doxycycline) for at least 60 days after the 2001 attacks. In May 2002, the Working Group on Civilian Biodefense concluded that antibiotic therapy in conjunction with vaccination would be optimal for exposed persons, and current recommendations incorporate that concept (see Official recommendations below).

Preexposure vaccination is based on a quantifiable risk for exposure and is not recommended for the general public. Although a vaccine has been licensed since 1970, it was in limited use until 1991 when the U.S. military immunized 150,000 service members deployed for the Gulf War. The Anthrax Vaccine Immunization Program was started in March 1998 with the routine immunization of personnel deployed to high-risk areas. In June 2002, the Department of Defense reintroduced the program, which had slowed because of dwindling vaccine supplies, because of intelligence assessments indicating possible risk of exposure to military personnel. Mandatory vaccination has been instituted for active military personnel, emergency-essential Department of Defense civilians, and mission-critical contractors. In January 2003, plans were announced to make the vaccine available to journalists accompanying U.S. forces to the Persian Gulf.

D. **Vaccines.** The only licensed anthrax vaccine in the United States is called BioThrax (anthrax vaccine, adsorbed) and is manufactured for the Department of Defense by BioPort. The manufacturing facility was acquired from the State of Michigan in 1998 and was temporarily closed for renovation. In January 2002, BioPort received FDA approval for the product label, packaging facility, and release of three lots of vaccine. The vaccine is made from cell-free filtrates of microaerophilic cultures of an avirulent, nonencapsulated strain of *B. anthracis* called V770-NP1-R. The filtrate includes three cellular proteins—protective antigen, edema factor, and lethal factor—that naturally combine to form toxins that are involved in pathogenesis. The proteins are adsorbed to aluminum hydroxide, and the final product contains benzethonium chloride and formaldehyde as preservatives. It is supplied in 5-mL multidose vials and is only labeled for preexposure immunization.

E. **Storage, handling, and administration**
- Maintain at 35° to 46°F (2° to 8°C)
- Do not freeze
- Shake well before use
- Each dose is 0.5 mL given subcutaneously [see Chapter 3(III)]

F. **Schedule.** The primary series consists of three doses given at 0, 2, and 4 weeks, and three booster doses are given at 6, 12, and 18 months. Annual booster doses are recommended thereafter.

G. **Efficacy.** Protection has been demonstrated in a macaque model of inhalational anthrax. Although correlates of protective immunity are not defined, 95% of adults receiving at least three doses of the vaccine develop a fourfold rise in antibodies to protective antigen. One controlled trial of a similar vaccine among 1,249 mill workers (379 were immunized) demonstrated 92.5% efficacy. No inhalational cases occurred among vaccinees, but three cutaneous cases occurred in incompletely vaccinated individuals. Case surveillance data from 1962 to 1974 suggest that anthrax in mill workers or those living near mills occurred exclusively in unvaccinated or incompletely vaccinated individuals. No data are available regarding efficacy in persons younger than 18 or older than 65 years of age, and current studies are examining intramuscular administration and alternative dosing schedules.

H. **Official recommendations.** ACIP recommendations for use of anthrax vaccine in the United States were published on December 15, 2000 and included the following:
- Routine vaccination of persons working with production quantities of *B. anthracis* cultures and in activities with the potential for aerosol dispersal
- Vaccination of persons working with imported animal hides, furs, bone meal, wool, animal hair, or bristles only if existing standards and restrictions would be insufficient to prevent exposure to spores
- Routine vaccination was not recommended for workers in clinical laboratories or veterinarians
- Routine vaccination was not recommended for emergency first responders, federal responders, medical practitioners, or private citizens

These recommendations were supplemented on September 6 and November 15, 2002, in the wake of the anthrax attacks, to include the following:
- *Preexposure vaccination*
  - Workers making repeated entries into known contaminated areas (with concomitant prophylactic antibiotic use during the period of risk and for 60

Table 9.7. Local reactogenicity of anthrax vaccine

Reaction	Dose 1 (%)	Dose 2 (%)	Dose 3 (%)
Tenderness	71	61	58
Erythema	43	32	12
Subcutaneous nodule	36	39	4
Induration	21	18	8
Warmth	11	11	19
Pruritus	7	14	19
Limitation of motion	—	7	12

Adapted from BioThrax package insert (n = 28).

days thereafter, unless the entire six-dose series is completed and annual boosters are updated)
- Laboratory workers handling environmental specimens and performing confirmatory testing for *B. anthracis* (excluding workers using standard Biosafety Level 2 practices in routine processing of clinical samples or environmental swabs)
- *Postexposure vaccination*
  - A three-dose regimen (0, 2, 4 weeks) was recommended under an investigational new drug protocol (with concomitant antibiotics until 7 to 14 days after the third dose)
  - Partially or fully vaccinated individuals should receive at least 30 days of antibiotics and should continue with the licensed vaccine regimen
  - Fully vaccinated persons working in Biosafety Level 3 laboratories under recommended conditions and those wearing appropriate personal protective equipment need not receive antibiotics

I. **Safety.** In an open-label safety study, 15,907 doses of BioThrax were administered to 7,000 at-risk individuals using the six-dose schedule. Mild local reactions (erythema only or induration less than 30 mm) occurred in 8.6% of doses, moderate reactions (edema or induration between 30 mm and 120 mm) in 0.9%, and severe reactions (edema or induration greater than 120 mm accompanied by limitation of motion or axillary lymph node tenderness) in 0.15%. There were only four reports of systemic reactions such as fever, chills, nausea, and general body aches. Local reactogenicity in a more recent study of 28 volunteers is given in Table 9.7. Fewer than 10% of these volunteers had notable systemic reactions, and all of these were transient.

In a study involving more than 4,300 service personnel in Korea, 2% of individuals reported limitation in work performance after the first or second dose of vaccine, but fewer than 1% lost one or more day of work. Surveillance for adverse events in the Department of Defense program between 1998 and 2000 involving more than 400,000 recipients of over 1.5 million doses revealed no unexpected patterns of reactogenicity but did note higher rates of local reactions in women than in men. In another series of more than 10,000 doses in U.S. Army Medical Research Institute of Infectious Diseases (USAMRIID) employees, local reactions were noted in 4% and systemic reactions in 1%, and there were no long-term sequelae. A recent Institute of Medicine study concluded that the anthrax vaccine is safe, and epidemiologic studies provide no evidence linking the vaccine to Gulf War Syndrome.

J. Contraindications
- Allergic reaction to anthrax vaccine or any vaccine components
- Previous anthrax disease

K. Precautions
- Moderate or severe acute illness
- Pregnancy
- The vial stopper contains dry natural rubber and may cause reactions if contacted by individuals with latex sensitivity

III. Other category A agents

A. Plague. Plague is caused by *Yersinia pestis*, a nonmotile, facultative, bipolar-staining gram-negative bacillus in the Enterobacteriaceae family. The infection is enzootic in rodents and is transmitted to humans by the bite of infected fleas. Most cases are *bubonic plague*, characterized by sudden onset of fever, chills, weakness and a swollen, tender, erythematous lymph node. *Secondary septicemic plague* can develop, leading to disseminated intravascular coagulation, small-vessel necrosis, purpura, and distal gangrene, the origin of the name *black death* given in medieval times. *Primary septicemic plague* also occurs and is marked by the absence of buboes. *Secondary pneumonic plague* may develop from hematogenous spread. *Primary pneumonic plague*, although rare in natural circumstances, would be the most likely presentation of disease after an attack. Cases would be expected 2 to 4 days after exposure and would present with fever, dyspnea, chest pain, cough, and hemoptysis. Gastrointestinal symptoms might be present. Rapid progression to severe bronchopneumonia with bilateral infiltrates would occur. Findings associated with severe systemic inflammatory response syndrome would include leukocytosis, coagulopathy, hepatopathy, azotemia, and multiorgan failure. Person-to-person spread could occur through respiratory droplets.

The plague pandemic that began in 1346 eventually killed one-third of the population of Europe. Advances in living conditions, public health, and antibiotic therapy have made modern pandemics very unlikely. In fact, in the last 50 years, fewer than 2,000 cases have been reported worldwide. The WHO estimated, however, that a 50-kg aerosol release of *Y. pestis* over a city of 5 million would cause pneumonic plague in 150,000 persons, with 36,000 deaths. The main response to a plague attack would be early treatment of cases with parenteral streptomycin or gentamicin (alternatively doxycycline, ciprofloxacin, or chloramphenicol) and prophylaxis of exposed persons with oral doxycycline, ciprofloxacin, or chloramphenicol.

A formaldehyde-inactivated whole-cell vaccine was licensed in the United States and available until 1999. Initially produced by Cutter Laboratories and then by Greer Laboratories (Lenoir, NC), this vaccine was only protective against bubonic plague. All remaining stocks have now expired, and no other vaccine is currently available in the United States. A live-attenuated vaccine called EV76 has been used in Russia but is also not protective against pneumonic disease. There is also a commercially available heat-inactivated whole-cell vaccine from CSL Limited (New Zealand) that is given subcutaneously in a primary series of two or three doses and booster doses every 6 months. Current approaches to vaccine development involve subunits of the organism, most notably the F1 and V antigens, derived by recombinant technology.

B. Tularemia. Tularemia is caused by *Francisella tularensis*, a nonmotile, aerobic gram-negative coccobacillus. The infection is enzootic in small mammals and is commonly transmitted to humans by ticks, causing *ulceroglandular* disease, characterized by an ulcer at the site of the bite, tender enlarged regional lymph nodes, and systemic symptoms. *Oropharyngeal* disease, characterized by pseudomembrane formation, follows ingestion of contaminated food or drink, as does gastrointestinal tularemia. *Oculoglandular* tularemia (*Parinaud's syndrome*), characterized by nodular conjunctivitis and painful preauricular lymphadenopathy, usually occurs through self-inoculation by contaminated fingers. A *typhoidal form* of the disease has also been described, with shock, disseminated intravascular coagulation, acute respiratory distress syndrome, and multisystem organ failure. Bioterrorism-related tularemia would most likely take the form of *pneumonic* disease, which occurs after aerosol transmission. Illness would begin with a nonspecific febrile illness 3 to 5 days after exposure and would progress to pleuropneumonitis and hilar lymphadenitis with systemic symptoms. Early radiographic findings would include peribronchial infiltrates that would advance to bronchopneumonia with pleural effusion and hilar adenopathy. The disease would be differentiated from plague, which would progress faster and be associated with hemoptysis, and from anthrax, which would progress despite antibiotic therapy and would be associated with characteristic mediastinal widening. Person-to-person spread would not be expected.

F. tularensis is one of the most infectious organisms known, requiring as few as ten organisms to cause disease. However, during the 1990s, fewer than 200 annual cases of tularemia were reported in the United States. The occurrence of a cluster of disease in an urban area should trigger concerns for an intentional release, as most natural cases occur in rural areas. The WHO estimated that a 50-kg aerosol release of *F. tularensis* over a city of 5 million would result in 250,000 incapacitating casualties and 19,000 deaths. The main response to an attack would be early antibiotic treatment of cases and prophylaxis of exposed persons using drug regimens similar to those used for plague.

A live-attenuated vaccine called LVS was developed in the United States and given under an investigational new drug protocol to more than 1,000 laboratorians working with the organism. The vaccine was shown to be safe and effective, reducing the incidence of laboratory-associated inhalational disease from 5.7 cases per 1,000 person years to 0.27 cases per 1,000 person years. Although the incidence of ulceroglandular disease did not change, the clinical findings were mitigated. The vaccine is not currently available but is under review by the FDA.

C. **Botulinum toxin.** Natural botulism is described in Chapter 11(VIII). Botulinum toxin is the most poisonous substance known—1 g, evenly dispersed, could kill more than 1 million people. After the Gulf War, it was discovered that Iraq had produced 19,000 L of concentrated toxin, enough to kill the entire current human population three times over. Botulinum toxin could be distributed by aerosol or through food contamination. Contamination of water supplies is less likely because the toxin is inactivated in fresh water within 3 to 6 days and is rapidly inactivated by standard water treatments. Intentional release would be expected to cause outbreaks of acute flaccid paralysis with prominent bulbar palsies.

Antitoxin and botulinum immune globulin [see Chapter 11(VIII)] can be used for therapy but do not represent viable options for preexposure prophylaxis. An investigational pentavalent (toxins type A, B, C, D, and E) botulinum toxoid vaccine is distributed by the CDC for laboratory workers at high risk of exposure and is also used by the U.S. military. The vaccine is administered subcutaneously at 0, 2, and 12 weeks, with a booster dose at 1 year. Antitoxin levels are measured every 2 years after the booster dose, and additional doses are given as needed. Studies have shown that all vaccinees develop antibodies to toxins A and B after the first booster dose. Although mass vaccination would theoretically eliminate the threat from the five toxins in the vaccine, this approach is not considered feasible. In addition, because antibodies take months to form, vaccination is not considered useful for postexposure prophylaxis.

D. **Viral hemorrhagic fevers.** Hemorrhagic fever viruses are enveloped, single-stranded RNA viruses that reside in animal hosts or arthropod vectors; humans are incidentally infected. They belong to four distinct families:

- *Filoviruses (e.g., Ebola, Marburg)*: Approximately 1,500 cases have been known to occur during a total of 18 described outbreaks, mostly in Africa. The natural reservoir is not known. Transmission occurs through direct contact with blood, secretions, or tissues of infected patients or primates, including needlestick injury and permucosal exposure. Mortality is as high as 90%.
- *Arenaviruses (e.g., Lassa, Machupo, Junin, Guanarito)*: These agents are transmitted to humans by aerosolization from rodent urine and feces or other contact with these materials. Person-to-person transmission occurs through contact with blood and body fluids. Mortality approaches 30%.
- *Bunyaviruses (e.g., Rift Valley fever)*: Transmission to humans occurs through the bite of infected mosquitoes, direct contact with animal tissues, or aerosolization from animal carcasses. Person-to-person transmission does not occur, and mortality is less than 1%.
- *Flaviviruses (e.g., yellow fever, Omsk hemorrhagic fever, Kyasanur Forest disease)*: Yellow fever is acquired from mosquitoes, whereas Omsk hemorrhagic fever and Kyasanur Forest disease are acquired from ticks. Person-to-person transmission does not occur, and mortality is as high as 20%.

Despite differences between these viruses, the clinical manifestations are similar. Illness begins with a prodrome of high fever, myalgia, arthralgia, headache, malaise, nausea, abdominal pain, and diarrhea. Rash develops in most cases. Later signs include progressive bleeding diathesis, disseminated intravascular coagulation, circulatory collapse, and evidence of encephalitis.

The only agent for which a vaccine currently exists is yellow fever [see Chapter 8(X)]. This would not be useful, however, in the postexposure setting because of the short incubation period of the disease.

IV. **Resources.** Table 9.8 lists excellent resources for more information about bioterrorism preparedness.

Table 9.8. Bioterrorism resources

Agency	Web site (accessed 02/01/03)
American Academy of Family Physicians	www.aafp.org/btresponse.xml
American Academy of Pediatrics	www.aap.org/terrorism/index.html
Centers for Disease Control and Prevention	www.bt.cdc.gov
U.S. Food and Drug Administration	www.fda.gov/oc/opacom/hottopics/ bioterrorism.html
Infectious Diseases Society of America	www.idsociety.org/BT/ToC.htm
National Institute of Allergy and Infectious Diseases	www.niaid.nih.gov/publications/ bioterrorism.htm

Vaccines in Development for General Use

I. 2000 Institute of Medicine report. In 1985, the Institute of Medicine (IOM) released a report entitled *New Vaccine Development: Establishing Priorities*, a project commissioned by the National Institutes of Health (NIH) as part of its planning for the future. The committee developed a quantitative model that could be used by policy makers to prioritize development of vaccines for infectious diseases that represented significant public health threats. Data on 14 candidate vaccines were analyzed; many of those candidates have been licensed and are in use today. Ten years later, the NIH asked for a progress assessment, a discussion of the barriers to vaccine research and development, and another quantitative model for prioritizing vaccine development. The resulting report, *Vaccines for the 21st Century: A Tool for Decisionmaking*, was issued in 2000 and is available at books.nap.edu/books/0309056462/html/index.html (accessed 02/21/03). The IOM used a cost-effectiveness model to compare potential new vaccines based on their anticipated impact on morbidity and mortality and the costs associated with health care of the disease, vaccine development, and vaccine use. Health benefits were measured in terms of quality-adjusted life years (QALYs) gained by use of the vaccine.

The committee selected 26 candidate vaccines to analyze—vaccines that were of interest to many people, directed against conditions of domestic importance, and capable of being brought to licensure within 20 years. These vaccines fell into four categories based on whether they saved money and also saved QALYs (most favorable) or cost money for each QALY gained (more favorable for the lowest cost, favorable for moderate cost, and less favorable for the highest cost). These categories, and the candidate vaccines that fit into them, are shown in Table 10.1. To some extent, this listing serves as a road map of what to expect in the coming years. The report also addressed a number of other important topics, including ethical issues in vaccine research and development, funding for research, vaccine implementation in specific populations, barriers to vaccine delivery, and combination vaccines.

The status of vaccine development at the beginning of the 21st century is best summarized in a report from the National Institute of Allergy and Infectious Diseases (NIAID) entitled *The Jordan Report 20th Anniversary: Accelerated Development of Vaccines 2002*, available at www.niaid.nih.gov/dmid/vaccines/jordan20 (accessed 02/19/03).

Table 10.1. Institute of Medicine vaccine development priorities

Category	Description	Candidate vaccines	Target group
Most favorable	Saves money and QALYs	Cytomegalovirus	12 yr olds
		Influenza	General population every 5 yr or 20% of population each yr
		Group B streptococcus	Routine prenatal care, women during first pregnancy, high-risk adults
		Streptococcus pneumoniae	Infants, 65 yr olds
More favorable	Costs <$10,000/ QALY saved	Chlamydia (genital)	12 yr olds
		Helicobacter pylori	Infants
		Hepatitis C	Infants
		Herpes simplex virus	12 yr olds
		Human papilloma virus	12 yr olds
		Tuberculosis	High-risk populations
		Neisseria gonorrhea	12 yr olds
		Respiratory syncytial virus	Infants, 12-yr-old females

(continued)

Table 10.1. *Continued*

Category	Description	Candidate vaccines	Target group
Favorable	Costs $10,000–$100,000/ QALY saved	Parainfluenza virus	Infants, women during first pregnancy
		Rotavirus	Infants
		Group A streptococcus	Infants
		Group B streptococcus	High-risk adults, 12-yr-old females or women during first pregnancy (low utilization)
Less favorable	Costs >$100,000/ QALY saved	*Borrelia burgdorferi*	Resident infants born in, and immigrants of any age to, high-risk areas
		Coccidioides immitis	Resident infants born in, and immigrants of any age to, high-risk areas
		Enterotoxigenic *E. coli*	Infants and travelers
		Epstein-Barr virus	12 yr olds
		Histoplasma capsulatum	Resident infants born in, and immigrants of any age to, high-risk areas
		Neisseria meningitidis serogroup B	Infants
		Shigella	Infants and travelers or travelers only

QALYs, quality-adjusted life years.
Adapted from Stratton KR, Durch JS, Lawrence RS, eds. *Vaccines for the 21st century: a tool for decisionmaking.* Washington, DC: National Academy Press, 2000.

II. New combinations

A. DTaP5/Hib/IPV.
This combination vaccine is licensed and widely used in Canada under the trade name PENTACEL. The manufacturer, Aventis Pasteur, intends to file for licensure in the United States in 2004. In analogy to TriHIBit [DTaP2/PRP-T; see Chapter 6(II)], PENTACEL is a mixture of two vaccines—ActHIB (lyophilized PRP-T) and QUADRACEL (liquid formulation DTaP5/IPV)—made by reconstituting the former with the latter immediately before administration. Each 0.5-mL dose contains pertussis toxin (PT, 20 μg), filamentous hemagglutinin (FHA, 20 μg), fimbriae or agglutinogens (FIM-2 and FIM-3, 5 μg total), pertactin (PRN, 3 μg), diphtheria toxoid [15 limit of flocculation (Lf) units], tetanus toxoid (5 Lf units), poliovirus type 1 [Mahoney, 40 D-antigen units (DU)], type 2 (MEF-1, 8 DU), and type 3 (Saukett, 32 DU), and polyribosylribotol phosphate (PRP, 10 μg) conjugated to tetanus toxoid (20 μg). Other constituents include aluminum phosphate; Tween 80; traces of bovine serum, neomycin, and polymyxin B; and 2-phenoxyethanol as preservative The vaccine is given intramuscularly at 2, 4, 6, and 15 to 18 months of age. It should be noted that QUADRACEL contains IPV components identical to IPOL [see Chapter 5(IV)], and although the DTaP constituents are the same as those in DAPTACEL [see Chapter 5(I)], the amounts of PT and FHA are higher.

Prior attempts at combining Hib with DTaP components resulted in lower PRP responses as compared to monovalent vaccines; PENTACEL appears to have overcome this difficulty. In a study of 135 Taiwanese infants, 68 were given a combined DTaP5/PRP-T vaccine, and 67 were given separate injections of the two vaccines. Antibody responses to each of the vaccine antigens were similar in the two groups. After the primary series, the geometric mean anti-PRP antibody concentration was 11.8 μg/mL in the combined group and 13.0 μg/mL in the separate group; 96% and 99% of subjects, respectively, achieved levels predictive of long-term protection. In a Canadian trial, 107 infants received ActHIB (PRP-T) reconstituted with QUADRACEL (DTaP5/IPV), and 108 infants received the separate vaccines at 2, 4, and 6 months of age. The proportion of children achieving protective levels of antibody to all antigens was similar, including PRP responses. Additional studies are under way to evaluate the safety and immunogenicity of DTaP5/Hib/IPV in expanded populations of U.S. infants and children.

B. MMRV.
In the United States, measles, mumps, and rubella vaccine (MMR) is routinely given at 12 to 15 months of age, and varicella vaccine is given at 12 to 18 months of age. Because these two live viral vaccines can be given simultaneously, it makes sense to con-

sider combining them into a single injection. As varicella vaccine uptake has lagged behind that of MMR, a combination would have the potential advantage of boosting varicella vaccination rates. In addition, there is some interest in giving two doses of varicella vaccine because of the continued occurrence of breakthrough disease (although it should be noted that breakthrough disease is universally mild). Because a second dose of MMR is routinely given at 4 to 6 years of age, a measles, mumps, rubella, and varicella (MMRV) vaccine would facilitate this without adding injections to the current schedule. Both GlaxoSmithKline and Merck have developed and tested MMRV vaccines; these candidate vaccines use the same strains of rubella and varicella but different strains of measles and mumps. The development process has been hindered by the phenomenon of *viral interference*, whereby the replication of one virus (most notably, measles) at the injection site interferes with the replication of another virus (most notably, varicella), resulting in decreased "take" of the latter.

The first studies of MMRV vaccine were published in 1986. Viral interference was noted with a GlaxoSmithKline candidate, for which seroconversion rates to low- and high-potency varicella were 42% and 79%, respectively, in subjects given MMRV but 78% and 98%, respectively, in those given separate MMR and varicella vaccines. Improved results were seen when low-potency MMR was used; 98% or more of subjects seroconverted to all MMRV components. In a Finnish study, the most immunogenic combination consisted of high-potency varicella and low-potency MMR, but no combination induced adequate responses to varicella.

Early studies of the Merck candidate involved children given MMR or MMRV vaccine followed 6 weeks later by varicella vaccine in both groups; nearly 100% seroconversion rates to all vaccine components were seen. In a second study, seroconversion rates were higher with a single dose of MMRV (90%) than with varicella vaccine alone (74%), but the dose of varicella virus was higher in the combination. Cell-mediated responses were similar in children given MMRV and those given the separate vaccines, even though humoral responses were significantly lower in children receiving the combination. In the largest study published so far, 812 children were enrolled into two trials evaluating MMRV versus separate MMR and varicella vaccines given either simultaneously or separated by 6 weeks [in the later study, DTaP and oral poliovirus vaccine (OPV) were given concurrently with MMRV or MMR]. Although more than 95% of children in both studies seroconverted to measles, mumps, rubella, and varicella, the magnitude of antibody responses to the varicella component was significantly lower in children given the combination. No differences were seen in the occurrence of varicella-like rashes between groups in either study. Most recently, no interference was demonstrated when MMRV and Hib vaccine (PRP-OMP) were given concurrently.

In ongoing clinical trials, it appears that viral interference can be overcome by increasing the amount of varicella in the MMRV combination, and this can be done without increasing adverse reactions.

C. **Other combinations.** HEXAVAC is a liquid DTaP2/Hep-B/IPV/PRP-T combination developed collaboratively by Aventis Pasteur and Merck and licensed outside the United States. There is a similar product made by GlaxoSmithKline that contains DTaP3 and is licensed in Germany. It is unlikely that these products will be licensed anytime soon in the United States because of immunologic interference between the DTaP and Hib components. Wyeth is studying combination vaccines designed to prevent meningitis and sepsis due to the most common pyogenic organisms, *Streptococcus pneumoniae*, *Neisseria meningitidis*, and Hib. A recent report indicated that PRP antibody responses were lower in infants given a combination of pneumococcal, meningococcal, and Hib conjugates, implicating immunologic interference. Other combination vaccines may target specific circumstances. For example, a travel vaccine combination might include yellow fever and typhoid fever.

III. **Cytomegalovirus.** Additional information on cytomegalovirus (CMV) disease is found in Chapter 11(I), which deals with passive immunoprophylaxis for immunocompromised patients. This section focuses primarily on active immunization to prevent congenital CMV disease.

A. **Disease.** *Symptomatic congenital CMV infection* is characterized by intrauterine growth retardation, jaundice, hepatosplenomegaly, thrombocytopenia, petechiae, purpura, and central nervous system damage manifest by microcephaly, intracerebral calcifications, chorioretinitis, seizures, and progressive sensorineural hearing loss. Up to 12% of infants with this condition die in infancy, and 90% of survivors have serious permanent sequelae. Infants with congenital CMV infection who are not symptomatic at birth are still at risk—10% to 20% may develop neurologic deficits later, particularly hearing loss. CMV also may be acquired *perinatally*, manifesting in the first few months with self-limited lymphadenopathy, hepatosplenomegaly, and pneumonitis.

CMV is the most important viral opportunistic cause of disease in immunocompromised individuals. Disease syndromes include hepatitis, meningoencephalitis, colitis, and pneumonitis; the latter can be particularly severe in bone marrow transplant recipients. In acquired immunodeficiency syndrome (AIDS) patients, CMV causes retinitis that can lead to blindness. Healthy indi-

viduals who acquire primary infection may develop het-
erophil-negative mononucleosis, characterized by fever,
malaise, atypical lymphocytosis, and elevation of liver
enzymes.

B. Epidemiology and transmission. CMV infection is
ubiquitous and is spread by close physical contact,
including sexual activity. In the United States, approximately 50% of adults in middle to upper socioeconomic
groups, and 80% of those in lower socioeconomic
groups, have been infected. The vast majority of these
infections are asymptomatic. However, like all herpesviruses, CMV establishes latency and can periodically
reactivate; when reactivation results from immunosuppression, disease can ensue.

Fetal infection rates approximate 40% if the mother
experiences a *primary infection* during pregnancy but
are closer to 2% if the mother experiences *reactivation*
or *reinfection*. The combined effect of all CMV infections during pregnancy results in 1% of babies being
born with CMV. Fortunately, fewer than 10% of these
infants are symptomatic, and most of these are born to
mothers experiencing primary infection. Sources of
transmission to pregnant women include close physical or sexual contact with infected adults and exposure
to body fluids or secretions of infected young children.
The high prevalence of asymptomatic shedding among
day care–attending infants and toddlers (greater than
60% in some centers) and the relatively low prevalence
of immunity in women in certain sociodemographic
groups make primary infections, and therefore symptomatic congenital disease, more likely. In addition,
although women from lower socioeconomic groups
tend to have higher rates of immunity, they acquire
CMV infection at a younger age, implying high transmission rates during adolescence. Thus, women in
these groups who become pregnant at a young age are
also at higher risk for experiencing primary infection
during pregnancy and giving birth to symptomatic
babies.

CMV can also be transmitted perinatally by exposure
to virus in the mother's vaginal secretions, saliva, and
breast milk. Toddlers and young children acquire the
infection horizontally through sharing secretions and
poor hygiene. Transmission may also occur through
blood product transfusion and organ transplantation.

C. Rationale for vaccine use. The public health burden
of congenital CMV infection is appreciable—8,000
affected babies born every year and approximately $4 bil-
lion in annual costs. In fact, CMV is the most common
microbial cause of birth handicap in developed countries
and is a major cause of hearing loss. It is clear that most
of the disease burden results from primary maternal
infection during pregnancy. Because natural immunity
before conception is not entirely protective against con-

genital *infection* per se but is protective against *disease*, a reasonable goal for a vaccine would be to reduce congenital *disease* by mimicking natural preconceptual immunity. If a vaccine were further able to prevent congenital *infection*, additional benefits would accrue from reducing the reservoir of virus in the community represented by asymptomatically infected infants.

CMV disease is less severe in organ transplant recipients who are seropositive before transplantation compared to those who are seronegative. In addition, passive immunization with CMV–IGIV immune globulin for intravenous administration [see Chapter 11(I)] can reduce the severity of CMV disease in seronegative transplant recipients who are given kidneys from seropositive donors. These observations suggest that vaccine-induced immunity might provide similar benefits to transplant patients. There might also be use in boosting immunity in seropositive patients as a way of preventing reactivation.

D. Target population. Ideally, girls would be vaccinated at puberty. Although this strategy is likely to be cost effective, it would only work if vaccine-induced immunity lasted into the childbearing years, unless periodic boosters were used. An alternative strategy would target seronegative women closer to the time of conception. Other targets for vaccination include seronegative transplant candidates. Incorporation of a CMV vaccine into the routine childhood schedule might be effective if vaccine-induced immunity were as long-lasting as natural immunity. Along these lines, it is likely that natural immunity is enhanced by periodic subclinical reactivation, and this mechanism might be operative for a live-attenuated CMV vaccine [a similar scenario has been proposed for varicella vaccine; see Chapter 5(VII)].

E. Candidate vaccines. A live-attenuated vaccine strain called Towne was derived from an infant with congenital CMV infection by 125 passages in human diploid fibroblasts. In early clinical studies, the vaccine was shown to induce humoral and cellular responses and to impart resistance to low-dose wild-type challenge. Vaccination was safe, did not result in shedding of virus, and did not result in detectable latency. Efficacy was evaluated in three large placebo-controlled trials involving more than 1,000 renal transplant patients. In seronegative subjects receiving kidneys from seropositive donors (the highest-risk situation), no effect was seen on the rate of infection, but efficacy against severe disease was estimated at 89%. In another placebo-controlled study, Towne vaccine failed to prevent infection in seronegative mothers whose children were shedding CMV. However, in this study, neutralizing antibody titers were much lower than those seen in naturally infected individuals, leading to thoughts that the dose of Towne vaccine used was too low; a higher dose is currently under study. One of the differences between Towne and more virulent natural isolates is a 13-kilobase deletion in the unique long region of the genome. An approach taken by Aviron (which was acquired by MedImmune in 2002) has been to engineer chimeric viruses that restore portions of this deletion using sequences from a low-passage clinical isolate called Toledo, hopefully enhancing immunogenicity without increasing virulence.

The most promising candidate for an inactivated subvirion CMV vaccine is the surface glycoprotein gB, which regularly induces neutralizing antibodies. A gB vaccine was produced by Chiron in the 1990s and is currently under development and testing by Aventis Pasteur. The vaccine consists of a modified gB molecule produced in mammalian cells and formulated with MF-59, an oil-in-water emulsion adjuvant. This vaccine induced strong humoral [including mucosal antibody and secretory IgA] and cellular immune responses in children and adults after multiple doses. A double-blind, placebo-controlled efficacy trial in seronegative women is currently underway in Birmingham, Alabama. The study has a primary endpoint of CMV infection and secondary endpoints of duration of shedding in women who acquire CMV and rate of congenital infection in their offspring. Another approach has been to use recombinant viral vectors to deliver gB. In fact, gB vaccination using a canarypox vector has been used to prime subjects for boosted antibody responses after Towne vaccination.

Other approaches to CMV vaccination include DNA vaccines and the use of defective subviral particles.

IV. Epstein-Barr virus

Epstein-Barr virus (EBV) has a large, double-stranded DNA genome and a protein nucleocapsid surrounded by a lipid envelope; it is tropic for B lymphocytes and, like all herpesviruses, establishes latency and periodically reactivates.

A. Disease. The prototypical EBV disease is *infectious mononucleosis*, characterized by fever, sore throat, fatigue, malaise, lymphadenopathy, and atypical lymphocytosis. The incubation period is 4 to 6 weeks. Fever typically lasts approximately 6 days, but it may continue for many weeks. Lymphadenopathy is most noticeable in the anterior and posterior cervical chains, but mesenteric, hilar, and mediastinal lymph nodes may be involved. Approximately one-half of patients develop splenomegaly that may last as long as 2 months; trauma can result in splenic hemorrhage or rupture. Most patients experience elevated hepatic transaminases, and some manifest hepatomegaly and jaundice. Rash may accompany the syndrome, especially after exposure to ampicillin and other antibiotics. Complications include meningitis, encephalitis, Guillain-Barré syndrome and other neurologic conditions, transient leucopenia or thrombocytopenia, orchitis, and renal complications. Rarely, patients may develop *chronic active infection* with hepatitis, pneumonitis, cardiomyopathy, neutropenia, thrombocytopenia, dysgammaglobulinemia, hemophagocytic syndrome, or lymphoma (this should not be confused with chronic fatigue syndrome, which is not caused by EBV).

EBV-infected transplant patients may develop *posttransplant lymphoproliferative disease* (PTLD), manifested by fever, generalized lymphadenopathy, and multiple tumors in the grafted organ, gastrointestinal tract, or central nervous system. These tumors consist of monoclonal or polyclonal EBV-infected B lymphocytes, and the pathogenesis is related to the ability of EBV to immortalize B cells. Patients with *X-linked lymphoproliferative syndrome* are unable to mount an effective cellular immune response to EBV and, although they are healthy before infection, develop serious and often fatal infectious mononucleosis after infection. There are a variety of EBV-associated diseases in human immunodeficiency virus (HIV)-infected individuals, including *lymphoid interstitial pneumonitis*, *non-Hodgkin's lymphoma*, *oral hairy leukoplakia*, and *leiomyosarcoma*. EBV also causes *Burkitt's lymphoma* (Central Africa) and *nasopharyngeal carcinoma* (Southeast Asia) and has been associated with *Hodgkin's disease*.

B. **Epidemiology and transmission.** In developing countries and in low socioeconomic groups, EBV infection in childhood is almost universal. In higher socioeconomic groups, only approximately half of adolescents are seropositive. The vast majority of infections are asymptomatic. Humans are the only source of EBV, and transmission occurs during prolonged close personal contact. The virus is shed in saliva for months after the acute infection, and this is a major source of spread to others. Occasionally, EBV is transmitted by blood transfusion or organ transplantation. Like all herpesviruses, EBV establishes latency and can periodically reactivate. Reactivations in healthy hosts are almost universally asymptomatic, but reactivations in immunocompromised hosts can result in disease.

C. **Rationale for vaccine use.** There are an estimated 118,000 new symptomatic EBV infections each year in the United States, the vast majority of which manifest as uncomplicated infectious mononucleosis. Because this illness is rarely fatal, the justification for a vaccination program lies in the prevention of morbidity and the associated medical (physician visits, diagnostic evaluations, medications) and societal (lost school or work) costs. The latter are significant because the illness affects young adults. The IOM estimated that a vaccine that was 100% efficacious and was given to 100% of pre-adolescents would save $12.6 million in annual health care costs but would cost $1.1 million per QALY gained. Theoretic benefits might derive from vaccine-induced immunity in patients who become immunosuppressed, and a vaccine that could prevent Burkitt's lymphoma and nasopharyngeal carcinoma would have great benefits outside the United States.

D. Target population. Universal immunization of infants or toddlers might prevent infectious mononucleosis later on, but delaying vaccination until puberty would have much the same effect, as infected children rarely manifest clinical disease. Puberty would be a reasonable time to institute universal immunization. High-risk individuals could also be targeted, such as those with primary or acquired immunodeficiencies, those with malignancy, and those awaiting solid organ or bone marrow transplantation.

E. Candidate vaccines. Vaccines for EBV are still in the early stages of development, and because of differences in pathogenesis, vaccines for mononucleosis may require different viral antigens and vaccination strategies than vaccines for PTLD, Burkitt's lymphoma, and nasopharyngeal carcinoma. The molecular mechanisms by which EBV causes these diseases are not fully understood, making vaccine development more problematic. There is also a theoretic concern that EBV vaccines administered in childhood may predispose to more severe clinical disease later in life. For example, vaccines that stimulate high IgA levels at mucosal surfaces could potentiate infection by enhancing virus adsorption rather than providing protection. In addition, some EBV proteins have oncogenic potential.

One candidate for prevention of infectious mononucleosis is the envelope glycoprotein gp350, which functions to bind the virus to the CD21 molecule (C3d complement receptor) on B cells, initiating infection. Like CMV gB, gp350 induces neutralizing antibodies. Vaccines based on gp350 have been protective against EBV-induced lymphomas in an animal model. A live recombinant vaccinia virus expressing gp350 was immunogenic in a study of 1 year olds in China. The vaccine prevented acquisition of EBV in six of nine children followed for 16 months, whereas all ten unimmunized controls became infected during the same period of time. gp350 also has been expressed in plasmid vectors and genetically altered Chinese hamster ovary cells. Other antigens such as gp340 and gp85 are being explored as immunogens either alone or in combination with gp350.

Another approach to vaccination uses peptides from antigens expressed in latently infected B cells to stimulate cytotoxic T cells. In fact, PTLD has been successfully treated in some transplant patients by stimulation of their cytotoxic T lymphocytes (CTLs) with EBV latent antigen epitopes. Vaccines for EBV-associated malignancies may require novel strategies because the pattern of viral gene and protein expression differs for each disease. For some diseases, therapeutic vaccines may be more effective than preventive vaccines. In addition, prevention of EBV-associated tumors will require an understanding of how they avoid immune surveillance. One novel strategy has been to infect dendritic cells with a recombinant adenovirus expressing latent membrane protein 2B; these cells have been used to stimulate EBV-specific CTLs.

V. Herpes simplex virus

Herpes simplex virus (HSV) has a large, double-stranded DNA genome and a protein nucleocapsid surrounded by a lipid envelope; it establishes latency in sensory neural ganglia and, like all herpesviruses, periodically reactivates.

A. Disease. HSV causes skin and mucosal lesions that are characterized as thin-walled vesicles on an erythematous base, often occurring in clusters and evolving into honey-colored crusts and scabs. The prototypical disease caused by HSV-1 is *orolabial herpes. Primary herpetic gingivostomatitis* occurs predominantly in children and is marked by extensive lesions throughout the mouth, fever, irritability, poor oral intake, and dehydration. Occasionally, there is autoinoculation of other sites; lesions that result on the distal phalanges are called *herpetic whitlow* and may be confused with bacterial infection because of fever, erythema, and swelling. Recurrent orolabial lesions, commonly known as *fever blisters* or *cold sores*, may be triggered by intercurrent illness, sun exposure, emotional stress, trauma, or fatigue. Itching, tingling, and pain may precede the appearance of grouped vesicles at the outer edge of the vermillion border, and the illness lasts as long as 10 days. Wrestlers and rugby players can spread herpes skin lesions to each other, causing *"herpes gladiatorum"* and *"scrum-pox,"* respectively. HSV-1 also can cause *keratoconjunctivitis*, characterized by tearing, pain, photophobia, chemosis, periorbital edema, and preauricular lymphadenopathy. Ulcers and dendritic lesions develop on the cornea, accompanied by blurred vision. HSV can be locally invasive or cause fulminant disseminated disease, particularly hepatitis, in immunocompromised hosts.

Approximately 75% of primary and 98% of recurrent cases of *genital herpes* are caused by HSV-2. Primary infection may be asymptomatic or may be manifest by lesions that evolve from vesicles and pustules to ulcers and last as long as 3 weeks. Women develop lesions over the labia, vaginal mucosa, and cervix, and men usually have lesions over the shaft of the penis. Accompanying symptoms include vaginal or penile discharge, dysuria, tender inguinal adenopathy, fever, headache, myalgia, and backache; up to one-third of women and 10% of men have associated aseptic meningitis. Recurrent genital lesions, which initially may occur monthly, may be associated with constitutional symptoms and last up to 10 days.

Neonatal herpes usually results from acquisition of HSV-2 from infected cervicovaginal secretions during delivery. The disease may manifest with skin, eye, and mucous membrane (SEM) involvement, CNS disease, or disseminated infection. SEM disease usually presents in the first 2 weeks of life, CNS disease at 2 to 3 weeks, and disseminated infection as early as the first few days. SEM disease can progress to more involved forms of disease if treatment is not initiated early. CNS disease is marked by fever, seizures, and high mortality rates. Disseminated disease presents with signs of sepsis, including cardiovascular instability, lethargy, bleeding, hepatomegaly, and respiratory failure.

HSV is also the most common cause of sporadic fatal *encephalitis* in the United States. Most cases outside of the neonatal period are caused by HSV-1. Hallmarks are fever, change in mental status, unusual behavior, focal neurologic abnormalities, and seizures. Electroencephalogram (EEG) may show paroxysmal lateralizing epileptiform discharges, and magnetic resonance imaging (MRI) usually demonstrates edema in the temporal lobes.

B. **Epidemiology and transmission.** Like all herpesviruses, HSV establishes latency and can periodically reactivate; the site of latency is the sensory neural ganglia. Humans are the only reservoir, and the virus is endemic worldwide. Primary infection may be asymptomatic but can lead to symptomatic reactivation later on, demonstrating that natural immunity is imperfect. Transmission requires close physical contact and may occur from individuals who are shedding the virus asymptomatically. Primary HSV-1 infection usually occurs during young childhood; in the United States, by 5 years of age, approximately 20% of white and 40% of black children have HSV-1 antibodies. HSV-2 infections rise with the onset of sexual activity and peak between 15 and 40 years of age. Seroprevalence in the general population increased from approximately 17% in 1978 to 22% in 1991.

The risk of neonatal disease is related to the serostatus of the mother. Symptomatic primary genital herpes at the time of delivery carries a 50% risk of transmission to the infant, whereas the risk with asymptomatic recurrent genital herpes is less than 5%. However, neonates also may acquire HSV horizontally from infected caretakers. Rarely, transplacental infection can result in a congenital infection syndrome.

C. **Rationale for vaccine use.** In the United States, more than 100 million individuals are infected with HSV-1 and 40 to 60 million with HSV-2. As many as 500,000 new orolabial, 20,000 ocular, and 300,000 genital infections occur each year; 1,000 to 1,500 annual cases of neonatal herpes and 1,500 to 2,000 cases of HSV encephalitis occur as well. The IOM estimated that a vaccine that was 100% efficacious and was given to 100% of preadolescents would save $850 million in annual health care costs and would save $6,000 per QALY gained. Under less-than-ideal conditions of utilization and factoring in other costs, a vaccine might cost as much as $3,000 per QALY gained.

D. **Target population.** Universal vaccination of infants could prevent or reduce the severity of primary herpetic gingivostomatitis, keratitis, whitlow, and other mucocutaneous infections. Childhood vaccination also might lead to decreased prevalence of serious herpetic infections in adulthood that result from reactivation, including encephalitis. A vaccine administered to adolescents that reduced asymptomatic shedding would decrease transmission between sexual partners and reduce the number of new primary infections, thereby reducing the incidence of neonatal herpes. A herpes vaccine also could be used to protect seronegative persons who are candidates for transplantation or who anticipate therapy with immunosuppressive medications.

   The ideal vaccine for genital herpes would entirely prevent infection, but this goal may not be achievable. A vaccine that prevented symptomatic disease and blocked the establishment of latency would still be useful, as would a vaccine that prevented severe manifestations of genital herpes. One caveat is that a partially protective vaccine could encourage people to engage in riskier sexual behaviors and facilitate the spread of the virus. A vaccine that boosted immunity in people with recurrent genital herpes might find use as a therapeutic agent.

E. **Candidate vaccines.** Concerns about genetic stability, latency, and the potential for oncogenicity have precluded development of live, classically attenuated (serially passaged) HSV vaccines. Other approaches to attenuation such as genetic manipulation have met with limited success so far, although one such candidate from Aviron (acquired by MedImmune in 2002) is undergoing testing in animals. There has been interest in replication-limited and replication-incompetent mutant viruses, which are immunogenic but cannot cause disease. One example is an HSV-2 strain developed by Xenova (Berkshire, UK; formerly Cantab Pharmaceuticals) and licensed to GlaxoSmithKline, which is lacking in the essential glycoprotein gH. This virus undergoes only one round of replication, producing progeny that are not infectious. During this round of replication, however, all viral antigens except gH are produced, stimulating broad immune responses. In another strategy, genes encoding immunogenic HSV proteins have been inserted into a variety of vectors that can replicate in humans and express heterologous proteins.

Inactivated HSV vaccines have fewer safety concerns but are less immunogenic than live vaccines. A number of inactivated vaccines have failed to provide efficacy against HSV in clinical trials dating back to the 1930s. More recently, subunit vaccines consisting of surface glycoproteins (analogous to CMV gB and EBV gp350) have been tested. These vaccines have used novel adjuvants to enhance humoral and cell-mediated immune responses. Chiron developed a recombinant, truncated HSV-2 glycoprotein gD (gD2) vaccine adsorbed to alum that was only modestly effective in preventing recurrent genital herpes. Another Chiron vaccine containing recombinant gD2 and gB2 with an adjuvant called MF-59 (composed of squalene, polysorbate 80, and sorbitan trioleate) was tested in clinical trials involving 2,393 seronegative subjects. Doses were given intramuscularly at 0, 1, and 6 months. Despite demonstrably high levels of neutralizing antibody postvaccination, overall efficacy was estimated at only 9%. Furthermore, the vaccine had no effect on the duration of first clinical episodes of genital herpes in those who became infected and no effect on the frequency of subsequent reactivation.

A gD2 vaccine was developed by GlaxoSmithKline and recently tested in two randomized controlled trials involving a total of 2,714 subjects. In this case, the adjuvant used was 3-O-deacylated monophosphoryl lipid A and alum, and the vaccine was given intramuscularly at 0, 1, and 6 months. The vaccine was well-tolerated and induced humoral and cellular responses. Efficacy for prevention of clinical genital herpes was 38% in adults who were seronegative for both HSV-1 and HSV-2. In women who were seronegative for HSV-2, efficacy was 42%. No efficacy was seen in men or in women who were seropositive for HSV-1, but slightly greater than 70% efficacy was seen in women who were seronegative for both HSV-1 and HSV-2. The gender differences may be related to differences in the portal of entry of HSV, and the vaccine may induce antibodies that bathe the vaginal mucosa but do not provide similar protection in men. In addition, it appears that prior infection with HSV-1 confers protection for women against acquisition of genital HSV-2 disease.

Nucleic acid–based vaccines represent another strategy for HSV prevention. Plasmid vectors expressing genes for herpes glycoproteins have been immunogenic and protective in animal studies.

VI. Human immunodeficiency virus

HIV is an enveloped RNA virus that, like all retroviruses, copies its RNA into DNA that then integrates into the host genome, from which viral messages are transcribed and translated into viral proteins.

A. Disease. HIV causes disease by infecting CD4-positive T cells, depleting their number and impairing their function, ultimately leading to downstream immunologic dysregulation and AIDS. Neonates with perinatally acquired HIV infection are usually asymptomatic. Some untreated infants develop symptoms early and die by 1 year of age, whereas others have few symptoms and survive beyond 5 years of age. Clinical manifestations in infants include failure to thrive, generalized lymphadenopathy, hepatosplenomegaly, parotitis, oral candidiasis, and lymphoid interstitial pneumonitis, as well as recurrent diarrhea, otitis media, sinopulmonary infections, and invasive bacterial infections; ultimately, life-threatening opportunistic infections such as pneumocystis pneumonia occur. Age-specific CD4 lymphopenia, thrombocytopenia, anemia, neutropenia, and hyperimmunoglobulinemia may be seen. Progressive encephalopathy can occur with developmental delay or regression, spastic paresis, dystonia, gait abnormalities, and language impairment. Malignancies are unusual but may include non-Hodgkin's lymphoma, leiomyosarcoma, leiomyoma, and Kaposi sarcoma. Cardiomyopathy, hepatitis, nephropathy, and dermatitis are frequently seen.

Adolescents and adults who acquire HIV infection often experience a self-limited mononucleosis- or flulike illness followed by an asymptomatic latent period that may last as long as 5 or 10 years. During this period of time, there is progressive loss of immune function, and eventually the development of signs and symptoms including lymphadenopathy, fatigue, weight loss, fevers and sweats, severe mucocutaneous herpes or shingles, and mucosal candidiasis. Opportunistic infections then ensue, including pneumocystis pneumonia, disseminated CMV, nontuberculous mycobacteria, toxoplasma, cryptosporidiosis, disseminated fungal infection, unusual viruses such as JC virus, and parasites such as cryptosporidium. Wasting syndrome is also seen, characterized by unexplained weight loss, chronic diarrhea, and fever. Malignancies such as Kaposi sarcoma, cervical cancer, and lymphomas can occur.

B. Epidemiology and transmission. As of December 2001, the cumulative number of AIDS cases in the United States was slightly greater than 800,000; 82% were in males, 42% in whites, 38% in blacks, and 18% in Hispanics. Approximately 360,000 persons were living with AIDS and 440,000 had died; this number is more Americans than died in World War I and World War II combined. An estimated 40,000 new HIV infections occur each year, the majority of which are in minority racial groups. Risk factors for women are heterosexual contact (75% of cases) and injecting drug use (25% of cases). For males, risk factors are homosexual contact (60%), injecting drug use (25%), and heterosexual contact (15%). The number of infected children under age 13 is approximately 9,000; more than 90% of these children were perinatally infected. By 2001, the annual number of new cases of pediatric AIDS had fallen to below 200, largely the result of identification and treatment of infected mothers. Fifty-six percent of all AIDS cases have been reported from five states: New York, California, Florida, Texas, and New Jersey.

The United Nations estimates that 42 million people worldwide are living with HIV infection or AIDS; this figure includes 19.2 million women and 3.2 million children younger than 15 years of age. An estimated 5 million individuals, including 800,000 children, acquire HIV each year, and 3.1 million people, including 610,000 children, die from the infection.

Transmission occurs through close contact with infected blood or secretions. In general, parenteral or mucous membrane inoculation is required, although mothers can also transmit to the fetus through the placenta. Most children acquire the infection perinatally through transplacental transmission, intrapartum exposure to maternal blood, or breast-feeding. The overall risk of transmission from an infected mother in the absence of preventive measures is between 13% and 30%. Factors associated with elevated transmission rates include maternal seroconversion during pregnancy, high maternal viral load, low maternal CD4 lymphocyte count, and prolonged rupture of the membranes.

Screening and testing of blood donors and treatment of blood products has all but eliminated the risk of transfusion-associated HIV infection in the United States—it is estimated that fewer than 1 in 600,000 units of blood may be contaminated. Among adolescents and adults, transmission occurs through male homosexual contact, heterosexual contact, and needle sharing. High-risk behaviors include early initiation of sexual activity, unprotected anal and vaginal sex, intravenous drug use, and tattooing; other risk factors include multiple sexual partners and high rates of other sexually transmitted diseases. HIV is rarely transmitted between household or other close contacts without sexual, parenteral, or direct skin or mucous membrane exposure to contaminated blood or bodily fluids. Transmission to health care workers can occur through needle-stick injuries or permucosal exposure to blood or secretions containing large amounts of virus.

C. **Rationale for vaccine use.** The HIV pandemic is one of the most devastating health events the world has experienced. More than 21 million people have already died, and the stability of nations and societies has been threatened, especially in sub-Saharan Africa. AIDS has led to the death of young parents, caretakers, and wage earners, and millions of children have become orphans. The need to control the spread of HIV has become a critical issue for the survival of a number of countries.

   HIV infection is entirely preventable by modification of behavior. Measures such as education, promotion and provision of condoms, treatment of other sexually transmitted diseases and drug abuse, and access to clean needles are effective. Moreover, antiretroviral therapy of mothers can prevent perinatal transmission, and the advent of highly active antiretroviral therapy itself has dramatically improved the natural history of HIV infection. However, many of these measures are costly, inefficient, partially effective, or otherwise difficult to implement on a global scale. The development of a safe, effective, and affordable vaccine is therefore the best hope for controlling the pandemic. An effective vaccine might also find use in the treatment of individuals who are already infected with HIV.

D. **Target population.** Ideally, a vaccine would be administered to persons at greatest risk of acquiring HIV. However, risk-targeted vaccination programs, exemplified by the one for hepatitis B implemented in the United States in the 1980s, are unlikely to be effective. Universal immunization of children or adolescents may be the only way to protect individuals before high-risk behaviors begin. This would also have the potential benefit of preventing perinatal transmission.

E. **Candidate vaccines.** The development of an effective HIV vaccine has proved to be an enormous challenge. Problems include a lack of understanding of the critical factors needed for protective immunity, genetic variation of HIV strains and the high rate of mutation, and the absence of a suitable animal model. Whereas humoral immunity plays some role in preventing infection, CTL responses appear to be critical in inhibiting HIV replication; it is very likely that mucosal immunity also plays an important role. HIV exhibits so much genetic variation that individuals may be infected simultaneously with thousands of "quasispecies," and analysis of envelope glycoprotein sequences demonstrates the existence of at least ten genetically distinct HIV subtypes or "clades." Unfortunately, chimpanzees are the only animals that can be infected with HIV, and the infection is usually asymptomatic. Important data have been generated, however, from vaccine experiments in macaques infected with simian immunodeficiency virus (SIV) and SIV/HIV chimeras. Although many HIV vaccines have been tested in clinical trials, there is no agreement on the optimal vaccine strategy or construct.

Inactivated whole HIV is not considered a viable vaccine candidate because of failures in chimpanzee experiments and because of safety concerns. Live-attenuated SIV vaccines have shown protection in rhesus monkeys. However, it is doubtful that live vaccines will ever be used in humans because of concerns over reversion to virulence and the possibility of inducing tumors through insertional oncogenesis.

A number of live recombinant vaccines have been produced using viral or bacterial vectors that carry genes encoding HIV antigens. Vectors expressing *env, gag, pol,* and *nef* genes have shown promising results. These vaccines have the capacity to elicit both humoral and cell-mediated immunity. Vaccinia virus vectors have shown protection in a macaque/SIV model, but there are significant safety concerns regarding vaccinia [see Chapter 9(I)]. Attenuated vaccinia viruses such as NYVAC (attenuated by deletional mutagenesis) and Ankara (passaged through chick embryo fibroblasts) may be safer for use as vectors in humans. Avian poxviruses such as canarypox, or ALVAC, do not replicate in mammalian cells but are capable of expressing heterologous genes after infection. Importantly, a canarypox vaccine has been shown to induce CTL responses across HIV clades. Other vectors being tested include adenoviruses, polio virus, influenza virus, Bacille Calmette-Guérin (BCG), and *Salmonella*.

Another approach is to use viruslike particles that contain the products of the *gag, pol,* and *env* genes but do not contain RNA. Vaccines based on these particles present HIV proteins in their native conformation but do not carry the risks associated with a whole-virus vaccine.

Subunit vaccines containing HIV envelope glycoproteins such as gp120, gp140, and gp160 have been studied extensively. These recombinant antigens have been generated in various vectors and mammalian cell cultures. Because the proteins are poorly immunogenic, they have been incorporated into novel delivery systems or complexed with new adjuvants. The immunogenicity of envelope protein vaccines may be limited because free glycoproteins differ conformationally from glycoproteins on the surface of the virion. In addition, neutralizing antibody responses are restricted to the homologous clade. Synthetic peptide vaccines representing part of the V3 loop (one of the variable regions) of gp120 have been linked to other HIV proteins and have been shown to induce high titers of neutralizing antibody but limited CTL responses. Core proteins such as p17 and p24 generate CTL responses and are better conserved across strains compared with envelope proteins.

Nucleic acid vaccines have also been developed. These are composed of segments of the HIV genome that, when administered intramuscularly or intradermally, undergo transcription and translation and express HIV antigens in cells (without producing infectious virions). DNA vaccine candidates consisting of *env/rev* and *gag/pol* have undergone evaluation in humans. Primary immune responses to these vaccines can be boosted by vaccination with protein or glycoprotein subunits.

In human trials, envelope glycoprotein subunit vaccines are good at inducing neutralizing antibodies but poor at inducing CTL responses. In contrast, live recombinant vectors expressing the same antigens induce strong CTL responses but low levels of neutralizing antibodies. For an optimal response, these vaccines can be used in a "prime-boost" immunization regimen wherein a live recombinant vaccine or a DNA vaccine is followed by a glycoprotein subunit vaccine.

Phase II clinical trials have been conducted with recombinant gp120 subunit vaccines in HIV seronegative persons. After three immunizations, more than 87% of subjects had neutralizing antibodies, but the proportion was lower in some groups, especially intravenous drug users. On February 24, 2003, VaxGen (Brisbane, CA) announced the results of a phase III trial of a bivalent gp120 vaccine called AIDSVAX B/B. The vaccine consists of gp120 from two clade B strains (MN and GNE8) produced in mammalian cells by recombinant DNA technology. The study enrolled 5,108 men who have sex with men and 309 at-risk women in the United States, Canada, Puerto Rico, and the Netherlands, and volunteers were randomized to vaccine or placebo at a ratio of 2:1. Injections were scheduled at 0, 1, 6, 12, 18, 24, and 30 months. Preliminary analysis included all subjects who had received at least three doses. In the study population as a whole, there was no reduction in HIV infection. However, subgroup analyses demonstrated 67% efficacy among nonwhites and 78% efficacy among blacks; efficacy rates correlated with higher titers of neutralizing antibodies. Importantly, study participants did not show increases in risk behaviors. Before firm conclusions can be drawn, the validity of these preliminary subgroup analyses must be assured, and further analysis of the complete dataset must be undertaken.

A similarly designed trial using AIDSVAX B/E (containing gp120 from a clade B and a clade E strain) is being conducted among 2,500 seronegative intravenous drug users in Thailand. In addition, a prime-boost efficacy study using a canarypox/gp120 vector vaccine followed by a recombinant gp120 vaccine is planned in the United States.

VII. Human papillomavirus

Human papillomavirus (HPV) is a small, nonenveloped, double-stranded DNA virus that produces proteins that interact with tumor suppressor proteins, causing malignant transformation.

A. Disease. HPV is one of the few human viruses unequivocally implicated as a cause of cancer (other members of this group include hepatitis B virus and EBV). *Cervical cancer* (squamous cell carcinoma), one of the most common female malignancies, is usually caused by HPV types 16 and 18 (less often types 31, 45, and others). The duration of time from the first intraepithelial lesion to invasive cancer is 15 to 20 years, although the majority of women who acquire genital HPV resolve their infection without the development of cancer. HIV-positive women are at especially high risk for progression.

Anogenital warts are associated with HPV types 6 and 11, although some children with genital warts acquire the infection by hand contact with nongenital lesions and might therefore have types 1 and 2. The incubation period is 3 weeks to 8 months. Women with anogenital warts, or *condyloma* (cauliflower-like clusters of lesions), may have lesions on the external genital area, in the vagina, cervix, and urethra, and on the inguinal areas or upper thighs. In males, the most common site is the shaft of the penis. Genital warts may appear as classic condyloma, smooth papular warts, cutaneous-like warts, and flat warts. Most individuals are asymptomatic, but some experience itching, burning, pain, and tenderness.

Recurrent respiratory papillomatosis is caused by HPV types 6 and 11 and is seen most commonly in infants and children younger than 5 years of age. The larynx is affected most commonly, but other sites can be involved, including the nasopharynx, oropharynx, trachea, and esophagus. Infants may present with hoarseness, weak cry, stridor, feeding difficulties, and failure to thrive. Airway obstruction can result from enlarged lesions, and rarely, malignancy can develop.

Cutaneous warts may appear as flat warts (HPV types 3 and 10), deep plantar warts (type 1), or "common warts" (type 2). These lesions almost never undergo malignant transformation in healthy hosts. Flat warts usually appear as multiple, slightly raised papules with a smooth surface on the face, neck, and hands. Plantar warts look like raised bundles of soft keratotic fibers. They may be found on the soles and/or palms and can be quite painful. Common warts are well-demarcated hyperkeratotic papules with a rough surface. The most common sites are the dorsum of the hands, between the fingers, in the periungual areas, on the palms and soles, and, rarely, on mucous membranes. Spontaneous resolution is often seen within 1 to 5 years.

HPV also causes *focal epithelial hyperplasia* in the oral cavity (types 13 and 32), primarily affecting indigenous populations of Central and South America, Alaska, and Greenland. *Epidermodysplasia verruciformis*, consisting of extensive cutaneous warts that remain for life, is caused by types 5 and 8. The disease begins in infancy or childhood with multiple lesions on the face, trunk, and extremities, and one-third of patients develop invasive squamous cell carcinoma.

B. Epidemiology and transmission. HPV is the most common pathogen transmitted by sexual contact, and anogenital warts are the most common viral sexually transmitted disease in the United States. The lifetime risk for genital HPV infection in women in developed countries is approximately 80%. The prevalence of genital HPV among sexually active college women is greater than 40% and is directly related to the number of lifetime sexual partners and to recent changes in sexual partners. The prevalence is higher among women who are HIV positive. Infected mothers can transmit the virus to newborns during the birth process, resulting in anogenital warts or recurrent respiratory papillomatosis. Only a few hundred cases of the latter are thought to occur annually in the United States; risk factors include first-order birth and young maternal age.

Cutaneous or so-called common warts are prevalent among school-aged children, whereas plantar warts are more common among adolescents and young adults. Persons at high risk because of frequent skin trauma include butchers, meat packers, and fish handlers. Cutaneous warts are transmitted by close personal contact, and minor trauma at the site of inoculation may be important.

C. Rationale for vaccine use. In the United States, well over 1 million HPV infections occur each year, resulting in approximately 13,000 cases of cervical cancer; as many as 500,000 annual cases are diagnosed worldwide. Although pap smear screening for preneoplastic lesions and appropriate treatment can prevent the development of most cervical cancers, an HPV vaccine that provided immunity to types 16 and 18 would be the most cost-effective prevention method. Such a vaccine would also impact the incidence of squamous cell cancers of the vulva, vagina, penis, and anus. Cost savings would be realized not only by disease prevention but also by the reduced need for screening. Therapeutic vaccines might have a role in treating established cervical cancers.

D. Target population. The most appropriate timing for vaccination would be before the onset of sexual activity, for example, at the middle school check-up or vaccination visit. Both females and males would be targeted, because males act as vectors. The infrastructure for delivery of such a vaccine is present in the United States but not in developing countries, where it may be easier to incorporate a vaccine into the routine infant schedule.

E. Candidate vaccines. In animal studies, neutralizing antibodies have been shown to protect against HPV infection. Viruslike particles (VLPs) containing surface proteins of HPV but lacking DNA induce neutralizing antibodies and are good candidates for prophylactic vaccines. VLPs consisting of type 16 alone or type 16 plus other types (6, 11, and 18) are being evaluated in clinical trials. These vaccines consist of capsid proteins (L1 and/or L2) or nonstructural proteins (E1, E2, E6, and/or E7). A VLP vaccine consisting of HPV type 11 was recently tested in seronegative women. The vaccine induced both humoral and cellular responses. Chimeric VLPs that incorporate structural proteins fused to a nonstructural protein induce both humoral and cellular immunity and are undergoing clinical evaluation.

In a recent double-blind study, 2,392 women 16 to 23 years of age were randomized to receive three doses of placebo or an HPV-16 VLP vaccine, consisting of a yeast-derived L1 capsid combined with alum adjuvant and developed by Merck. The vaccine was given at 0, 2, and 6 months, and the women were followed for a median of 17.4 months. The vaccine was well tolerated and induced strong antibody responses. Among 1,533 women whose baseline studies were negative, the incidence of HPV infection was 3.8 per 100 woman years in the placebo group and 0 per 100 woman years in the vaccine group; the calculated efficacy was 100%, with the lower limit of the 95% confidence interval being 90%.

Therapeutic vaccines are directed against oncogenic proteins such as E6 and E7, which are expressed in all HPV-associated cancers and premalignant lesions. CTL responses to these proteins may be important in clearance of the infection and prevention of progression to cancer. Recombinant vaccinia viruses encoding HPV-16 and HPV-18 E6 and E7 oncogenes have been evaluated in clinical studies. The vaccines were apparently safe but induced CTLs in only a minority of patients with preinvasive and invasive cancers. An alternative approach using dendritic cells that express HPV-16 E7 peptide is being evaluated.

Challenges to effective HPV vaccines include the development of better protection at the mucosal surface and induction of long-lasting immunity. In addition, whereas most cervical cancers are caused by four HPV types, the remaining 20% are due to many other types. The optimal vaccine valency, route of administration, and type of the vaccine are all unresolved. Therapeutic vaccines face even greater challenges because the immune mechanisms responsible for regression of established cancerous lesions are not well understood, and cancerous epithelial cells are efficient at avoiding interaction with the immune system.

VIII. **Live-attenuated influenza.** Discussion of the disease, epidemiology and transmission, and target populations can be found in Chapter 7(III). The rationale for an intranasal influenza vaccine is predominantly ease of administration, increased use, broader immune response, induction of mucosal immunity, ability to rapidly update the vaccine in the event of antigenic changes, and the possibility of cross-strain protection. The recent appearance of virulent strains of influenza A(H5N1) in Southeast Asia and the potential for pandemic spread underscore the need for vaccines with these advantages.

Cold-adapted strains of influenza virus were developed by serial passage in chick embryo cells at successively lower temperatures. These temperature-sensitive mutants grow at 77°F (25°C), but their replication is restricted at 100.4° to 102.2°F (38° to 39°C). The strains have been used as the basis for live-attenuated influenza vaccines (LAIVs) because they replicate in the cooler temperatures of the upper airway, inducing broad systemic and mucosal immune responses but few symptoms. However, they do not replicate in the warmer environment of the lower airways and are therefore incapable of causing pneumonia or other more serious influenza syndromes. To prepare vaccine for a given season, the parental cold-adapted strain is cocultured with the prevailing epidemic strains; reassortants that contain six internal genes from the cold-adapted strain plus the hemagglutinin and neuraminidase genes from the prevailing strains are selected. These reassortants have the temperature-sensitive and cold-adapted phenotype of the parental strain but induce immunity to the prevailing strains. One potential concern is that LAIVs could reassort with wild-type influenza viruses, acquiring internal genes that would result in reversion to virulence or the introduction of new phenotypes into the community.

Since 1976, monovalent, bivalent, and trivalent LAIVs have been evaluated in individuals of all ages. These studies have confirmed that the vaccines are genetically stable and well tolerated. Although the vaccine virus is shed in low titer for as long as 9 days, horizontal transmission is very unusual. Reversion to virulence or wild phenotype has not been observed. Demonstrable immune responses include serum antibodies, IgA in nasal secretions, T-cell responses, and interferon production. Cell-mediated responses against heterologous strains of influenza have been seen, something which does not occur with the inactivated vaccine.

In 1985, a controlled trial comparing one candidate LAIV for strains A(H1N1) and A(H3N2) to a trivalent inactivated vaccine was initiated. A total of 5,210 subjects aged 1 to 65 years were enrolled. Efficacy of the live and inactivated vaccines against culture-proved influenza A(H1N1) was 85% and 76%, respectively, and efficacy against influenza A(H3N2) was 58% and 74%, respectively. Efficacy in vaccinees younger than 16 years of age was somewhat better but still comparable. Some studies do show, however, better and longer-lasting efficacy of LAIV in children as compared to that of inactivated vaccine.

In experiments using LAIV as a challenge, subjects previously immunized with LAIV shed less virus than those previously immunized with inactivated vaccine. These results suggest that LAIV may reduce carriage of natural influenza virus and help to control spread of infection in the community. In an ongoing open-label study in central Texas, greater than 16,000 children between 18 months and 18 years of age are targeted for immunization with LAIV to determine whether herd immunity will be operative. Safety data from the first 2 years of the study (7,448 children given 9,548 doses) have demonstrated no increase in health care use during the first 14 days after vaccination and no reports of serious adverse reactions.

LAIVs appear to be safe in high-risk adults with chronic obstructive pulmonary disease. A controlled trial conducted in 662 elderly residents of long-term care facilities showed better protection in subjects given both LAIV and inactivated vaccine compared to inactivated vaccine alone. Other studies have demonstrated the safety of LAIV in patients with cystic fibrosis.

In a controlled study of seronegative adults who were subsequently challenged with wild-type viruses, efficacy of trivalent LAIV against infection was 85%, and efficacy of inactivated vaccine was 71%. Trivalent LAIV was then evaluated in a multicenter placebo-controlled study involving 1,602 children 15 to 71 months of age; most of them received two doses 60 days apart. Low-grade fever was more common 2 days after the first dose of vaccine, and rhinorrhea or nasal congestion was more common on days 2, 3, 8, and 9 postvaccination. Efficacy was 93% against culture-proved influenza A(H3N2) and B [there was no circulation of influenza A(H1N1)]. Febrile otitis media, antibiotic usage, and medical visits were also reduced. Approximately 85% of the subjects returned for vaccination the next year, when the circulating influenza A virus was A/Sydney/5/97-like (H3N2) [the vaccine contained A/Wuhan/359/95 (H3N2)]. Despite the mismatch between vaccine and circulating strains, efficacy against influenza A that year was 92%, indicating *cross-strain protection*. Efficacy against pneumonia, other lower respiratory tract disease, and influenza-associated otitis media was also demonstrated. Children who received vaccine in the second year did not experience increased adverse reactions compared to placebo. To test for efficacy against influenza A(H1N1), vaccinated children were challenged with a monovalent cold-adapted strain. LAIV provided 83% protection against nasopharyngeal shedding of the challenge virus. A large safety trial has been conducted among 9,700 healthy children 1 to 17 years of age enrolled in the Kaiser Permanente Medical Program of Northern California. There appeared to be an increase in asthma events in LAIV recipients in children 18 to 35 months of age; none of these was considered serious and many occurred in children with a history of wheezing, even though asthma was an exclusion criterion for the study.

LAIV was developed by Aviron during the 1990s, and a biologic license application was filed with the U.S. Food and Drug Administration (FDA) in October 2000. In 2002, MedImmune acquired Aviron and partnered with Wyeth for global marketing of LAIV, with the trade name FluMist, after licensure. At the initial meeting of the Vaccines and Related Biological Products Advisory Committee (VRBPAC) in July 2002, concerns were raised about availability of efficacy data in infants and older patients, safety and efficacy with concomitant use of other vaccines, possible association with adverse respiratory events, transmissibility, and the possibility of reversion to virulence. By November 2002, data were available from 20 clinical trials including 20,228 individuals who had received at least one dose of vaccine and 8,469 who had received placebo. Based on these data, on December 17, 2002, VRBPAC recommended that the vaccine be licensed for use in healthy persons 5 to 49 years of age, and licensure was granted on June 17, 2003. Additional studies are planned to evaluate FluMist in asthmatic patients and in patients receiving other routine childhood vaccines.

FluMist contains approximately $10^{6.5-7.5}$ infective units of LAIV (50% tissue culture–infective doses, or $TCID_{50}$) per 0.5-mL dose; each of the three influenza strains (two influenza A and one influenza B) recommended each year by the FDA is included. The vaccine is grown in eggs, harvested, purified, and stabilized with buffer containing sucrose, potassium phosphate, and monosodium glutamate. FluMist is packaged in spray applicators and must be stored frozen. When properly dispensed, the syringelike applicator sprays 0.25 mL of vaccine into each nostril. As with the inactivated vaccine, children 5 to 8 years of age receiving FluMist for the first time should receive two doses separated by at least 6 weeks. FluMist has not been tested in immunocompromised individuals or in pregnant women and is contraindicated for use in these groups. The vaccine is also contraindicated in egg-allergic individuals, those receiving aspirin therapy (because of the theoretical risk of Reye syndrome), those with a history of Guillain-Barré syndrome, and those with asthma or other medical conditions that put them at high risk for severe wild-type influenza. FluMist should not be administered concurrently with other vaccines.

IX. Meningococcal polysaccharide conjugate. Discussion of the disease, epidemiology and transmission, and target populations can be found in Chapter 8(VII). The main rationale for a meningococcal conjugate vaccine (MCV) is the ability to introduce routine immunization into infancy. Additional benefits would include better immunogenicity in high-risk individuals, robust immunologic memory, and the possibility of eliminating nasopharyngeal carriage and interrupting spread.

Covalent linkage of polysaccharides to carrier proteins imparts *T-cell dependent* properties, including immunogenicity in infants, induction of memory, and booster responses with subsequent doses. None of these beneficial phenomena occur with polysaccharide antigens alone, because they behave as *T-cell independent* antigens. Hib conjugate vaccines [see Chapter 5(II)] have virtually eliminated invasive Hib disease in the United States, and pneumococcal conjugates [Chapter 5(VI)] hold similar promise. Part of the success of Hib conjugates has been their ability to reduce nasopharyngeal carriage, thus interrupting transmission and protecting unvaccinated persons through herd immunity. The highest-risk period for meningococcal disease is during the first 2 years of life, a time when the licensed quadrivalent Men-PS vaccine is not very effective, especially for serogroups C, Y, and W-135. For these reasons, there has been great interest in conjugate vaccines linking the serogroup A, C, Y, and W-135 polysaccharides to carrier proteins. Unfortunately, this approach will probably not work for serogroup B because it is inherently not immunogenic.

Candidate vaccines use serogroup A and C polysaccharides conjugated to CRM_{197} (cross-reactive material, a mutant diphtheria toxin), the same protein used in HibTITER (HbOC) and Prevnar (PCV-7), or tetanus toxoid, as in ActHIB (PRP-T). In phase II studies, MCV-A/C and MCV-C have demonstrated excellent safety, improved immunogenicity, and the ability to induce immunologic memory and elicit booster responses. After immunization with MCV-C at 2, 3, and 4 months of age, 75% of infants tested at 12 months of age had adequate levels of bactericidal antibody. In a separate study, 5-year-old children had low levels of antibody after infant immunization with MCV-A/C, but immunologic memory was demonstrated by booster responses to pure polysaccharide. Mucosal IgG, but not IgA, has been demonstrated in saliva samples taken after infant immunization with MCV-C. The most common reactions to MCVs are mild injection-site redness, tenderness, and swelling; irritability and fever in infants; and headache and malaise in adolescents and adults.

Administration of MCVs concurrently with other routine childhood immunizations has not resulted in interference with antibody responses. There have been some concerns that repeated exposure to pure polysaccharides, particularly serogroups A and C, can result in *immunologic hyporesponsiveness*; that is, the rise in antibody after the second dose is significantly lower than the rise after the first dose (even though a rise *does* occur). In adults, this hyporesponsiveness can be overcome with MCVs. Infants younger than 1 year of age at the time of polysaccharide immunization may still demonstrate hyporesponsiveness even after MCV, but this does not appear to be the case for older children. The clinical implications of hyporesponsiveness are not clear.

During the 1990s, increased serogroup C disease was seen in the United Kingdom, with a disproportionate number of cases in adolescents, attracting considerable public concern and media interest. Manufacturers of MCV-C were solicited by the government, and three new vaccines were licensed in 1999 based on immunogenicity data alone: Meningitec (CRM_{197} conjugate, Wyeth), Menjugate (CRM_{197} conjugate, Chiron), and Neisvac (tetanus toxoid conjugate, Baxter). In November 1999, the United Kingdom became the first country to institute universal immunization of children with MCV-C. The target population was 15 million children in the first 12 months. First priority was given to adolescents between 15 and 17 years of age, followed by school-based immunization of 5 to 17 year olds and then practice-based immunization of children younger than 5 years of age. The youngest infants were given three doses at 2, 3, and 4 months of age; infants aged 5 to 11 months were given two doses; and children 12 months of age or older were given a single dose. For all age groups combined, the incidence of serogroup C disease decreased 87% between 1999 and 2001, and the number of deaths decreased from 67 in 1999 to five in 2001. Vaccine coverage has exceeded 80% in all of the targeted age groups. Efficacy over a 21-month period has been estimated at 92% in infants, 89% in toddlers, and at least 92% in older children and adolescents. There is also evidence for herd immunity, in that serogroup C disease decreased 34% and 61% in unvaccinated 9 to 14 year olds and 15 to 17 year olds, respectively. Nasopharyngeal carriage of *N. meningitidis* serogroup C decreased by 70% in children younger than 18 years of age, and there has been no evidence of strain replacement or capsular switching to other serogroups. The vaccine has been well tolerated.

It is hoped that MCVs will be available in the United States in the next few years. Recently, the proportion of cases due to serogroup Y has increased, and outbreaks of W-135 disease have occurred; therefore a conjugate vaccine including these serogroups would be preferable. A vaccine containing polysaccharides from serogroups A, C, Y, and W-135 conjugated to diphtheria toxoid (Menactra, Aventis Pasteur) has been tested in adults. Only 1 of 89 subjects reported fever, and one reported severe reactogenicity; 65% to 100% of subjects had a fourfold increase in serum bactericidal antibody, depending on dose and serogroup analyzed.

In the meningitis belt of Africa, MCV-A would help reduce both endemic and epidemic disease. MCVs also may be used to control community or regional outbreaks. Ongoing studies are evaluating the effects of different protein carriers on immunogenicity, efficacy against invasive disease, duration of protection, and effect on nasopharyngeal carriage. Duration of protection is critical because meningococcal disease may occur at any age, and vaccination in infancy must provide decades-long protection. Alternatively, periodic boosters may be necessary. Other concerns include the possibility of increased carriage of meningococcal strains not included in the vaccine.

Combination meningitis vaccines comprised of meningococcal, pneumococcal, and Hib conjugates are being evaluated. However, immunologic interference caused by the administration of multiple vaccines using the same carrier protein (*carrier-induced epitopic suppression*) may become a problem [see Chapter 6(I)].

Immunization against serogroup B disease represents a special problem. The polysaccharide is homologous to glycopeptides of human neuronal adhesion molecules and is therefore not recognized as "nonself" by the immune system. Approaches to a serogroup B vaccine include chemical modification of the polysaccharide molecule, the use of outer membrane proteins, and vesicles made up of bacterial lipid membranes containing outer membrane proteins. Outer membrane vesicle vaccines have been tested in Brazil (in combination with C polysaccharide), Norway, and the Netherlands. Variable immunogenicity has been seen, but memory can be demonstrated. In Cuba, an outer membrane vesicle vaccine called VA-MENGOC-BC was developed to control clonal serogroup B disease. The incidence of serogroup B disease dropped from 14 per 100,000 in 1984 to less than 2 per 100,000 in 1999, and the vaccine is now part of the routine infant immunization schedule.

X. **Increased valency pneumococcal polysaccharide conjugates.** Discussion of the disease, epidemiology and transmission, and target populations can be found in Chapters 5(VI) and 7(II). The main rationale for increasing the valency of pneumococcal conjugate vaccines is to protect more infants and, potentially, more adults from invasive pneumococcal infection.

More than 90 serotypes of *S. pneumoniae* have been described, but a relatively limited number cause the majority of invasive infections in children. Prevnar (PCV-7) contains the seven serotypes (4, 6B, 9V, 14, 18C, 19F, and 23F) that account for 80% of invasive disease in children younger than 6 years of age in the United States. However, serotype prevalence differs by age group and geographic location. For example, these same seven serotypes account for only 50% to 60% of isolates among persons aged 6 years or older. Types 1 and 5 account for some cases in the United States but are more common in Western Europe and in certain developing countries. In many developing countries, only half of invasive childhood isolates are covered by PCV-7, and in Asia only 30% are covered. In addition, serotype distribution differs by clinical syndrome. For example, PCV-7 serotypes account for only 60% to 70% of middle-ear isolates from children younger than 24 months of age.

In young children, a 9-valent vaccine that includes serotypes 1 and 5 would cover 85% of invasive isolates in developed countries and 70% in developing countries. An 11-valent vaccine that, in addition, includes serotypes 3 and 7F would result in greater than 80% coverage in all regions except Asia, where coverage would still be a respectable 76%. In older children and adults, a 9-valent vaccine would cover greater than 60% in nearly all regions except Asia, where coverage would be approximately 55%. An 11-valent vaccine would cover greater than 70% of invasive strains, even in Asia.

Wyeth is evaluating a 9-valent vaccine (PCV-9) that is similar to Prevnar (PCV-7) but includes serotypes 1 and 5. As in PCV-7, the protein carrier is CRM_{197}. In a double-blind study, 500 South African children were given PCV-9 or placebo at 6, 10, and 14 weeks of age. The vaccine was well tolerated and immunogenic for all nine serotypes. Importantly, at 9 months of age, nasopharyngeal carriage rates of vaccine serotypes were 18% and 36% in the vaccine and placebo groups, respectively, and carriage rates of penicillin-resistant pneumococci were 21% and 41%, respectively. In contrast, carriage of nonvaccine serotypes was higher in the vaccine group. Two studies conducted in Gambian infants have confirmed the safety and immunogenicity of the vaccine when administered at 2, 3, and 4 months of age. In the first study, there was no significant reduction of nasopharyngeal carriage of vaccine serotypes. In the second study, there was no interference with antibody response due to coadministration of DTP/HbOC (Tetramune), except possibly some interference with responses to pertussis toxoid.

In a controlled study in eight day care centers in Israel, 264 toddlers 12 to 35 months of age were given one or two doses of PCV-9 or a control vaccine. During a 2-year surveillance period, nasopharyngeal carriage of vaccine serotypes was significantly lower in vaccinees compared with controls (13.0% vs. 21.3%, respectively), but carriage of nonvaccine serotypes was significantly higher in the vaccinees (43.7% vs. 34.1%). Reductions of 15% to 17% were seen in upper respiratory infections, lower respiratory diseases, otitis media, and antibiotic days in the vaccine group compared with the control group. Children younger than 36 months of age appeared to benefit more from vaccination than older children.

In a recent U.S. study, 948 infants were randomized to receive one of the following vaccine regimens at 2, 4, and 6 months of age: (a) Prevnar (PCV-7) coadministered with HibTITER (HbOC), (b) PCV-9-MCV-C (nine pneumococcal serotypes and meningococcal serogroup C polysaccharide conjugated to CRM_{197}) coadministered with HibTITER (HbOC), or (c) PCV-9-MCV-C combined with HbOC (PCV-9-MCV-C/HbOC). Antibody responses to the pneumococcal serotypes were similar in each group, but the responses to the Hib component were inferior in infants given PCV-9-MCV-C/HbOC compared to responses in those given HbOC separately. The mechanism of interference may be carrier-induced epitopic suppression [see Chapter 6(I)].

Another candidate vaccine manufactured by Aventis Pasteur consists of 11 serotypes (PCV-11): all of those in PCV-9 plus serotypes 3 and 7F. To reduce the risk of carrier-induced epitopic suppression, this vaccine is produced using two different protein carriers. Serotypes 1, 4, 5, 7F, 9V, 19F, and 23F are conjugated to tetanus toxoid, and serotypes 3, 6B, 14, and 18C are conjugated to diphtheria toxoid. A single dose of the vaccine given to Finnish and Israeli toddlers was well tolerated and induced adequate antibody responses to most of the serotypes, although the responses to 6B, 14, and 23F were weak. In another study, PCV-11 was administered to 50 Filipino infants at ages 6, 10, and 14 weeks, with a booster dose at 9 months. Antibody responses to most of the serotypes were adequate, except for responses to serotypes 6B, 14, and 18C.

XI. Parainfluenza virus

Parainfluenza virus (PIV) is an enveloped virus with a single-stranded, nonsegmented RNA genome that is closely related to respiratory syncytial virus (RSV).

A. **Disease.** PIV causes a variety of respiratory illnesses in persons of all ages. PIV is responsible for up to one-fourth of lower respiratory infections (LRIs) and tracheobronchitis, one-half of upper respiratory infections (URIs) and laryngitis, and two-thirds of cases of croup. Four serotypes have been described (PIV1, PIV2, PIV3, and PIV4), and these have substantial serologic cross-reactivity. URI, or the *common cold*, is caused by all serotypes and presents with rhinorrhea, sneezing, pharyngitis, and cough, usually lasting 3 or 4 days. *Laryngitis*, characterized by loss of voice, is common. *Croup*, or *laryngotracheobronchitis*, is most often caused by PIV1. The peak age is 6 months to 2 years, and typical symptoms include a barking or brassy cough, inspiratory stridor, and retractions. The onset may be sudden and the cough may be *spasmodic*. Some children with a history of croup have abnormalities of lung function for years after the infection. PIV3 is the second most common cause of *bronchiolitis*, characterized by URI symptoms and wheezing of somewhat lesser severity than that seen with RSV. The peak age is 6 to 12 months. *Pneumonia* may occur in immunocompromised children and adults. PIV may cause apnea in neonates and has been associated with sudden infant death syndrome. PIV also may cause serious respiratory infections in adults, especially the elderly and those with underlying medical conditions. Complications of PIV infection include otitis media and bacterial sinusitis, and rare manifestations include parotitis, myopericarditis, and encephalitis.

B. **Epidemiology and transmission.** PIV infections typically occur early in life, but reinfections may occur at any age. Virtually all children acquire the infection by 3 to 5 years of age. Infection with PIV3 usually occurs at an earlier age than PIV1 or PIV2. Primary infection in the first 2 years of life is often associated with lower respiratory tract disease. In contrast, reinfections are usually mild, resulting only in cold symptoms. PIV4 is the least common reported serotype causing illness, but this may be due to difficulties in laboratory diagnosis. Outbreaks of PIV3 have been described in neonatal nurseries and pediatric wards. Seasonal patterns have been observed with some of the serotypes—PIV1 occurs in the fall of odd-numbered years, and PIV2 has demonstrated periodicity unique to each geographic region—but PIV3 occurs year-round (although in some areas it may be seen more often between spring and fall).

Transmission occurs by exposure to large droplets of infected respiratory secretions. Autoinoculation of mucous membranes commonly occurs from contaminated hands. Children exposed to PIV3 in closed settings are nearly universally infected; exposure to PIV1 and PIV2 causes infection in two-thirds to three-fourths of children. PIV1 is shed for 4 to 7 days after primary infection, but PIV3 may be shed for as long as 4 weeks. PIV can survive for up to 4 hours on porous surfaces and 10 hours on nonporous surfaces.

C. **Rationale for vaccine use.** As many as 6 million PIV infections occur annually in the United States. In one estimate, these infections result in 250,000 annual visits to the emergency department (with costs exceeding $50 million) and 70,000 hospitalizations (with costs exceeding $140 million). Epidemics of PIV1-induced croup may result in 77,000 emergency department visits, subsequent hospitalizations, and costs of $27 million. Substantial morbidity would be prevented and medical and societal costs saved by an effective vaccine.

D. **Target population.** Infants younger than one year of age would benefit most from vaccination against PIV3. However, protection would be difficult to achieve in the first few months of life unless pregnant women were vaccinated and babies were protected by passive antibodies. Toddlers would benefit most from PIV1 and PIV2 vaccines. Adults with chronic underlying medical conditions and the elderly also would benefit from an effective PIV vaccine.

E. **Candidate vaccines.** The first vaccines developed for prevention of PIV were formalin inactivated and contained one, two, or three PIV serotypes. These vaccines were highly immunogenic in seronegative children and induced fourfold rises in neutralizing antibodies in seropositive children. Unfortunately, the vaccines were not protective against PIV infection in clinical trials. Subunit vaccines have been developed using the surface hemagglutinin-neuraminidase (HN) and fusion (F) glycoproteins. Specifically, PIV3 vaccine candidates with HN and F proteins were immunogenic in animals and provided protection against live-virus challenge. However, progress with these subunit vaccines has been slowed by evidence of relatively poor immunogenicity in seronegative subjects.

Recently, live-attenuated PIV vaccine candidates have been tested using intranasal administration, similar to the live-attenuated influenza vaccine. Wild-type PIV was adapted to growth at low temperatures to allow for replication in the cooler upper airway but not in the warmer lower airways. One such cold-adapted strain called HPIV3cp18 was protective in animal models but caused rhinorrhea and wheezing in some seronegative children. A further attenuated strain called HPIV3cp45 was administered intranasally to infants older than 6 months of age. The vaccine was well tolerated, infected 86% of the recipients, and induced serum antibody titers in 81% of vaccinees. HPIV3cp45 will be further studied in phase II trials.

Another approach uses a live bovine PIV3 strain (BPIV3) administered intranasally. BPIV3 is closely related to human PIV3 and is naturally attenuated in the human host. Restricted replication of this virus was confirmed in an adult study. Intranasal BPIV3 vaccine was well tolerated and immunogenic in seronegative and seropositive children as young as 2 months of age. BPIV3 successfully infected 92% of children 6 to 60 months of age, and 92% and 61% developed antibody responses to bovine and human PIV3, respectively. In another study, the vaccine infected 92% of infants younger than 6 months of age, and antibody responses to BPIV3 were induced in 67% and to HPIV3 in 42%. When present, maternal antibody interfered with antibody responses. Recently, BPIV3 vaccine was administered to infants at 2, 4, 6, and 12 months of age. The vaccine was well tolerated and induced antibody responses in the majority of recipients. Larger scale studies of BPIV3 vaccine are planned.

Sendai virus has been explored as a possible vaccine candidate for protection against PIV1 because of its antigenic relatedness and because Sendai virus is attenuated, stable, and immunogenic in a mouse model.

Reverse genetics has been used to identify regions of cold-passaged PIV that contribute to attenuation. These mutations can be inserted into cDNA to produce attenuated vaccine candidates. One such chimeric virus consists of BPIV3 in which the genes encoding the HN and F proteins have been replaced by those of human PIV3. This vaccine, designated rB/HPIV3, demonstrated attenuation and immunogenicity in rhesus monkeys. Another vaccine candidate has the HPIV3cp45 backbone with the HN and F proteins of human PIV1 inserted. This recombinant chimeric virus, rHPIV3-1cp45, was attenuated and immunogenic in African green monkeys and demonstrated protection against challenge with wild-type PIV1. In addition, the HN and F genes of PIV1 and PIV2 have been inserted into an infectious clone of the PIV3 genome to produce a vaccine that might protect against all three serotypes.

XII. Respiratory syncytial virus. Discussion of the disease, epidemiology and transmission, and target populations can be found in Chapter 11(IV). Although passive prophylaxis is available in the form of RSV-mAb (palivizumab), this approach is only targeted to infants at the highest risk for complicated RSV disease, and it is extremely expensive. In the United States each year, 3.5 to 4 million children younger than 4 years of age acquire RSV infection, and more than 100,000 are hospitalized, resulting in costs of approximately $300 million. Worldwide, acute respiratory infections are responsible for an estimated 4 million annual deaths in children younger than 5 years of age, and RSV is responsible for most of this mortality. Although infants with predisposing conditions have high rates of morbidity and mortality, the overall burden of RSV disease at the population level falls on healthy children, as virtually all children are infected. For this reason, universal vaccination represents the only viable option for significant reduction of morbidity. Recent epidemiologic data suggest that RSV contributes to more than 17,000 adult deaths each year, the majority in individuals 65 years of age or older.

Primary benefits of a universal vaccine program would be prevention of lower respiratory tract disease, hospitalization, and death. Secondary goals would include decreases in otitis media and reduction of antibiotic use in children with respiratory illnesses. Priority targets would include infants and prepregnant or pregnant women (to provide protection to newborns). Special target populations would include older children and adults with chronic respiratory conditions, including asthma, cystic fibrosis, bronchopulmonary dysplasia, premature birth, congenital heart disease, congenital immunodeficiencies, secondary immunosuppression, malnutrition, and advanced age. Prevention of *infection* would be an ideal outcome, but this may not be achievable; prevention of *disease* alone would be acceptable, but would be less likely to provide protection at the population level through herd immunity.

Targeting an RSV vaccine does present major challenges. The most severe infections occur in infants younger than 6 months of age. Multiple doses of a vaccine will probably be required during this period of immunologic immaturity. In addition, maternal antibodies may interfere with vaccine response. High-risk populations, such as premature infants, patients with congenital heart disease or chronic lung conditions, immunosuppressed patients, and the elderly present other unique challenges, especially for live vaccines. Concern for the safety of vaccine testing in infants, especially with live-attenuated candidates, requires a slow progression of clinical trials.

There are other challenges to the development of an effective vaccine for RSV. Preclinical testing of vaccine candidates has been hampered by the lack of an ideal animal model. Perhaps the most important reason for the delay in bringing a vaccine to licensure is the early experience with formalin-inactivated RSV vaccines. Infants and children given these vaccine candidates in the late 1960s developed more severe infection, and even death, when subsequently exposed to wild-type RSV. Depending on the age of vaccination, RSV pneumonia occurred in 69% to 80% of vaccinees as compared with only 4% to 5% of unvaccinated controls. The inactivated vaccine induced high titers of antibody to the fusion protein but relatively low titers of virus-neutralizing antibodies. Vaccinees also developed abnormal *in vitro* lymphocyte responses to RSV. In a mouse model, inactivated RSV induced stronger T–helper cell type 2 (Th-2) responses than cytotoxic Th-1 responses. This immunologic imbalance may have led to enhanced disease by delaying the clearance of wild-type virus. This experience and the lack of a compete immunologic explanation inhibited vaccine development for many years.

RSV contains two surface components—the G (attachment) and F glycoproteins—that have been used in subunit vaccines. Antibody to the F glycoprotein is cross-reactive between RSV subgroups (RSV is divided in A and B subgroups), but antibody to the G protein is subgroup specific. Purified F protein (PFP) subunit vaccine candidates have been developed by Wyeth. In a study of seropositive children 18 to 36 months of age, a first-generation vaccine (purified 90% to 95% by affinity chromatography), PFP-1, was well tolerated and immunogenic, and it protected vaccinees against clinical RSV disease during a 6-month follow-up period. A second-generation vaccine (purified more than 99.9% by ion-exchange chromatography), PFP-2, was shown to be safe, immunogenic, and protective in patients with BPD. PFP-2 has also been given to women during the third trimester of pregnancy. The vaccine was well tolerated, had no adverse effects on the newborn, and was immunogenic; in addition, maternal antibodies were efficiently transferred to the infant. Recently, a third-generation vaccine (made from the attenuated 248/404 strain), PFP-3, was tested in healthy adults and children with cystic fibrosis. Unlike formalin-inactivated vaccines, PFP vaccines induce strong F-protein responses as well as neutralizing antibodies, and there has been no evidence of enhancement of wild-type disease.

A novel recombinant subunit vaccine has been produced by the Centre d'Immunologie Pierre Fabre (Saint-Julien-en-Genevois, France). It consists of the conserved central domain of the RSV G protein (G2Na) fused to the albumin-binding region of streptococcal G protein. This vaccine, designated BBG2Na, was well tolerated and immunogenic in a study of 108 adults. Aventis Pasteur also has developed a subunit vaccine containing the F, G, and M proteins of RSV. Two phase I trials have been conducted in adults comparing an aluminum phosphate adjuvant and a novel adjuvant called poly[di(carboxylatophenoxy)phosphazene]. Both formulations were well tolerated and immunogenic, and phase II trials are planned. A number of other subunit vaccines using combinations of the F and G proteins and new adjuvants are in preclinical development. Both parenteral and intranasal administration are being tested.

Live-attenuated vaccine candidates developed at the NIH and Wyeth have undergone extensive testing in animals and humans. As with the live-attenuated influenza vaccine, candidate strains have been cold-passaged (*cp*) and/or have undergone chemical mutagenesis to produce temperature-sensitive (*ts*) strains that replicate only below

98.6°F (37°C). Candidate vaccines are selected for genetic stability and attenuated phenotype in animal models. These vaccines are administered intranasally, replicate on mucosal surfaces (even in the presence of maternal antibodies), do not replicate in the lower airways, and induce humoral, cellular, and mucosal immune responses.

Two vaccines, designated *cpts*530/1009 and *cpts*248/955, are genetically stable, immunogenic in animal models, highly attenuated in adult volunteers, and immunogenic in seronegative children. However, these strains are shed at high titers and are transmitted to seronegative contacts with a frequency of 20% to 25%. A more attenuated strain called *cpts*248/404 was evaluated in infants and children. Although it was well tolerated and immunogenic in infants older than 6 months of age, it caused unacceptable nasal congestion in younger infants. Live-attenuated vaccines will continue to be tested in children. However, safety issues in seronegative infants must be addressed. Immune responses may be insufficient to prevent severe RSV disease in the youngest infants, and genetic stability may not be fully elucidated until these vaccines are used in large populations.

Other approaches to vaccine development include site-directed mutagenesis to produce strains that are ideally attenuated and genetically stable, as well as the creation of chimeric live viruses that contain proteins from both RSV subgroups or from different viruses. For example, the genes for human RSV G and F proteins have been placed into a recombinant bovine-human parainfluenza virus. Such a vaccine might be used to protect infants against both RSV and PIV infections.

XIII. Rotavirus

Rotavirus is a nonenveloped, double-stranded RNA virus whose genome is divided into 11 segments, each of which encodes a different viral protein.

A. Disease. Rotavirus gastroenteritis has an incubation period of 1 to 4 days. Illness begins suddenly with vomiting, diarrhea, and fever and lasts for 4 to 8 days. There may be more than 20 daily episodes of vomiting and/or diarrhea during the peak of the illness. Severe vomiting may lead to dehydration even before the diarrhea begins. Associated symptoms include irritability, lethargy, pharyngitis, rhinitis, cervical lymphadenopathy, and otitis media. Two-thirds of patients hospitalized with rotavirus experience a transient rise of hepatic transaminase levels. Common complications include isotonic dehydration, electrolyte disturbances, metabolic acidosis, and temporary milk intolerance. Rare complications include necrotizing enterocolitis and hemorrhagic gastroenteritis. Immunocompromised patients may develop particularly severe or fatal illness and may shed virus in the stool for months. When infected, adults are usually asymptomatic, but outbreaks in nursing homes have led to symptomatic disease and several fatalities in the elderly.

B. Epidemiology and transmission. Worldwide, rotavirus is the most common cause of severe gastroenteritis in children, responsible for 20% to 50% of hospitalizations for vomiting and diarrhea. In developed countries, virtually all children experience at least one rotaviral infection by 4 years of age. In developing countries, the first infection occurs earlier. For example, in Mexico, one-third of children experience their first infection by 3 months of age. For unknown reasons, infections before this age are usually asymptomatic, but after 3 months of age, initial infection is usually symptomatic and the illness may be severe. Reinfections with rotavirus are common and are usually mild or asymptomatic. Outbreaks and nosocomial spread occur frequently in day care centers, pediatric hospital wards, and nurseries.

In most areas of the world, rotavirus has a distinct seasonal pattern. In the United States, for example, annual epidemics begin in the late fall in the Southwest and spread to the North and East by the end of winter or early spring. In the tropics, rotavirus may occur at any time of the year. Multiple rotavirus strains occur worldwide, but the most common types (based on VP7 serotypes, as below) are G1, G2, G3, and G4, accounting for 90% of infections.

Transmission occurs through the fecal-oral route, airborne droplets, and contaminated fomites. Infected children shed the virus in high quantities. Rotavirus is highly contagious and survives well in the environment. Because rotavirus is not spread by fecally contaminated food or water, improvements in water sanitation and hygiene do not affect the incidence of disease.

C. Rationale for vaccine use. The tremendous burden of rotavirus disease justifies development of an effective vaccine. In the United States, approximately 2.7 million episodes of rotaviral gastroenteritis occur annually, resulting in 600,000 medical visits, 50,000 hospitalizations, and 20 to 40 deaths. The annual direct and indirect medical costs are estimated at $1.1 billion. In developing countries as a whole, there are an estimated 100 million episodes of rotaviral illness each year, of which 16 million can be characterized as moderate or severe. As many as 1 million deaths occur annually.

D. Target population. Infants younger than 2 years of age would benefit the most from a vaccine, because infections are most severe at this age. Older children and adults experience few, if any, symptoms with reinfection, although they may contribute to the spread of virus to susceptible infants. It is possible that the elderly may benefit from vaccination as well.

E. Candidate vaccines. Rotavirus consists of two major surface proteins, VP4 and VP7, which elicit serotype-specific neutralizing antibodies. VP7 is also called the *G protein* and has four predominant serotypes, designated G1, G2, G3, and G4. Any effective vaccine must provide protection against all four of these serotypes. VP4 is also called the *P protein* and is more difficult to differentiate serologically between strains. All of the vaccines discussed below are administered by the oral route.

The first rotavirus vaccine was produced from Nebraska calf diarrhea virus (a bovine rotavirus). In clinical trials, it provided marginal benefit with efficacy rates of 40% to 58%. Another bovine rotavirus vaccine called WC3 demonstrated 100% protection against severe rotavirus disease in an efficacy study in Philadelphia, but poor efficacy was demonstrated in subsequent studies. The first rhesus rotavirus vaccine (RRV), called MMU 18006, was notable for the development of fevers 3 to 4 days after vaccination in some studies and for efficacy rates that varied from 0% to 65%. All of these vaccine candidates were withdrawn from further development because of disappointing efficacy. Recently, a lamb strain of rotavirus produced by the Lanzhou Institute of Biological Products was licensed in China.

Second generation live vaccines have been constructed by generating reassortants between animal and human rotaviruses. In essence, these vaccines have the genetic backbone and phenotype of the animal strain but, because they contain a gene segment from human rotavirus, they express antigenic proteins that elicit neutralizing antibodies to the human virus. The first of these vaccines to be brought to market was produced by Wyeth and was called RotaShield [see Chapter 13(III)]. It was based on a rhesus rotavirus (strain MMU 18006, passaged nine times in monkey kidney cells and seven times in fetal rhesus diploid cells) into which the human VP7 gene (G protein) had been substituted. The vaccine was actually a mixture of four viruses; the unaltered rhesus rotavirus, which provided cross-protection for human G3 rotavirus infection, plus three rhesus-human reassortant strains bearing the human G1, G2, and G4 proteins. This tetravalent vaccine contained 1×10^5 plaque-forming units of each strain and was administered orally at 2, 4, and 6 months of age. Efficacy in prelicensure trials, which involved nearly 18,000 infants, ranged from 48% to 68% against all rotavirus disease and 70% to 100% against severe rotavirus disease. Mild adverse reactions, which occurred more often after the first dose, included fever, irritability, and decreased appetite and activity. Chapter 11(III) describes events occurring postlicensure that led to the finding that RotaShield caused intussusception at a frequency of approximately 1 per 11,000 vaccinees. Several hypotheses have been proposed to explain this association. One possibility involves the relative virulence of rhesus rotavirus, which causes diarrhea in several mammalian species, hepatitis in some strains of mice, and invades gut-associated lymphoid tissue in animal models. In human infants, vaccination was associated with fever, and the virus was shed in stool. These observations taken together suggest that rhesus rotavirus is not completely attenuated; intussusception may have resulted from invasion and inflammation of lymphoid tissue in the gut, creating a lead point for intussusception. Intussusception does not appear to be associated with wild-type rotavirus infection.

Another reassortant rotavirus vaccine called RotaTeq has been developed by Merck. This is a pentavalent reassortant based on the WC3 bovine rotavirus strain consisting of a mixture of five different reassortants—four of these express different human VP7 genes (serotypes G1, G2, G3, and G4) and one expresses a human VP4 gene (serotype P1a, which is present in nearly all G1, G3, and G4 strains and some G9 strains). Clinical studies of a prototype G1 bovine-human reassortant vaccine demonstrated efficacy of 64% to 100% against all rotavirus disease and 84% to 100% against severe disease. Another prototype quadrivalent vaccine (G1, G2, G3, and P1a) demonstrated 75% efficacy against all rotavirus and 100% efficacy against severe disease.

In contrast to the rhesus reassortant vaccine (RotaShield), the bovine reassortant does not cause serious adverse events in animals. In addition, it is not associated with fever, decreased appetite, vomiting, diarrhea, or irritability in infants. Less than 5% of infants shed the vaccine in the stool after the first dose (shedding has not been seen after subsequent doses). These observations suggest that RotaTeq is more attenuated than RotaShield; hopefully, this will translate into no association with intussusception. As of July 2003, more than 50,000 infants had been enrolled in a phase III trial in the United States, Europe, and Latin America. Although there were some cases of intussusception, the characteristics of cases were consistent with background disease. Each case had been reviewed by a data safety monitoring board, which had recommended continuation of the study. Based on observations to date, a sample size of 60,000 should be adequate to determine that the vaccine is clinically acceptable for licensure.

A quadrivalent (G1 through G4) reassortant using a different bovine backbone (UK strain) is currently undergoing clinical trials. Early results show that it is well tolerated and immunogenic. Another live vaccine candidate uses a human rotavirus strain (originally designated 89-12 but now referred to as RIX-4414) that was attenuated by 33 *in vitro* passages. The vaccine, produced by GlaxoSmithKline with the trade name Rotarix, has a

VP7 serotype of G1 and a VP4 serotype of P1a. Although it consists of only one strain, it provides protection against G3 and G4 strains because they usually contain P1a. Rotarix does not replicate as well in the small intestine of infants as wild-type virus does, but it does induce rotavirus-specific neutralizing antibodies. In an efficacy trial, two doses of strain 89-12 were given to 108 children 10 to 16 months of age. During a 2-year surveillance period, efficacy was 76% against any rotavirus disease, 83% against severe disease, and 100% against rotaviral disease requiring medical intervention. Fever was noted more often in vaccinees compared with placebo recipients. Additional clinical trials are currently underway. Because wild-type rotavirus is not associated with intussusception, it is hoped that this attenuated human strain will also not cause intussusception.

Several neonatal strains of human rotavirus also are being evaluated in early clinical trials, including strain RV3 (University of Melbourne, Australia), and strains 116E and 1321 (Bharat Biotech, India). These strains are thought to be naturally attenuated because they were collected from asymptomatic neonates, but they have also been passaged in tissue culture.

Factors that may affect the reactogenicity, immunogenicity, and efficacy of orally administered live rotavirus vaccines include potential interference from OPV in regions of the world where it is still used, the quantity of infective viral particles in each dose of vaccine, and the number of doses given. All rotaviruses are rapidly inactivated in the acid environment of the stomach, so vaccines must be administered with a buffer. Maternally derived serum antibody may interfere with immunogenicity. Concern has also been raised regarding potential interference from breast-feeding, but so far there is no evidence that this affects protective efficacy.

XIV. Group A streptococcus

Group A streptococcus (GAS), also known as *Streptococcus pyogenes*, is a facultatively anaerobic, encapsulated, β-hemolytic, gram-positive coccus that produces a variety of hemolysins, streptokinases, DNAses, proteinases, and pyrogenic exotoxins.

A. Disease. GAS is best known as a cause of *exudative pharyngitis*, marked by sudden onset of fever and sore throat, frequently associated with cervical lymphadenopathy, headache, malaise, and abdominal pain. *Suppurative complications* such as tonsillar abscess can occur, and the illness may be accompanied by *scarlet fever*, marked by the development of a diffuse sandpaper-like exanthem caused by erythrogenic exotoxins. GAS also is a common cause of skin and soft tissue infections, most notably *impetigo*, *cellulitis*, and *lymphadenitis*. *Erysipelas* refers to a rapidly advancing superficial cellulitis with lymphatic involvement, characterized by bright red skin and well-demarcated induration.

Several severe, life-threatening GAS syndromes are well recognized. *Necrotizing fasciitis* is a deep soft tissue infection associated with tissue destruction and systemic toxicity; common sites of initiation include surgical wounds and varicella lesions. Deep suppurative infections such as pyomyositis, septic arthritis, and pneumonia with empyema also occur. *Severe invasive streptococcal syndrome* refers to septicemia with GAS, with or without a localized focus of infection. GAS also is a cause of *toxic shock syndrome*, characterized by hypotension and multiorgan dysfunction, a condition mediated by exotoxins that act as superantigens. Of historical note, *puerperal sepsis* was a fulminant infection of the reproductive tract in postpartum women, acquired from the contaminated hands of examiners. Semmelweis' demonstration that handwashing prevented the disease was a landmark in infection control.

Acute rheumatic fever (ARF) is the classic nonsuppurative sequela of GAS upper respiratory tract infection. Major manifestations include carditis (valvulitis), migratory large joint polyarthritis, Sydenham chorea, erythema marginatum (a serpiginous macular erythematous rash), and subcutaneous nodules along the extensor surfaces of tendons and bony prominences. Associated findings (which constitute minor diagnostic criteria) include arthralgia, fever, acute phase reaction, and first-degree heart block. Long-term complications are limited to the heart and consist of valvular dysfunction, most notably mitral insufficiency. GAS also causes *poststreptococcal arthritis*, a reactive phenomenon that falls short of the full diagnostic criteria for ARF. ARF is probably an autoimmune disease that arises in genetically predisposed hosts as the result of molecular mimicry between components of GAS and mammalian tissues. This explains the long latent period between infection and disease manifestations and the fact that only a very small proportion of individuals with GAS pharyngitis develop ARF. The diagnosis of rheumatic fever necessitates lifelong antibiotic prophylaxis to prevent recurrent GAS infection, which can trigger recurrent rheumatic fever.

The other major nonsuppurative sequela of GAS infection is *poststreptococcal glomerulonephritis* (PSGN, also known as *Bright disease*). Unlike ARF, PSGN can occur after pharyngitis or pyoderma. Renal injury probably results from deposition of immune complexes in the kidney. Hematuria and periorbital edema are the first signs, often accompanied by fever, anorexia, lethargy, and abdominal pain. Most patients develop hypertension and fluid overload, but the syndrome is usually self-limited. Occasionally complications related to severe hypertension ensue, but chronic glomerulonephritis is rare.

B. Epidemiology and transmission. GAS infections are ubiquitous, distributed worldwide, and confined to humans. Asymptomatic pharyngeal carriage rates in school children during the winter and spring range from 15% to 50%, and the organism causes approximately 20% of all cases of pharyngitis, with peak age incidence between 5 and 14 years. Overall, it is estimated that 4 million noninvasive GAS infections occur each year in the United States. In addition, there may be as many as 15,000 invasive cases, with case-fatality rates of 30% to 80% in adults. Pharyngeal infection is transmitted by respiratory droplets, and skin infection is transmitted by direct contact; fomites are not thought to play a role. Transmission of pharyngitis is facilitated in the winter when children are confined to closed spaces, and transmission of pyoderma is facilitated by warm weather and incidental breaks in the skin. There is evidence that household contacts of cases of severe invasive disease have a 200-fold increased risk of invasive disease compared to the general community; despite this evidence, a role for chemoprophylaxis has not yet been defined.

In some developing countries, the incidence of ARF approaches 300 per 100,000 population, and ARF is the most common form of acquired heart disease. Rates this high were seen in the United States until the 1940s, when, for unclear reasons, the incidence began to decline. By the early 1980s, the incidence was less than 0.5 per 100,000. However, in the mid-1980s there was a resurgence of disease in certain geographic locations, linked to the circulation of "rheumatogenic" serotypes. Antibiotic therapy for acute GAS pharyngitis is very effective in preventing ARF. Because many cases of PSGN are asymptomatic, the incidence is difficult to estimate, but it is clearly the most common cause of glomerulonephritis in children. Certain GAS strains appear to be "nephritogenic," but unlike ARF, there is no evidence that antibiotic therapy of the antecedent infection can prevent the disease.

C. Rationale for vaccine use. The burden of invasive disease alone constitutes a rationale for vaccine development, as it is comparable to the burden of other pyogenic infections such as invasive Hib disease in the prevaccine era. The morbidity and societal costs of noninvasive GAS disease add tremendously to the value of a vaccine program. Although most cases of ARF can be prevented by antibiotic therapy, it should be noted that up to a third of patients do not have antecedent symptomatic pharyngitis and, therefore, have no opportunity for treatment. The IOM estimated that a 100% effective GAS vaccine universally given in infancy would cost approximately $14,000 per QALY saved.

D. Target population. Immunization would need to occur before school age to prevent the majority of cases of pharyngitis. Vaccines targeted to invasive infections as well would need to be given in infancy.

E. Candidate vaccines. The development of a GAS vaccine has been hampered by concerns that immune responses to the organism can cause disease. In fact, early trials with crude vaccines caused ARF in some patients. One current approach is to exploit antigens that are shared among strains. For example, many strains produce a C5a peptidase, which inactivates C5a, a potent chemoattractant for neutrophils. A vaccine that induced antibodies to the peptidase would promote infiltration of neutrophils to the site of infection and perhaps limit spread. Other targets might include fibronectin binding proteins, which mediate adherence to mucosal surfaces, and the conserved C-terminal regions of surface M proteins. Streptococcal exotoxins also represent potential targets for vaccine development; although these vaccines might prevent severe invasive disease, they would be unlikely to prevent less severe infections. Unfortunately, the hyaluronate capsule is identical to the hyaluronic acid in human tissues and is therefore not immunogenic.

Type-specific immunity to GAS appears to be mediated by M-type proteins, of which there are more than 90. Early attempts at M protein vaccines were hampered by contamination of preparations with exotoxins and the demonstration that vaccinated animals developed antibodies reactive with human myocardium. More recent work has shown that the epitopes that elicit bactericidal antibodies are located on the N-terminal part of the molecule and can be separated from the epitopes that generate tissue-reactive antibodies. Thus, one approach has been to construct recombinant hybrid proteins containing N-terminal peptides of several strains linked in series. Immunization of rabbits with such hybrid molecules demonstrated type-specific M protein antibodies as well as opsonizing antibodies to the corresponding GAS strains, although responses to different serotypes were not uniform. Cross-reactive antibodies to human heart tissue were not demonstrated. Lethal challenge experiments in mice using a hexavalent hybrid peptide vaccine demonstrated significant protection, and phase I trials in humans have started.

Derivative approaches include peptides expressed by commensal vectors or linked to haptens and delivered at mucosal surfaces. There are also efforts to develop conjugate vaccines that link the group A polysaccharide to tetanus toxoid, in analogy to ActHIB (PRP-T).

XV. Group B streptococcus

Group B streptococcus (GBS), also known as *Streptococcus agalactiae*, is a facultatively anaerobic, encapsulated, β-hemolytic, gram-positive coccus that can be subdivided into serotypes based on cell-wall carbohydrate antigens.

A. Disease. GBS is best known as a cause of perinatal infection, which is divided into three distinct time periods. *Early-onset disease* usually presents within hours of birth (80% to 90% of cases) but may present as late as seven days after birth. Before the institution of maternal screening and antibiotic prophylaxis, this was the most common perinatal manifestation of GBS infection. Clinical features are indistinguishable from sepsis caused by other organisms—apnea and bradycardia, lethargy, irritability, poor feeding, pallor, decreased perfusion, respiratory distress, and, ultimately, shock. Common serotypes are I, II, III, and V. Meningitis is seen in 5% to 10% of cases, and mortality rates are as high as 10%. *Late-onset disease* commonly occurs at 3 to 4 weeks of age and presents as bacteremia or sepsis syndrome with or without meningitis. Occasionally, musculoskeletal or deep soft tissue infection is seen. Serotype III predominates, and mortality is approximately 5%. *Very late–onset disease* occurs after 3 months of age and accounts for 20% of cases beyond the immediate newborn period. Bacteremia without a focus of infection predominates, and the prognosis is good. GBS also causes *chorioamnionitis* and *postpartum endometritis*.

GBS causes invasive disease in nonpregnant adults. Manifestations include bacteremia without focus, sepsis, pneumonia, septic arthritis, soft tissue infection, urinary tract infection, and endocarditis. Case-fatality rates are higher than in newborns and increase significantly beyond age 65 years. Patients with underlying medical problems such as diabetes, chronic liver disease, renal failure, cardiovascular disease, and cancer are also at higher risk for infection. Nonsuppurative sequelae such as those seen with GAS are not seen with GBS.

B. Epidemiology and transmission. Between 10% and 30% of pregnant women are colonized with GBS in the birth canal. The reservoir of infection is probably the gastrointestinal tract, and these women are usually asymptomatic. Transmission may occur *in utero* through ascending infection or may occur at the time of birth; not surprisingly, the risk of early-onset disease is increased with premature or prolonged rupture of the membranes, high maternal organism burden, preterm delivery, intrapartum fever, chorioamnionitis, bacteruria, and low levels of maternal antibody. Other risk factors include young maternal age, a previous infant with invasive GBS disease, and black race. Rarely, horizontal transmission can occur after birth.

In the late 1980s in the United States, the incidence of neonatal GBS infection was 2 to 3 cases per 1,000 live births. Beginning in the mid 1990s, two approaches to antibiotic prophylaxis were taken—a screening-based approach, whereby vaginal-rectal cultures were done at 35 to 37 weeks gestation and penicillin was given to GBS carriers as well as those women delivering before

37 weeks, and a risk-based approach, whereby screening was not done, but penicillin was offered to women with certain risk factors. As a result, a 70% decline in early-onset disease was documented; in 1999 alone, 4,500 cases and 225 deaths were prevented. In August 2002, the Centers for Disease Control and Prevention (CDC) released revised guidelines for the prevention of perinatal GBS disease, calling for screening cultures on all pregnant women and intrapartum antibiotic therapy for all carriers, regardless of risk factors.

The incidence of late-onset disease has not been affected by maternal chemoprophylaxis. Modes of acquisition for this form of disease, as well as adult infection, are not well understood.

C. **Rationale for vaccine use.** Screening-based maternal prophylaxis may not prevent infections in fetuses and premature infants, would not affect late-onset disease in infants, and would have no effect on nonpregnant adults. Maternal vaccination represents a cost-effective way to protect pregnant women and their newborns. The paradigm of protecting newborns by active maternal immunization was established by the prevention of neonatal tetanus through administration of tetanus toxoid to pregnant women. Protection is mediated by transplacental antibody and, because these antibodies may be present for several months, there is the possibility that late-onset disease would be prevented or modified in addition to early-onset disease. A vaccine would eliminate the need for screening programs and would minimize antibiotic exposure for mothers and the possibility that antibiotic resistance would increase. Furthermore, it would eliminate the clinical dilemma represented by sick infants born to carrier mothers who are treated with antibiotics intrapartum; bacterial cultures in these infants may be falsely negative, a concern that often leads to prolonged empiric antibiotic therapy. Although medical and medicolegal concerns have been raised about the advisability of immunizing during pregnancy, a precedent for this approach has clearly been set by tetanus and influenza vaccination, both of which are recommended during pregnancy [see Chapter 12(II)].

D. **Target population.** Potential targets for immunization include pregnant women, nonpregnant adults 65 years of age or older, and adults with chronic disease. Another potential strategy includes immunization of all girls at 12 years of age, but vaccination at this age would need to produce immunity that lasts through the childbearing years.

E. **Candidate vaccines.** GBS has two distinct polysaccharides on the cell surface—the group B antigen that is common to all strains but poorly immunogenic and the serotype-specific capsular polysaccharides (Ia, Ib, II, III, IV, V, VI, VII, and VIII) that are major virulence factors and elicit protective antibody responses. Purified capsular polysaccharides were well tolerated when tested as vaccines in adults. They elicited IgG1 and IgG2 antibodies, subclasses that are readily transported across the placenta. In a 1988 study, 20 of 35 pregnant women who had low levels of type III antibody responded to a single dose of a purified type III capsular polysaccharide vaccine. Infant antibody levels correlated with maternal levels at delivery, and 80% and 64% of infants had protective levels at 1 month and at 3 months of age, respectively. In general, however, response rates to pure polysaccharide vaccines have been disappointing, varying anywhere from 40% to 90%.

As with Hib, pneumococcus, and meningococcus, the immunogenicity of GBS capsular polysaccharides is enhanced by conjugation to protein carriers. Conjugates of several different serotypes to tetanus toxoid have been developed, and in each case, the conjugates have been more immunogenic in animals compared to the pure polysaccharide. Factors that appear to be important in the immunogenicity of GBS conjugates are high molecular mass of the polysaccharide and high degrees of polysaccharide-to-protein cross-linking. Vaccines consisting of types Ia or Ib polysaccharide coupled to tetanus toxoid were well tolerated in a study of 190 healthy nonpregnant women between 18 and 40 years of age. Rapid IgG responses were seen after a single intramuscular injection, and more than 90% of women had protective antibody levels 8 weeks postvaccination. Furthermore, effective opsonization, phagocytosis, and *in vitro* killing of homologous strains were demonstrated. Similar results were seen with a serotype II conjugate vaccine, an important finding because the type II polysaccharide is structurally more complex than other serotypes. Significant IgM and IgA responses were seen, in contrast to the predominantly IgG responses seen with other serotypes. Conjugation of GBS polysaccharides to other carrier proteins, such as cholera toxin B subunit, has been studied.

Another approach to increasing the immunogenicity of GBS polysaccharides is to encapsulate them within biodegradable microspheres, which present multiple copies of the antigen in particulate form, protect it from degradation, promote uptake by antigen-presenting cells and retention in lymph nodes, have adjuvant effects, and enhance uptake at mucosal surfaces. Studies have shown robust serum and mucosal antibody responses (after parenteral and mucosal delivery, respectively) in animals vaccinated with GBS polysaccharides encapsulated in poly (D, L-lactic-coglycolic acid) microparticles (essentially an oil-in-water emulsion) that also contained CpG, a synthetic oligodeoxynucleotide with cytidine-phosphate-guanosine motifs that acts as a potent adjuvant.

Protein vaccines have several possible advantages, including T-cell dependence, memory responses, and the ability to be produced by recombinant DNA technology or to be delivered by a DNA vaccine. One candidate surface protein is the C protein, which is common to two-thirds of maternal and neonatal strains and confers resistance to opsonization and intracellular killing. Antibodies to C proteins are protective in animal challenge experiments using C-bearing GBS strains. Approximately 90% of strains express either Rib or α, members of a novel family of cell surface proteins with repetitive amino acid sequences. A recent study in mice demonstrated the immunogenicity of a bivalent vaccine containing these two proteins with alum as adjuvant. Protection from lethal challenge with four serotypes of GBS was also demonstrated.

Passive Immunization

I. Cytomegalovirus immune globulin intravenous

> Cytomegalovirus (CMV) has a large, double-stranded DNA genome and a protein nucleocapsid surrounded by a lipid envelope; like all herpesviruses, it can establish latency and periodically reactivate.

A. Disease. The vast majority of infections in immunocompetent individuals are completely asymptomatic, although a self-limited mononucleosis-like syndrome has been described. In contrast, CMV causes birth defects in fetuses and disease in immunocompromised patients, including low-birth-weight preterm infants, organ transplant patients, human immunodeficiency virus (HIV)-infected individuals, and those receiving immunosuppressive chemotherapy. *Primary infections* occur in immunologically naïve (seronegative and without CMV-specific T-cell immunity) hosts; *secondary infections* occur in previously infected individuals and can result from *reactivation* of latent virus or *reinfection* with exogenous strains. The risk of severe disease is directly related to the *degree of immunosuppression* (more immunosuppression confers higher risk) and whether the infection is primary or secondary (primary infection confers higher risk). The fact that secondary infections are less severe attests to the protective effect of prior immunity and raises the possibility that vaccination may be useful [see Chapter 10(III)].

CMV syndrome is characterized by fever, anorexia, and malaise that may last as long as 4 weeks. Associated findings include myalgia, arthralgia and arthritis, leucopenia, and thrombocytopenia. Serious manifestations of CMV infection include pneumonitis, colitis, hepatitis, and chorioretinitis. Transplant recipients frequently experience focal involvement of the transplanted organ. Transplant patients may experience opportunistic superinfections due to the immunosuppressive effects of CMV. CMV infection is associated with allograft dysfunction and rejection, although the pathogenesis of this association is not clear.

B. Epidemiology and transmission. Humans are the only hosts for CMV (animals have their own strains), and the virus is ubiquitous; the majority of persons in every culture become infected at some point in their lives. The virus is transmitted in three ways: (a) horizontally, by close person-to-person contact with virus-transmission from mother to infant before birth (through the placenta), during birth (through contact with genital tract secretions), or after birth (through ingestion of infected human milk). Approximately 1% of all live-born infants are infected *in utero*, but the vast majority of these infants are asymptomatic. Serious sequelae such as sensorineural deafness and mental retardation are most commonly seen when the mother has had a primary infection during pregnancy.

As many as half of all solid organ transplant and two-thirds of all bone marrow transplant patients develop CMV infection. Disease incidence peaks 2 to 3 months after transplantation, and the highest risk is in seronegative recipients who receive organs from seropositive donors (referred to as *donor-positive/recipient-negative*, or *D+/R–*, situations). As might be expected from the degree of immunosuppression, disease is most severe in bone marrow recipients (the case-fatality rate for pneumonitis approached 90% before the availability of treatment) and least severe in renal transplant patients. CMV is also the most common viral opportunistic cause of death in acquired immunodeficiency syndrome (AIDS) patients.

C. Rationale for passive immunoprophylaxis. The most promising approach to prevention of congenital infection is vaccination of women before conception [see Chapter 10(III)]. Because nearly all HIV-infected individuals are CMV positive (especially men who have sex with men) and experience secondary infections, control of disease involves immune restoration through highly active antiretroviral therapy, monitoring for disease, and early, or in some cases prophylactic, antiviral therapy. CMV infection in seronegative transplant patients can be avoided by selecting seronegative donors, avoiding exogenous horizontal exposures, and using filtered, leukoreduced (CMV is carried in white cells) blood products. However, the practicality of the first two measures is limited by the ubiquity of CMV in the general population, and these measures would not dramatically impact seropositive recipients who are at risk for reactivation of endogenous virus. Although vaccination shows promise, other modes of prevention include antiviral prophylaxis, surveillance for infection and preemptive antiviral therapy, and passive immunoprophylaxis.

D. Passive immunoprophylactics. The only product available in the United States is CytoGam [cytomegalovirus immune globulin intravenous, human (CMV-IGIV)], manufactured by the Massachusetts Public Health Biologic Laboratories and distributed by MedImmune. It consists of IgG derived from pooled human plasma selected for high titers of antibody to CMV and is, therefore, polyclonal (contains a variety of antibodies, including antibodies to other organisms). The immune globulin is purified by cold ethanol fractionation, solvent/detergent treated to inactivate potential contaminating bloodborne pathogens, and formulated for intravenous administration. Each milliliter contains approximately 50 mg of IgG with trace amounts of IgA and IgM, 50 mg sucrose, and 10 mg human albumin. The sodium content is 20 to 30 mEq/L and there is no preservative. It is supplied as liquid in one-dose vials containing approximately 1,000 mg in 20 mL or 2,500 mg in 50 mL (the concentration for both is 50 mg/mL). CytoGam (CMV-IGIV) is labeled for prophylaxis of CMV *disease* (not *infection*) in patients receiving kidney, lung, liver, pancreas, and heart transplants.

E. Storage, handling, and administration
   - Maintain temperature at 35° to 46°F (2° to 8°C)
   - Use within 6 hours of entering the vial, and complete infusion within 12 hours
   - Do not shake vial
   - Administer intravenously [see Chapter 3(III)]
      - Use separate intravenous line with a constant infusion pump and in-line filter (pore size 15 μ or smaller)
      - May be piggybacked into a preexisting line running sodium chloride or dextrose solutions (2.5%, 5%, 10%, or 20% in water, with or without sodium chloride); should not be diluted more than 1:2 with any of these solutions
      - *Initial dose*: 15 mg/kg/h; if tolerated after 30 minutes, increase to 30 mg/kg/h; if tolerated after a subsequent 30 minutes, increase to 60 mg/kg/h (infusion rate should not exceed 75 mL/h)
      - *Subsequent doses*: 15 mg/kg/h; if tolerated after 15 minutes, increase to 30 mg/kg/h; if tolerated after a subsequent 15 minutes, increase to 60 mg/kg/h (infusion rate should not exceed 75 mL/h)
   - Maximum dose per infusion is 150 mg/kg (Table 11.1)

F. Schedule. Table 11.1 gives recommended doses and schedules.

G. Efficacy. Table 11.2 summarizes the results of several studies of prophylaxis with CMV-IGIV in kidney and liver transplant patients. In general, there is moderate efficacy in preventing CMV disease, reducing disease severity, preventing opportunistic infections, and preventing death in solid organ transplant patients. The greatest benefit appears to be in high-risk renal transplants. Efficacy appears to be diminished when antilymphocyte antibodies are used and is marginal in high-risk liver transplant patients. The issue of efficacy of CMV-IGIV in bone marrow transplant patients is somewhat controversial. For the highest risk patients (D+/R–), the combination of antiviral agents plus CMV-IGIV appears to offer an advantage over monotherapy, and there is some evidence that the combination may be synergistic. Therapy is usually started immediately after transplant and continued for several months.

CMV-IGIV used in combination with antiviral agents also has demonstrated efficacy in the treatment of

Table 11.1.   Dose and schedule for CMV-IGIV

Timing with respect to transplant	Type of transplant	
	Kidney (mg/kg)	Liver, pancreas, lung, heart (mg/kg)
Within 72 h	150	150
2 wk post	100	150
4 wk post	100	150
6 wk post	100	150
8 wk post	100	150
12 wk post	50	100
16 wk post	50	100

Table 11.2.   Studies of CMV-IGIV prophylaxis in solid organ transplant patients

Transplant	Number of subjects (number high risk[a])		Control type	Outcomes
	Treatment	Control		
Kidney	24	24	No treatment	Disease decreased 17% to 0% in patients receiving cyclosporin
	24 (24)	35 (35)	No treatment	Disease decreased 60% to 21% Mortality decreased 14% to 4% Reduced opportunistic infections
Liver	22 (15)	12 (7)	No treatment	Disease decreased 86% to 27% in high-risk patients
	69 (19)	72 (19)	Placebo	Disease decreased 31% to 19% but no effect in high-risk patients
	21 (9)	44 (19)	Placebo	Disease decreased 32% to 14%

[a]Refers to situation in which donor is CMV seropositive and recipient is CMV seronegative.
Adapted from Sia IG, Patel R. New strategies for prevention and therapy of cytomegalovirus infection and disease in solid-organ transplant recipients. *Clin Microbiol Rev* 2000;13:83–121.

established CMV disease in both solid organ and bone marrow transplant patients.

H. Official recommendations. Most centers use the same rules for solid organ and bone marrow transplants. If both donor and recipient are CMV seronegative, CMV-IGIV is not necessary. If the donor is seropositive and the recipient is seronegative, most centers use CMV-IGIV as well as prophylactic ganciclovir. In situations in which the recipient is seropositive, CMV-IGIV is often used without ganciclovir, regardless of donor serostatus. However, practice in this area varies widely from institution to institution.

Antibodies in CytoGam (CMV-IGIV) may interfere with the immune response to live virus vaccines such as measles, mumps, and rubella (MMR) and varicella [see Chapter 1(I)]. These vaccinations should therefore be deferred at least 6 months, although most patients have contraindications to live virus vaccines because of immunosuppression.

I. Safety. Flushing, chills, muscle cramps, back pain, fever, nausea, vomiting, arthralgia, and wheezing were reported in less than 6% of infusions during clinical trials. Most reactions were related to the infusion rate. Certain safety issues are common to all intravenous immune globulin products, including the possibility of renal failure, sensitization of IgA-deficient individuals, aseptic meningitis, and transmission of bloodborne pathogens [see Chapter 11(III)].

J. Contraindications
- Anaphylactic reaction to a prior dose or to any immune globulin product
- Selective IgA deficiency

K. Precautions. Renal insufficiency, volume depletion, or concomitant nephrotoxic drugs.

KEY CONCEPTS: CMV IMMUNE GLOBULIN INTRAVENOUS

- CMV is a major cause of disease in transplant patients
- Highest risk when donor is seropositive and recipient is seronegative
- CMV-IGIV reduces primary CMV disease in renal transplant patients by 50%
- Shows modest benefits in other solid-organ transplant patients
- Benefits for bone marrow transplantation not clear
- Combination with antivirals may have added benefits

II. Hepatitis B immune globulin

Hepatitis B virus is a nonenveloped, partially double-stranded DNA virus that is tropic for the liver, can establish chronic infection, and has oncogenic properties.

The disease and its epidemiology and transmission are discussed in Chapter 5(III).

A. Rationale for passive immunoprophylaxis. The rationale for active vaccination against hepatitis B is given in Chapter 5(III). In situations in which exposure has occurred, the long incubation period allows for postexposure prophylaxis with vaccine. However, even an accelerated vaccination series requires a minimum of 4 months to complete, and neonates cannot complete the series until 6 months of age. Therefore, passive immunization is a necessary adjunct to active vaccination for immediate protection after exposure.

B. Passive immunoprophylactics. Two hepatitis B immune globulin (HBIG) products are available in the United States: BayHep B (HBIG; Bayer Corporation) and Nabi-HB [HBIG; Nabi (North American Biologicals, Inc.)]. These products consist of IgG derived from pooled human plasma selected for high titers of antibody to hepatitis B; they are therefore polyclonal (they contain a variety of antibodies, including antibodies to other organisms). The immune globulin is purified by cold ethanol fractionation, solvent/detergent treated to inactivate potential contaminating bloodborne pathogens, ultrafiltered to further reduce the risk of viral infection, and formulated for intramuscular administration. Both products contain anti–hepatitis B virus surface antigen (HBsAg) antibody equal to or exceeding the HBIG reference standard of the U.S. Food and Drug Administration (FDA), and both are preservative free. BayHep B (HBIG) contains 15% to 18% protein, and excipients present include glycine. It is supplied as a liquid in a neonatal dose (0.5 mL in a prefilled syringe with needle and UltraSafe Needle Guard), as a 1.0-mL prefilled syringe with needle and UltraSafe Needle Guard, and a 5.0-mL one-dose vial. Nabi-HB (HBIG) contains 5% protein, and excipients present include glycine and polysorbate 80. It is supplied as a liquid in 1.0-mL and 5.0-mL one-dose vials.

BayHep B (HBIG) and Nabi-HB (HBIG) are labeled for postexposure prophylaxis in the following situations: acute exposure to blood containing HBsAg, perinatal exposure of infants born to HBsAg-positive mothers, sexual exposure to HBsAg-positive persons, and household exposure of infants younger than 12 months of age to persons with acute hepatitis B infection.

C. Storage, handling, and administration
- Maintain temperature at 35° to 46°F (2° to 8°C)
- Freezing can cause loss of potency
- Each dose for neonates (perinatal exposure) and infants younger than 12 months of age (household exposure) is 0.5 mL given intramuscularly [see Chapter 3(III)]
- Each dose for children and adults (exposures to contaminated blood or sexual contact) is 0.06 mL/kg

D. Schedule. In cases of perinatal exposure, HBIG should be given within 12 hours of birth; efficacy diminishes markedly after 48 hours. For blood exposure, HBIG should be given as soon as possible, preferably within 24 hours; efficacy beyond 7 days is not clear. For sexual exposure, HBIG should be given within 14 days of the most recent contact. In most exposures of previously unvaccinated individuals, the hepatitis B vaccine (Hep-B) series should be initiated. If vaccine is refused, a second dose of HBIG should be given 1 month after the first dose.

E. Efficacy. Antibodies to HBsAg appear within days of administration and peak in approximately 1 week; the half-life is approximately 3 weeks, and antibodies can be detected in the blood for several months. Protective efficacy after sexual or blood exposure is approximately 75%. For perinatal exposure, one dose of HBIG plus the Hep-B series is 85% to 95% effective.

F. Official recommendations. HBIG is recommended as follows:

- *Perinatal exposure (infants born to HBsAg-positive mothers)*
  - Give within 12 hours of birth
  - Initiate three-dose vaccine series (use separate site from HBIG) within 12 hours of birth
  - Third dose of vaccine should be given at 6 months of age (as opposed to 6 to 18 months of age)
  - An alternative vaccine schedule at birth, 1, 2, and 12 months is approved for Engerix-B (Hep-B) only
  - Test for HBsAg and anti-HBsAg antibody 1 to 3 months after completion of the vaccine series or at 9 to 15 months of age; if both tests are negative, repeat three-dose vaccine series using two-month intervals and repeat testing
  - For preterm infants weighing less than 2 kg, the birth dose of vaccine should still be given, but it *should not count* toward completion of the primary series; the series should be continued with doses at 1, 2 to 3, and 6 to 7 months of age
  - HBIG should not be given routinely if the mother's HBsAg status is *unknown* (unless the infant weighs less than 2 kg and the mother's status cannot be determined within 12 hours; rather, the mother should be tested at delivery and HBIG should be given if the test is positive (vaccine should be given regardless of the results)
- *Sexual contact with a person with acute hepatitis B*
  - Give within 14 days of most recent contact
  - Initiate vaccine series if person is unimmunized
  - HBIG is not recommended in cases of sexual abuse or rape unless the offender is known to have *acute* hepatitis B infection; vaccine series should be given if victim is unimmunized
- *Household contact of person with acute hepatitis B*

- Unimmunized infants younger than 12 months of age whose primary caregiver has acute hepatitis B should receive HBIG (and complete the vaccine series as soon as possible); if one dose of vaccine has already been received, the second dose should be given if due, or give HBIG if vaccine is not due (if two doses have been received, HBIG is not indicated)
- HBIG is *not* indicated for older household members with casual contact
- HBIG *is* indicated for older household members who have exposure to blood or secretions (e.g., sharing toothbrushes or razors) or sexual contact)
- Persons (even, for example, adopted infants) entering households with a chronic hepatitis B virus–infected person should receive a primary vaccine series but not HBIG

- *Percutaneous or permucosal exposure to blood*: Table 11.3 provides guidelines for management of these types of exposures
- *Protection of liver transplantation patients from severe recurrent hepatitis B infection*
  - HBIG in combination with lamivudine can prevent recurrent hepatitis B infection in patients who undergo liver transplantation for chronic hepatitis B infection
  - Recurrence rates can be reduced to 0% to 10%
  - HBIG or lamivudine monotherapy has been shown to delay but not prevent recurrent hepatitis B infection, and lamivudine monotherapy may result in the development of drug resistance
  - Experimental protocols have used intramuscular formulations of HBIG administered intravenously in doses ranging from 10,000 to 80,000 IU during the first month posttransplant, followed by 1,500 to 5,000 IU per month. Other regimens include 10,000 IU at surgery then daily for 7 days, followed by doses to titrate anti-HBsAg levels to greater than 100 IU/L.

HBIG does not interfere with inactivated vaccines (including Hep-B) when given at separate sites, but live virus vaccines such as MMR and varicella should be deferred at least 3 months [see Chapter 1(I)].

- **G. Safety.** Local reactions such as pain and erythema at the injection site, and systemic reactions such as headache, malaise, nausea, diarrhea, joint stiffness, and myalgia occur in fewer than 15% of patients. Greater than 90% of reactions are characterized as mild. Fewer than 5% of patients may have elevated alkaline phosphatase, hepatic transaminases, or creatinine. Certain safety issues are common to all immune globulin products, including sensitization of IgA-deficient individuals and transmission of bloodborne pathogens [see Chapter 11(III)].
- **H. Contraindications.** Anaphylactic reaction to a prior dose or to any immune globulin product.

Table 11.3. Management of percutaneous and permucosal hepatitis B exposures[a]

Status of exposed person	HBsAg status of source individual		
	Positive	Negative	Unknown[b]
Not immunized	HBIG Initiate vaccination	Initiate vaccination	Initiate vaccination
Immunized; adequate antibody level[c]	No treatment	No treatment	No treatment
Immunized; inadequate antibody level	HBIG[d] Reinitiate vaccination[d]	No treatment	If high risk, assume HBsAg positive and treat accordingly
Immunized; antibody level unknown	Test exposed person for antibody If adequate,[c] no treatment If inadequate, give HBIG and initiate vaccination[d]	No treatment	Test exposed person for antibody If adequate,[c] no treatment If inadequate, give booster dose of vaccine[e]

[a]Examples of percutaneous injuries include needle sticks, lacerations, and bites. Permucosal exposures include splashes of blood, any fluid containing visible blood, or other potentially infectious fluid (including semen; vaginal secretions; CSF; synovial, pleural, peritoneal, pericardial, or amniotic fluids; tracheal secretions; and saliva) or tissue on to any mucosal site including conjunctivae and oral and buccal mucosa. The Hep-B series should be initiated in an unimmunized child who is injured by a discarded needle in the community. If the child received two doses of vaccine 4 months or more previously, the third dose should be given immediately. Opinions differ about the need for HBIG in children who have not completed the Hep-B series, but fully immunized children clearly do not need HBIG.
[b]Efforts should be made to test the source individual for HBsAg.
[c]Anti-HBsAg antibody 10 mIU/mL or more; routine postvaccination testing is only recommended for certain individuals [see Chapter 5(III)].
[d]If the exposed person is known not to have responded to two series of three doses, give two doses of HBIG separated by 1 month (no further vaccine is indicated); if only one three-dose vaccine series has been received, give one dose of HBIG and reinitiate a three-dose vaccine series.
[e]If patient has previously received only one three-dose series, test for antibody 1 to 2 months after booster; if level is inadequate, complete three-dose series.
Adapted from AAP. Hepatitis B. In: Pickering LK, ed. *Red book: 2003 report of the Committee on Infectious Diseases*, 26th ed. Elk Grove Village, IL: American Academy of Pediatrics; 2003:318–336.

I. Precautions
- Selective IgA deficiency (risk of sensitization due to minute amounts of IgA in HBIG)
- Severe thrombocytopenia or any coagulation disorder that would contraindicate intramuscular administration

---

KEY CONCEPTS: HEPATITIS B IMMUNE GLOBULIN
- Long incubation period of hepatitis B allows for postexposure prophylaxis
- Used as adjunct to active vaccination
- Administer within 12 hours of birth to infants of HBsAg-positive mothers
- May interfere with live virus vaccines

III. Immune globulin.
Immune globulin intramuscular (IGIM) has two principal uses: postexposure prophylaxis for measles [see Chapter 5(V)] and hepatitis A [see Chapter 8(IV)]. Immune globulin intravenous (IGIV) is used for routine passive immunization of patients with humoral immune deficiencies against all pathogens to which healthy donors produce antibodies (although IGIM also has indications for replacement therapy, its use has been largely been supplanted by IGIV). IGIV also has immunomodulatory properties and is used to treat a variety of diseases including Kawasaki disease, idiopathic (immune-mediated) thrombocytopenic purpura (ITP), Guillain-Barré syndrome, chronic inflammatory demyelinating polyradiculoneuropathy, myasthenia gravis, multifocal motor neuropathy, dermatomyositis, autoimmune vasculitis and uveitis, and multiple sclerosis. These uses are not discussed here.

A. Passive immunoprophylactics.
Table 11.4 gives the immune globulin products currently available in the United States, including details on their constitution and labeled indications. Although there are some differences between products, they share the following characteristics:
- Made from human plasma pooled from thousands of donors
- Provide biologically active antibodies to a broad spectrum of human pathogens that may vary in quantity and quality from product to product and lot to lot
- Contain IgG with varying trace amounts of other immunoglobulin classes
- Purified by Cohn-Oncley cold ethanol fractionation
- Undergo additional virus inactivation steps
- Formulated without preservatives

  The late 1990s were marked by severe shortages of IGIV in the United States, related in part to safety concerns (see Safety below). Current availability appears to be adequate.

B. Storage, handling, administration, and schedule
- See Table 11.4 for storage requirements; products should not be frozen

Table 11.4. Immune globulin preparations available in the United States

Trade name	Distributor (manufacturer)	Principal viral inactivation	Labeled indications	Excipients/sugars/stabilizers	IgA content	Formulation	Packaging and storage
Intramuscular (IGIM)							
BayGam	Bayer	Solvent/detergent	Hepatitis A Measles Varicella Rubella Immunoglobulin deficiency[a]	Glycine	<64 μg/mL	Liquid 15–18% protein	2-mL vial (1 or 10/pk) 10-mL vial (1 or 10/pk) Store at 35–46°F (2–8°C)
Immune Globulin (Human) USP	FFF Enterprises[b] (Massachusetts Public Health Biologic Laboratories)	Solvent/detergent	Hepatitis A Measles Varicella Rubella Immunoglobulin deficiency[a]	Glycine	Trace	Liquid 16.5% protein	2-mL vial Store at 35–46°F (2–8°C)
Intravenous (IGIV)							
Carimune	ZLB Bioplasma, Inc. (ZLB Bioplasma AG)	Low pH Pepsin	Immune deficiency ITP	Sucrose	720 μg/mL	Lyophilized Reconstituted with 5% dextrose or 0.9% saline to 3–12% protein solution	1-, 3-, 6-, 12-g vial with diluent Store at room temperature

(continued)

Table 11.4. *Continued*

Trade name	Distributor (manufacturer)	Principal viral inactivation	Labeled indications	Excipients/sugars/stabilizers	IgA content	Formulation	Packaging and storage
Gamimune N 10%	Bayer	Low pH Solvent/detergent	Immune deficiency ITP BMT Pediatric HIV	Glycine	152 μg/mL	Liquid 9–11% protein	1-g (10 mL), 2.5-g (25 mL), 5-g (50 mL), 10-g (100 mL), or 20-g (200 mL) vial Store at 35–46°F (2–8°C)
GAMMA-GARD S/D	Baxter	Solvent/detergent	Immune deficiency CLL ITP Kawasaki disease	Glycine Glucose Human albumin Polyethylene glycol Tri-n-butyl phosphate octoxynol Polysorbate 80	≤1.2 μg/mL in 5% solution	Lyophilized Reconstituted with sterile water to 5–10% protein solution	2.5-, 5-, or 10-g vial with diluent Store at or below room temperature
Gammar-P I.V.	Aventis Behring	Heat treatment	Immune deficiency	Sucrose Human albumin	<25 μg/mL	Lyophilized Reconstituted in sterile water to 5% protein solution	1-, 2.5-, 5-, or 10-g vial with diluent Store at or below room temperature

Iveegam EN	Baxter	Trypsin Polyethylene glycol	Immune deficiency Kawasaki disease	Glucose Polyethylene glycol	<10 μg/mL	Lyophilized Reconstituted with sterile water to 5% protein solution	0.5-, 1-, 2.5-, or 5-g vial with diluent Store at 35–46°F (2–8°C)
Panglobulin	American Red Cross (ZLB Bioplasma)	Low pH Pepsin	Immune deficiency ITP	Sucrose	720 μg/mL	Lyophilized Reconstituted with 5% dextrose or 0.9% saline to 3–12% protein solution	1-, 3-, 6-, or 12-g vial with diluent Store at room temperature
Polygam S/D	American Red Cross (Baxter)	Solvent/detergent	Immune deficiency CLL ITP Kawasaki disease	Glycine Glucose Human albumin Polyethylene glycol Tri-n-butyl phosphate-octoxynol Polysorbate 80	<3.7 μg/mL	Lyophilized Reconstituted with sterile water to 5–10% protein solution	2.5-, 5-, or 10-g vial with diluent Store at or below room temperature

(continued)

Table 11.4. Continued

Trade name	Distributor (manufacturer)	Principal viral inactivation	Labeled indications	Excipients/sugars/stabilizers	IgA content	Formulation	Packaging and storage
Venoglobulin-S (5% and 10%)	Alpha Therapeutic	Solvent/detergent Polyethylene glycol/bentonite fractionation	Immune deficiency ITP Kawasaki disease	D-sorbitol Human albumin Polyethylene glycol Polysorbate 80 Tri-n-butyl phosphate	5% product: 15.1 μg/mL 10% product: 20–50 μg/mL	Liquid 5% or 10% protein	5% product: 2.5-g (50 mL), 5-g (100 mL), or 10-g (200 mL) vial Store at or below room temperature 10% product: 5-g (50 mL), 10-g (100 mL), or 20-g (200 mL) vial Store at 35–46°F (2–8°C)

BMT, bone marrow transplant; CLL, B-cell chronic lymphocytic leukemia; ITP, idiopathic thrombocytopenic purpura; pk, package.

Note: Sandoglobulin, manufactured by ZLB Bioplasma AG (Swiss Red Cross) and distributed by Novartis is no longer available in the United States.

[a]IGIV is used more commonly for this indication.

[b]Formerly distributed by American Red Cross.

Adapted from package inserts, manufacturers, and Seigel J. Intravenous immune globulins: therapeutic, pharmaceutical, and cost considerations. *Pharm Pract News* 2002;29:13–15.

- See package insert for details on reconstitution of lyophilized products; in general, do not shake vigorously because doing so causes foaming
- IGIM is given intramuscularly [see Chapter 3(III)] as follows:
  - Immune deficiency (IGIV is favored for this indication): 0.6 mL/kg (100 mg/kg) every 3 to 4 weeks, but this can be titrated (by varying the dosing interval) to the patient's trough IgG level (aiming for approximately 700 mg/dL)
  - Hepatitis A—*preexposure prophylaxis*:
    - Length of stay less than 3 months: 0.02 mL/kg (3.3 mg/kg)
    - Length of stay 3 months or more: 0.06 mL/kg (10 mg/kg), repeat every 5 months unless immunization series can be completed (individuals 2 years of age or older)
  - Hepatitis A—*postexposure prophylaxis* (give within 2 weeks): 0.02 mL/kg (3.3 mg/kg)
  - Measles postexposure prophylaxis (give within 6 days):
    - *Immunocompetent*: 0.25 mL/kg (40 mg/kg; maximum, 15 mL)
    - *Immunocompromised*: 0.50 mL/kg (80 mg/kg; maximum, 15 mL); if the individual regularly receives IGIV and the last dose was within 3 weeks of exposure, IGIM is not necessary; if more than 3 weeks have elapsed since the last infusion, the next infusion can be given early
  - In general, maximum dose *at a single site* is 3 mL for infants and children and 5 mL for larger children and adults
- IGIV is given intravenously as follows:
  - *Humoral immune deficiency*: usual dose is 400 mg/kg every month, but this can be titrated (by varying the amount and/or dosing interval) to the patient's trough IgG level (aiming for approximately 700 mg/dL)
  - *Pediatric HIV*: usual dose is 400 mg/kg every month, but this can be titrated (by varying the amount and/or dosing interval) to the patient's clinical condition (trough IgG levels may not be helpful because patients may have *qualitative* rather than *quantitative* humoral immune deficiency)
  - *Chronic lymphocytic leukemia*: usual dose is 400 mg/kg every month
  - *Bone marrow transplantation*: usual dose is 500 mg/kg given 7 and 2 days before transplant (or at the time conditioning therapy is started) and weekly through the 90-day posttransplant period
  - *Kawasaki disease*: 2 g/kg; a second infusion 48 to 72 hours later can be considered in refractory cases

- *ITP*: dosing regimens vary, but some centers give 1 g/kg on as many as three alternating days for induction therapy
- Technique for administration is given in Chapter 3(III)

C. **Efficacy.** Serum IgG levels in peak 2 to 5 days after administration of IGIM. After administration of IGIV, 100% of the dose is immediately available in the patient's circulation. The mean half-life of circulating IgG is approximately 23 days. The benefits of replacement therapy for immune-deficient individuals are clear. In unvaccinated individuals, efficacy of IGIM against symptomatic hepatitis A infection (when given within 2 weeks of exposure) is greater than 85%; efficacy in preventing or modifying measles disease (when given within 6 days of exposure) is 80%.

A controlled trial of IGIV in 372 HIV-infected children was conducted by the National Institute of Child Health and Human Development in the late 1980s and early 1990s. Among children with CD4 counts 200/mL or higher, the proportion who were free of serious bacterial infections 2 years out was 67% in the IGIV group and 48% in the placebo group; the relative risk of both minor and serious bacterial infections was 0.68. No benefits were seen in children with CD4 counts lower than 200/mL, and this trial was conducted at a time when zidovudine was not yet established as standard therapy. In a subsequent open-label study, placebo recipients who crossed over to IGIV therapy had a reduction in serious bacterial infections from 32.1 episodes per 100 patient years to 16.3 episodes. Another study conducted by the Pediatric AIDS Clinical Trials Group in the early 1990s involved children who were all receiving zidovudine. Serious bacterial infections were reduced only among the 174 children who were not also receiving trimethoprim/sulfamethoxazole prophylaxis, and there was no difference in survival.

Although it is generally accepted that low immunoglobulin levels in premature neonates contribute to a high incidence of infection, the issue of IGIV prophylaxis has been controversial. Studies have yielded conflicting results, and even metaanalyses of published data have reached different conclusions. Table 11.5 gives the results of some recent noteworthy trials.

D. **Official recommendations.** Although important differences exist between immune globulin products, including manufacturing processes, stabilizers, excipients, IgA content, and antibody titers, IGIM and IGIV products are viewed as essentially equivalent in terms of efficacy. In addition, labeled indications differ, but many clinicians use these products interchangeably, except in patients who have reactions to particular brands.

IGIM is recommended for preexposure prophylaxis against hepatitis A for persons traveling to or working in countries with high or intermediate endemicity, including Africa, Asia (except Japan), the Mediterranean

Table 11.5. Selected controlled trials of IGIV prophylaxis in premature neonates

Year	Regimen	Treated		Not treated		Comments
		n	Infection rate (%)	n	Infection rate (%)	
1992[a]	500 mg/kg at weeks 0, 1, 3, 5, and 7	287	32.4[e]	297	46.8[e]	Differences statistically significant No effect on mortality
1994[b]	500 mg/kg on day 1	372	10.8[f]	381	10.2[f]	Only single dose given Differences not statistically significant No effect on mortality
1994[c]	700–900 mg/kg every 14 d until weight = 1,800 g	1,204	15.5[f]	1,212	17.2[f]	Differences not statistically significant No effect on mortality
2000[d]	1 g/kg on days 0, 3, 7, 14, and 21–81	40	47.5[f]	41	31.7[f]	Only infants with cord blood IgG levels ≤400 mg/dL were treated Differences not statistically significant No effect on mortality

[a]Baker CJ, Melish ME, Hall RT, et al. Intravenous immune globulin for the prevention of nosocomial infection in low-birth-weight neonates. *N Engl J Med* 1992;327:213–219.
[b]Weisman LE, Stoll BJ, Kueser TJ, et al. Intravenous immune globulin prophylaxis of late-onset sepsis in premature neonates. *J Pediatr* 1994;125:922–930.
[c]Fanaroff AA, Korones SB, Wright LL, et al. A controlled trial of intravenous immune globulin to reduce nosocomial infections in very-low-birth-weight infants. *N Engl J Med* 1994;330:1107–1113.
[d]Sandberg K, Fasth A, Berger A, et al. Preterm infants with low immunoglobulin G levels have increased risk of neonatal sepsis but do not benefit from prophylactic immunoglobulin G. *J Pediatr* 2000;137:623–628.
[e]All infections.
[f]Bacterial sepsis.

basin, Eastern Europe, the Middle East, Central and South America, Mexico, and parts of the Caribbean, *if* travel will occur before 4 weeks. The vaccine series should also be initiated [see Chapter 8(IV)] except in children younger than 2 years of age, who should receive IGIM alone because the vaccine is not approved in this age group. IGIM is also recommended for postexposure prophylaxis in *unimmunized* people in the following settings (*immunized* individuals do not need IGIM):

- Close contact (household or sexual) with index case
- *Day care center where children are toilet trained*: employees and children in the same room as an adult or child index case
- *Day care center where children are not toilet trained*: employees and children in the whole facility where the index case occurred; this also applies if two or more household contacts of children in the center have hepatitis A
- Residents and staff of custodial care institutions in close contact with an index case during an institutional outbreak
- Consider for
  - Infants whose mothers develop symptoms between 2 weeks before and 1 week after delivery
  - Documented transmission in a school setting
  - Food- or waterborne outbreaks

IGIM is also recommended for postexposure prophylaxis of measles in *unimmunized* household contacts, especially infants younger than 1 year of age (although infants less than 5 months of age are usually protected by maternal antibody) and pregnant women. Immunocompromised persons should receive IGIM *regardless of immunization status*, unless they regularly receive IGIV.

There are no specific infectious disease recommendations for IGIV other than passive immunization against a variety of diseases in immune-deficient individuals. For HIV-infected children, the benefits of IGIV therapy may not exceed those afforded by routine prophylaxis with trimethoprim/sulfamethoxazole and may be minimal in the era of highly active antiretroviral therapy. However, the following guidelines for use have been offered:

- Significant recurrent bacterial infections in patients with hypo- or hypergammaglobulinemia
- Absence of measles antibody despite two immunizations in children who live in high-prevalence regions
- HIV-associated thrombocytopenia (platelet count less than 20×10^9/L; regimen similar to that for ITP)
- Chronic bronchiectasis

IGIV is not routinely recommended for prophylaxis in low-birth-weight infants. Use of IGIV as adjunctive therapy for established neonatal sepsis is controversial but supported by several small studies.

Immune globulin products do not interfere with inactivated vaccines, as long as they are not given simulta-

Table 11.6. Adverse effects of IGIV

Symptoms	Clinical syndromes	Laboratory abnormalities
Headache	Migraine	Hyperglycemia
Fever	Aseptic meningitis	Pseudohyponatremia
Chills	Encephalopathy	Elevated hepatic
Myalgia	Immune complex arthritis	transaminases
Arthralgia	Hemolytic anemia	Leukopenia
Nausea	Renal failure	Neutropenia
Vomiting	Uveitis	Proteinuria
Tachycardia	Anaphylaxis	
Hypertension	Stroke	
Hypotension	Pulmonary embolism	
Pruritus	Cardiac failure	
Rash	Allergic myocarditis	
Alopecia		

Adapted from Anderson MS. Intravenous gammaglobulin for pediatric infectious diseases. *Pediatr Ann* 1999;28:499–506.

neously at the same site. They can, however, interfere with live-attenuated vaccines [see Chapter 1(I)]. Recommended intervals between receipt of immune globulin products and measles and varicella vaccines are given in Table 1.4. It should be noted that the intervals depend on the product and dose given.

E. Safety. Local reactions to IGIM include tenderness, pain, and muscle stiffness at the injection site. Systemic reactions include urticaria, angioedema, malaise, nausea, diarrhea, headache, chills, and fever. Less frequently reported reactions include emesis, fatigue, lightheadedness, flushing, diaphoresis, abdominal cramping, retching, myalgia, lethargy, and chest tightness.

Approximately 5% of patients receiving IGIV experience some side effect (Table 11.6). Most of these are mild and can be ameliorated by slowing or stopping the infusion; premedication can lower the incidence [see Chapter 3(III)].

The following adverse effects, which are common to all immune globulin products (including hyperimmune products), deserve special mention:

• IGIM and IGIV
  • *Sensitization of IgA-deficient individuals*: Individuals with selective IgA deficiency may interpret the trace amounts of IgA that contaminate immune globulin products as foreign proteins and respond by making IgE antibodies, leading to anaphylaxis on further exposure. IGIV products differ in IgA content (Table 11.4), but even trace amounts can cause reactions.
  • *Transmission of bloodborne pathogens*: Because immune globulin products are made from blood pooled from thousands of donors, transmission of

bloodborne pathogens is a possibility (despite the fact that donors are screened). In fact, a cluster of hepatitis C cases in 1994 related to IGIV prompted manufacturers to add more steps to inactivate pathogens. The Cohn-Oncley cold ethanol fractionation procedure itself inactivates most, if not all, viruses, but added measures include solvent/detergent treatment, incubation at acid pH, enzyme digestion, polyethylene glycol/bentonite fractionation, ultrafiltration, and heat treatment (Table 11.4). The efficacy of these procedures is routinely tested by spiking premanufacture material with known viruses. Despite these procedures, prions (such as those that cause Creutzfeldt-Jakob disease) could still theoretically be transmitted. There has not been a case of HIV transmission through immune globulin.

- IGIV
  - *Aseptic meningitis syndrome*: Symptoms begin during or within 2 days of the infusion and include severe headache, nuchal rigidity, drowsiness, fever, photophobia, painful eye movements, nausea, and vomiting. Cerebrospinal fluid (CSF) shows a granulocytic pleocytosis and elevated protein level. The syndrome may occur in up to 10% of recipients and may be more common in patients with a history of migraine and those receiving high doses of IGIV. Discontinuation of treatment results in remission of symptoms within a few days, and there are no sequelae. The pathogenesis is unknown.
  - *Acute renal failure*: Renal insufficiency and renal failure have been reported after IGIV infusions, mostly with products that have a high sucrose content. Histopathology suggests osmotic injury to the proximal tubule. Renal effects are more common in patients being treated for ITP than for primary immune deficiency, possibly because of the higher doses used for ITP. Patients should not be volume depleted before initiation of IGIV infusions. Those who deserve special caution and monitoring include patients with preexisting renal insufficiency, diabetes, sepsis, or paraproteinemia, as well as those over 65 years of age and those taking nephrotoxic drugs. Predisposed individuals might benefit from a reduction in dose, concentration, and/or rate of infusion.

F. Contraindications
- Anaphylactic reaction to a prior dose or to any immune globulin product
- Selective IgA deficiency
- IGIM only: severe thrombocytopenia or any coagulation disorder that would contraindicate intramuscular administration

G. Precautions
- Renal insufficiency, volume depletion, or concomitant nephrotoxic drugs

- Seriously ill patients with compromised cardiac function who might be sensitive to large-volume infusions

---

KEY CONCEPTS: IMMUNE GLOBULIN

- Made from pooled plasma from thousands of donors
- Products may be hyperimmune, but all are polyclonal
- IGIM indicated for prophylaxis against hepatitis A and measles
- IGIV indicated for replacement therapy and for several noninfectious conditions
- May compromise efficacy of live-attenuated vaccines

IV. Palivizumab [humanized murine monoclonal antibody to respiratory syncytial virus (RSV-mAb)] and RSV-IGIV

RSV is a paramyxovirus with a nonsegmented single-stranded RNA genome that forms syncytia in tissue culture.

A. **Disease.** The most distinctive clinical syndrome is *bronchiolitis*, seen predominantly in the first year of life. The first symptoms are usually rhinorrhea, low-grade fever, irritability, lethargy, and poor feeding, but very young infants can present with apnea alone. The illness progresses to lower respiratory tract disease manifest by cough, wheezing, increased work of breathing, retractions, and varying degrees of respiratory distress. Examination shows prolonged expiration, nasal flaring, grunting, accessory muscle use, rales, and rhonchi. Chest x-ray may show hyperinflation and right upper lobe atelectasis, and hypoxia and hypercarbia may develop. The illness is monophasic, and the typical infant admitted to the hospital spends 2 or 3 days. Prolonged wheezing, and recurrent wheezing with subsequent respiratory infections, are common in the weeks or months that follow recovery.

Occasionally, RSV causes *pneumonia* without bronchiolitis. Older children can have *upper respiratory tract disease* including rhinorrhea, cough, congestion, and pharyngitis that do not progress. RSV may also contribute to the development of otitis media, but systemic bacterial superinfections are rare.

B. **Epidemiology and transmission.** RSV occurs in annual epidemics during the winter and early spring. Humans are the only source of infection, and transmission occurs through close contact with contaminated secretions, including droplets and fomites. The virus can persist for longer than 30 minutes on hands and for hours on environmental surfaces; this helps explain the frequency of hospital-acquired infections. Most children are infected with RSV in the first year of life, and almost all have been infected by 2 years of age. One-third of infections in young infants progress to lower respiratory tract disease; reinfections in older children usually remain confined to the upper respiratory tract.

RSV is one of the most common serious infections of infants. Between 1980 and 1996 in the United States, 1.65 million hospitalizations for bronchiolitis occurred in children younger than 5 years of age; 81% of these were in infants younger than 1 year. Approximately 2% of all children in the first year of life are hospitalized, making this the single most common reason for pediatric hospitalization during the winter months. Approximately 4,500 deaths are attributed to RSV each year. Premature infants, particularly those younger than 32 weeks' gestation, are at risk for severe RSV infection, as are infants with chronic lung disease (CLD, or bronchopulmonary dysplasia), complicated or cyanotic congenital heart disease (CHD), and immunodeficiency or immunosuppressive therapy.

C. **Rationale for passive immunoprophylaxis.** The tremendous public health burden of RSV disease in infants has sparked interest in active vaccination. However, early trials with a formalin-inactivated vaccine led to enhancement of disease, and trials of live-attenuated vaccines were disappointing [see Chapter 10(XII)]. Although current approaches using subunit vaccines composed of surface glycoproteins from the virus are promising, recent attention has focused on provision of passive immunity to the highest-risk infants. Approximately 80,000 infants younger than 32 weeks' gestation are born in the United States each year, and hospitalization rates for RSV disease approach one-third in some studies; 30% may require intensive care, and 3% may die. Similar degrees of morbidity and mortality are seen with CHD. Because the risk of RSV disease continues through the second year of life, several hundred thousand infants are candidates for prophylaxis.

D. **Passive immunoprophylactics.** Two products are available in the United States for prevention of RSV disease:

- *Synagis (Palivizumab; RSV-mAb)*: This is a monoclonal antibody to the F protein of RSV manufactured by MedImmune and comarketed by the Ross Products Division of Abbott Laboratories. It was made by linking genes for the antigen-combining site of a murine monoclonal antibody to the effector region genes of a human antibody. It is composed of two heavy chains and two light chains and, in total, contains 95% human and 5% murine sequences. It is produced in a murine myeloma cell line and is supplied lyophilized in 50-mg (0.5 mL) and 100-mg (1.0 mL) vials for reconstitution with sterile water. Potential contaminants and excipients include histidine, glycine, and mannitol, but the product is preservative free. As Synagis (RSV-mAb) is a monoclonal product, it does not contain antibodies to any agents other than RSV, and it does not contain IgA. Synagis (RSV-mAb) is indicated for the prevention of serious lower respiratory tract disease caused by RSV in high-risk infants and children, including those with CLD or prematurity (younger than 35 weeks' gestation). The product is not currently labeled for use in patients with CHD.

- *RespiGam (RSV-IGIV)*: This is a hyperimmune globulin manufactured by the Massachusetts Public Health Biologic Laboratories and distributed by MedImmune. It consists of IgG derived from pooled human plasma selected for high titers of antibody to RSV and is therefore polyclonal (it contains a variety of antibodies, including antibodies to other organisms). The immune globulin is purified by cold ethanol fractionation, solvent/detergent treated to inactivate potential contaminating bloodborne pathogens, and formulated for intravenous administration. Each milliliter contains approximately 50 mg of IgG with trace amounts of IgA and IgM, 50 mg sucrose, and 10 mg human albumin. Sodium content is 20 to 30 mEq/L and there is no preservative. It is supplied as a liquid in one-dose vials containing approximately 1,000 mg in 20 mL or 2,500 mg in 50 mL (the concentration for both is 50 mg/mL). RespiGam (RSV-IGIV) is labeled for prevention of serious lower respiratory tract infection caused by RSV in children younger than 24 months of age with CLD or a history of premature birth (younger than 35 weeks' gestation), but it is not labeled for use in patients with CHD (see Official recommendations below).

Neither product is indicated for treatment of established RSV disease.

E. Storage, handling, and administration
- *Synagis (RSV-mAb)*
  - Maintain temperature at 35° to 46°F (2° to 8°C)
  - Do not freeze
  - Swirl gently to reconstitute (do not shake)
  - Reconstituted product should stand at room temperature for a minimum of 20 minutes until the solution is clear and should be administered within 6 hours of reconstitution
  - Each dose is 15 mg/kg given intramuscularly [see Chapter 3(III); volumes greater than 1 mL should be divided]
- *RespiGam (RSV-IGIV)*
  - Maintain temperature at 35° to 46°F (2° to 8°C)
  - Do not freeze
  - Do not shake vial because this causes foaming
  - Administer intravenously [see Chapter 3(III)]

- Use separate intravenous line with a constant infusion pump and in-line filter (pore size 15 μ or smaller)
- May be piggybacked into a preexisting line running sodium chloride or dextrose solutions (2.5%, 5%, 10%, or 20% in water, with or without sodium chloride); should not be diluted more than 1:2 with any of these solutions
- *Initial dose*: 1.5 mL/kg/h (75 mg/kg/h)
- *Subsequent doses*: if tolerated after 15 minutes, increase to 3.6 mL/kg/h (180 mg/kg/h) for remainder of infusion
- Maximum total dose per monthly infusion is 15 mL/kg (750 mg/kg)

F. Schedule. Monthly doses of either product are initiated before the onset of the RSV season and terminated at the end of the season. In most parts of the United States, this means starting in November and ending in March.

G. Efficacy

- *Synagis (RSV-mAb).* The safety and efficacy of RSV-mAb were assessed in a clinical trial (referred to as the IMpact-RSV Study) conducted in high-risk pediatric patients at 139 centers in the United States, Canada, and the United Kingdom during the 1996 to 1997 season. Patients were 24 months of age or younger with CLD or 6 months of age or younger and born at 35 weeks' gestation or less. Patients with uncorrected CHD were excluded from enrollment. Approximately 1,000 patients received RSV-mAb and 500 received placebo; five monthly injections were given. RSV hospitalization occurred in 10.6% of placebo recipients and 4.8% of RSV-mAb recipients, for an efficacy of 55%. Efficacy in children with CLD was 39% and in premature infants without CLD was 78%, and total hospital days were reduced by 42%. No difference in RSV mortality was seen. These results were the first to demonstrate efficacy of a monoclonal antibody in preventing disease in humans. Postmarketing data from nine pediatric centers during the 1998 to 1999 season showed hospitalization rates in treated patients with CLD or prematurity of 4% or less.

  In late 2002, the results of a large controlled trial in children with hemodynamically significant CHD were released. A total of 1,287 children 2 years of age or younger were enrolled at 76 centers worldwide over four RSV seasons. There was a 45% reduction in RSV hospitalization in children who received RSV-mAb (29% in cyanotic and 58% in acyanotic patients) compared to those who received placebo. The frequency of adverse events was similar between the two groups. Based on these data, RSV-mAb is felt to be safe and effective in this population.

- *RespiGam (RSV-IGIV).* Three main studies have looked at the safety and efficacy of RSV-IGIV. The first enrolled 249 children, including 102 with CLD and 87 with CHD who were younger than 48 months of age, as well as 60 infants 6 months of age or younger and born at 35 weeks' gestation or less. A 63% reduction in RSV hospitalization was demonstrated, but five of the six deaths occurred in children with CHD. A second trial, referred to as the PREVENT Study, was conducted in high-risk pediatric patients at 54 centers in the United States during the 1994 to 1995 season. Patients were 24 months of age or younger with CLD or 6 months of age or younger and born at 35 weeks' gestation or less. Approximately 250 patients received RSV-IGIV and 260 received placebo; monthly infusions were given beginning in November or December through April. RSV hospitalization occurred in 13.5% of placebo recipients and 8.0% of RSV-IGIV recipients, for an efficacy of 41%. The total number of hospital days was reduced by 53%, and the number of hospital days with oxygen requirement was reduced by 60%. Hospitalizations for respiratory illness of any cause were reduced by 38%. In a third study conducted between 1992 and 1995 in children younger than 48 months of age with CHD, 58% efficacy was observed in infants younger than 6 months of age. However, increased cyanotic episodes and cardiac surgery–related deaths were seen in treated subjects.

H. Official recommendations. Passive immunoprophylaxis for RSV *should be considered* for the following persons:
- Children younger than 2 years of age with CLD who have required medical therapy (e.g., supplemental oxygen) for this condition within 6 months before the anticipated RSV season (patients with severe CLD may benefit from prophylaxis for two RSV seasons)
- Infants born at 32 weeks' gestation or less without CLD: decision must be individualized to the patient and the prevailing epidemiology of RSV disease in the community
  - 28 weeks' gestation or less: consider up to 12 months of age
  - 29 to 32 weeks' gestation: consider up to 6 months of age
- Infants 32 to 35 weeks' gestation with additional risk factors, including neurologic disease in very-low-birth-weight infants, large number of young siblings, child care attendance, exposure to tobacco smoke in the home, anticipated cardiac surgery, anticipated problems in availability of hospital care for serious respiratory disease
- Patients meeting the above criteria with asymptomatic, acyanotic CHD
- Patients with severe immunodeficiencies
- Patients 24 months of age or younger with *hemodynamically significant* CHD

- Use of Synagis (RSV-mAb) may be considered based on results of recent clinical trial
- Candidates include patients receiving medication for congestive heart failure, those with pulmonary artery hypertension, and those with cyanotic lesions
- Infants with *hemodynamically insignificant* CHD and those with surgically corrected lesions do not need prophylaxis unless they still require medication for congestive heart failure
- A dose should be considered when stable after bypass because antibody levels decline substantially after surgery
- RespiGam (RSV-IGIV) is *contraindicated* in this patient population
- No recommendations can be made regarding the use of passive immunoprophylaxis in RSV outbreaks in high-risk settings (e.g., pediatric intensive care unit)

Synagis (RSV-mAb) is preferred in most patients because of ease of administration, safety, and effectiveness. However, RespiGam (RSV-IGIV) may be preferred in certain situations. For example, immune-deficient patients who receive IGIV replacement therapy might benefit from substitution of RSV-IGIV for IGIV during the respiratory season.

Synagis (RSV-mAb) can be administered concomitantly with any vaccines. Children receiving RespiGam (RSV-IGIV) can receive inactivated vaccines at any time, but live-attenuated vaccines should be deferred at least 9 months after the last dose [see Chapter 1(I)].

I. **Safety.** In the IMpact-RSV trial, there were no statistically significant differences in adverse events between placebo and Synagis (RSV-mAb) recipients. Transient local reactions were reported in approximately 3% of Synagis (RSV-mAb) recipients, including erythema, pain, induration, and bruising. Approximately 3% of patients reported fever. There are certain safety issues for RespiGam (RSV-IGIV) that are common to all intravenous immune globulin products, including the possibility of renal failure, sensitization of IgA-deficient individuals, aseptic meningitis, and transmission of bloodborne pathogens [see Chapter 11(III)]. Children with CLD may be sensitive to the volume of RespiGam (RSV-IGIV) infusion and may need added diuretic therapy. In the PREVENT trial, adverse events thought to be related to the study drug occurred in approximately 3% of subjects and included respiratory distress, fever, and acrocyanosis.

J. **Contraindications**
- *Synagis (RSV-mAb)*: anaphylactic reaction to a prior dose or to any component
- *RespiGam (RSV-IGIV)*
  - Anaphylactic reaction to a prior dose or to any immune globulin product

- Selective IgA deficiency
- Cyanotic CHD

K. Precautions
- *Synagis (RSV-mAb)*: severe thrombocytopenia or any coagulation disorder that would contraindicate intramuscular administration
- *RespiGam (RSV-IGIV)*: renal insufficiency, volume depletion, or concomitant nephrotoxic drugs

---

KEY CONCEPTS: RSV IMMUNE GLOBULINS

- RSV is a major cause of pediatric hospitalization in the winter
- Prematurity and CLD are risk factors for serious disease
- Prophylaxis available through monthly intramuscular injections of RSV-mAb or intravenous infusions of RSV-IGIV
- Indicated for high-risk children
- RSV-IGIV contraindicated in CHD

V. Rabies immune globulin

Rabies virus is a bullet-shaped, enveloped, single-stranded RNA virus in the Rhabdoviridae family that infects animals and is neurotropic.

The disease, epidemiology and transmission, and rationale for active vaccination are discussed in Chapter 8(VIII).

A. Rationale for passive immunoprophylaxis. The long incubation period makes rabies uniquely suited to postexposure prophylaxis through both active and passive immunization. Because rabies in humans is nearly always fatal, any encounter with a potentially rabid animal should lead to vaccination and, depending on prior vaccination status, administration of human rabies immune globulin (RIG). RIG provides immediate passive antibodies for a short period of time and protects the patient until antibodies are produced in response to the vaccine.

B. Passive immunoprophylactics. Two hyperimmune globulin preparations are available in the United States: BayRab (RIG; Bayer Corporation) and Imogam Rabies HT (RIG; Aventis Pasteur). These products consist of IgG derived from pooled human plasma from donors who have been hyperimmunized with rabies vaccine; they are therefore polyclonal (they contain a variety of antibodies, including antibodies to other organisms). Both products are purified by cold ethanol fractionation and are formulated for intramuscular administration; further virus inactivation steps for BayRab (RIG) include solvent/detergent treatment and for Imogam

Rabies HT (RIG) include heat treatment. Both products contain antirabies antibody of at least 150 IU/mL, and both are preservative free. BayRab (RIG) contains 15% to 18% protein, and Imogam Rabies HT (RIG) contains 10% to 18% protein; both products contain glycine. They are each supplied as a liquid in 2-mL (300 IU) and 10-mL (1,500 IU) vials and are indicated for postexposure prophylaxis in previously unimmunized individuals (RIG is always used in conjunction with active vaccination in such individuals).

C. Storage, handling, and administration
- Maintain temperature at 35° to 46°F (2° to 8°C)
- Do not freeze
- Each dose is 20 IU/kg (0.133 mL/kg), given at the same time as the first dose of vaccine (simultaneous administration is preferred, but if this does not occur, RIG can be given up to 7 days after vaccination is instituted); as much of the dose as possible should be thoroughly infiltrated into the wound and the surrounding tissues, and any remaining RIG should be given intramuscularly at a separate site from the vaccine

D. Schedule. RIG should be given as soon as possible after exposure, ideally within 24 hours, along with the first dose of rabies vaccine (*which is given at a separate site*). Only one dose should be administered. If initiation of treatment is delayed for any reason, RIG and the first dose of vaccine should still be given, regardless of the interval between exposure and treatment. RIG may be given up to 7 days after the first dose of vaccine was given.

E. Efficacy. RIG has a half-life of approximately 24 days. Adequate serum titers are present 24 hours after injection and peak within 2 to 13 days. Properly executed, postexposure prophylaxis with local wound care, vaccine, and RIG is probably 100% effective.

F. Official recommendations. For postexposure prophylaxis recommendations, see Chapter 8(VIII). Live viral vaccines such as MMR and varicella should not be given for 4 months after administration of RIG [see Chapter 1(I)].

G. Safety. Certain safety issues are common to all immune globulin products, including the sensitization of IgA-deficient individuals and transmission of bloodborne pathogens [see Chapter 11(III)]. Local reactions at the injection site include tenderness, pain, soreness, and muscle stiffness. Systemic reactions include headache and malaise.

H. Contraindications. None known.

I. Precautions
- Anaphylactic reaction to a prior dose or to any immune globulin product
- Selective IgA deficiency (risk of sensitization due to minute amounts of IgA in RIG)

- Severe thrombocytopenia or any coagulation disorder that would contraindicate intramuscular administration

---

KEY CONCEPTS: RIG

- Two products available in United States
- Vaccine series should always be initiated at same time (at separate site)
- As much of dose as possible is given into wound

VI. Tetanus immune globulin

Clostridium tetani is a nonencapsulated, gram-positive, obligately anaerobic bacillus that produces a potent neurotoxin.

The disease, epidemiology and transmission, and rationale for active vaccination are discussed in Chapters 5(I) and 7(I).

A. Rationale for passive immunoprophylaxis. In high-risk situations, such as deep, contaminated wounds in incompletely immunized persons, active vaccination alone may not provide enough toxin-neutralizing antibody in time to prevent tetanus. Passive immunization is therefore indicated.

B. Passive immunoprophylactics. The only hyperimmune globulin available in the United States is BayTet (human tetanus immune globulin, TIG), manufactured by Bayer Corporation. It consists of IgG derived from pooled human plasma from donors who have been immunized with tetanus toxoid vaccine, and is therefore polyclonal (it contains a variety of antibodies, including antibodies to other organisms). BayTet (TIG) is purified by cold ethanol fractionation, solvent/detergent treated for virus inactivation, and formulated for intramuscular administration without preservative. The product contains 15% to 18% protein as well as glycine and is supplied as a liquid in prefilled syringes (250 units) with a needle and UltraSafe Needle Guard. BayTet (TIG) is indicated for prophylaxis against tetanus after injury in patients with incomplete or uncertain immunization history. It is also indicated as part of a treatment regimen for active cases of tetanus, although evidence of effectiveness is limited. Simultaneous vaccination (at a separate site) is always indicated when TIG is given.

C. Storage, handling, and administration
- Maintain temperature at 35° to 46°F (2° to 8°C)
- Do not freeze (discard if frozen)
- Each dose for wound prophylaxis is 250 units given intramuscularly; for treatment of active disease, a single dose of 3,000 to 6,000 units is given intramus-

cularly (some authorities recommend infiltration of the wound)

D. Schedule. TIG should be given as soon as possible after exposure, along with a dose of a tetanus toxoid vaccine (*given at a separate site*). Only one dose should be administered.

E. Efficacy. Antibody is detectable within 24 hours of administration and peaks at 48 hours. TIG has a half-life of 3.5 to 4.5 weeks, and protective antibody concentrations (0.01 antitoxin units/mL) persist for approximately 4 weeks. Efficacy is high. Therapeutic use does not inactivate toxin already bound to nerve tissue, but it may modify the effects of circulating toxin.

F. Official recommendations. For wound prophylaxis recommendations, see Chapter 7(I) and Table 7.2. Live viral vaccines such as MMR and varicella should not be given for 3 months after administration of TIG [see Chapter 1(I)].

G. Safety. Certain safety issues are common to all immune globulin products, including the sensitization of IgA-deficient individuals and transmission of bloodborne pathogens [see Chapter 11(III)]. Reactions include slight soreness at the injection site and mild fever.

H. Contraindications. None known.

I. Precautions
- Anaphylactic reaction to a prior dose or to any immune globulin product
- Selective IgA deficiency (risk of sensitization due to minute amounts of IgA in TIG)
- Severe thrombocytopenia or any coagulation disorder that would contraindicate intramuscular administration

---

KEY CONCEPTS: TIG

- One product available in United States
- Indicated only when vaccination is incomplete or unknown
- Always used in conjunction with vaccine (at separate site) for prophylaxis
- Can be part of regimen for treatment of disease

VII. Varicella-zoster immune globulin

Varicella-zoster virus is a large, enveloped, double-stranded DNA virus capable of establishing latency.

The disease, epidemiology and transmission, and rationale for active vaccination are discussed in Chapter 5(VII).

A. Rationale for passive immunoprophylaxis. Active vaccination is available to immunocompetent individuals both pre- and postexposure. However, receipt of this live-attenuated vaccine is contraindicated in the very individuals who are at risk for complicated natural varicella, namely, those who are immunocompromised or pregnant. Passive immunization represents an alternative for individuals in these groups who are exposed and do not have natural immunity.

B. Passive immunoprophylactics. The only hyperimmune globulin available in the United States is varicella-zoster immune globulin (VZIG; no trade name), manufactured by the Massachusetts Public Health Biologic Laboratories and distributed by FFF Enterprises (formerly distributed by the American Red Cross). It consists of IgG derived from pooled human plasma from donors selected for high titers of antibody to varicella; as such, VZIG is polyclonal (it contains a variety of antibodies, including antibodies to other organisms). VZIG is purified by cold ethanol fractionation, solvent/detergent treated for virus inactivation, and formulated for intramuscular administration without preservative. The product contains 10% to 18% protein as well as glycine and is supplied as a liquid in 1.25-mL (125 units) and 6.25-mL (625 units) vials. VZIG is indicated for prophylaxis of exposed, susceptible individuals at high risk for complications of varicella, including immunocompromised children, newborns of mothers with varicella shortly before or after delivery, premature infants, immunocompromised and healthy susceptible adults, pregnant women, and full-term infants less than 1 year of age.

C. Storage, handling, and administration
- Maintain temperature at 35° to 46°F (2° to 8°C)
- Do not freeze
- Administered intramuscularly [see Chapter 3(III)] using dose given in Table 11.7
- For patients greater than 10 kg, the maximum volume at a single injection site is 2.5 mL

D. Schedule. VZIG should be given as soon as possible after exposure and within 96 hours. If a second exposure occurs more than 3 weeks after one dose, a second dose should be given.

E. Efficacy. VZIG contains 10 to 20 times the amount of varicella antibody than ordinary immune globulin, and

Table 11.7.   Dose of VZIG

Weight (kg)	Units	Number of vials
0–10	125	1 (125 unit)
10.1–20	250	2 (125 unit)
20.1–30	375	3 (125 unit)
30.1–40	500	4 (125 unit)
>40	625	1 (625 unit) or 5 (125 unit)

varicella antibodies persist for 1 month or longer after administration. Onset of action is very prompt, but the duration of protection is unknown. When given within 96 hours of exposure, VZIG has been shown to significantly reduce the morbidity and mortality from varicella among immunocompromised individuals. Attack rates among VZIG recipients vary from 20% to 65%, compared to 90% after household exposure. The majority of treated children who develop infection have very mild disease with complication rates of 7% or lower.

F. **Official recommendations.** VZIG is recommended for *susceptible, high-risk individuals* who are *exposed* to varicella. *Susceptibility* can reasonably be ascertained by the following criteria: no personal history of varicella or shingles and no history of immunization, or no detectable antibody despite a history of varicella and/or immunization (this definition is imperfect, because the absence of antibody by commercial assays does not necessarily mean the absence of immunity). Bone marrow transplant patients are considered susceptible regardless of disease and immunization status. In immunocompromised patients, receipt of blood products can give false-positive serologic results, and administration of VZIG may be indicated regardless of serologic results.

Exposure is considered to have occurred in the following situations:
- Residence in same household as index case
- Face-to-face play for greater than 1 hour (some experts say 5 minutes is enough) with index case
- Index case in a hospital
  - Staying in same two- or four-bed room
  - Staying in adjacent bed on a large ward
  - Face-to-face contact for greater than 1 hour (some experts say 5 minutes is enough)
- Hospital visitation by a contagious person
- Intimate contact (hugging or touching) with a person who has zoster
- Infant born to a mother with onset of varicella 5 days or less before or 48 hours or less after delivery

High-risk individuals who *should receive* VZIG if *susceptible* to varicella include the following:
- Immunocompromised children and adults, including those with HIV infection [see Chapter 12(I)]
- Pregnant women (VZIG can prevent serious disease in the mother; it is not known if it can prevent fetal varicella syndrome) [see Chapter 12(II)]

Other *high-risk individuals* who *should receive* VZIG include the following:
  • Infants born to mothers with onset of varicella 5 days or less before or 48 hours or less after delivery
  • Hospitalized premature infants 28 weeks' gestation or more whose mothers lack a reliable history of chickenpox or varicella antibody

• Hospitalized premature infants less than 28 weeks' gestation or 1,000 g birth weight or less regardless of the mother's history or serostatus

VZIG *may be considered* for healthy *susceptible* adults but is not routinely recommended. Most adults without a history of chickenpox are actually immune, and for those who are not, acyclovir treatment represents an alternative way to avert severe disease.

VZIG does not interfere with inactivated vaccines when given at separate sites, but live virus vaccines such as MMR and varicella should be deferred at least 5 months [see Chapter 1(I)]. Persons who receive VZIG within 14 days after live virus vaccination should be revaccinated 5 months later. Administration of VZIG results in false-positive tests for varicella immunity for approximately 2 months.

G. **Safety.** The most frequent local adverse reactions are pain, redness, and swelling at the injection site, occurring in approximately 1% of patients. Systemic reactions are less frequent and include gastrointestinal symptoms, malaise, headache, rash, and respiratory symptoms. Certain safety issues are common to all immune globulin products, including the sensitization of IgA-deficient individuals and transmission of blood-borne pathogens [see Chapter 11(III)].

H. **Contraindications.** Anaphylactic reaction to a prior dose or to any immune globulin product.

I. **Precautions**
   • Selective IgA deficiency (risk of sensitization due to minute amounts of IgA in VZIG)
   • Severe thrombocytopenia or any coagulation disorder that would contraindicate intramuscular administration

---

KEY CONCEPTS: VZIG

• One product available in United States
• Indicated for susceptible high-risk individuals
• Given within 96 hours of exposure

VIII. Human botulinum immune globulin and equine botulinum antitoxin

---

Clostridium botulinum is a gram-positive, anaerobic, spore-forming bacillus that produces one of the most potent neurotoxins known.

A. **Disease.** Botulism is a paralytic disorder caused by neurotoxins (predominantly types A and B) elaborated by *C. botulinum*. These toxins are systemically absorbed and bind irreversibly to receptors on presynaptic nerve endings, preventing the release of acetylcholine. *Infant botu-*

lism results from ingestion of spores and growth of the organism in the gastrointestinal tract. Symptoms begin 3 to 30 days after exposure and include constipation, lethargy, weak cry, poor feeding, diminished gag reflex, cranial nerve palsies, generalized weakness, and floppiness. Physical examination is remarkable for alertness, good color, and nontoxic appearance despite hypotonia, hyporeflexia, disconjugate gaze, and signs of autonomic dysfunction. Progression to respiratory failure can occur.

Foodborne botulism is due to the ingestion of preformed toxin in foods. Symptoms usually begin 12 to 36 hours after ingestion and initially involve the bulbar musculature, with double vision, difficulty swallowing, difficulty speaking, and dry mouth. Symmetric paralysis can descend rapidly, ultimately resulting in respiratory failure. *Wound botulism* resembles foodborne disease clinically but results from toxin elaborated by *C. botulinum* in traumatic wounds that are contaminated with soil. The onset of symptoms occurs 4 to 14 days after injury.

B. Epidemiology and transmission. *C. botulinum* spores are ubiquitous in soil. Most infant botulism cases can be related to spores in the immediate environment, including those carried by family members from soil (e.g., construction sites) into the home. Approximately 15% of cases are caused by spores contaminating honey fed to the infant. Clusters of cases may reflect a local high density of spores in the soil. Foodborne disease occurs when contaminated, improperly prepared food is stored under anaerobic conditions that permit germination, multiplication, and toxin production. Classically implicated are home-canned foods and ethnic foods prepared in the home and preserved under oil, which provides the anaerobic environment. High heat under high pressure can destroy spores before foods are canned; heating to 212°F (100°C) can destroy preformed toxin. In recent years, most cases of wound botulism have been in drug abusers who inject black tar heroin. In the United States an average of 110 cases of botulism are reported each year—25% foodborne, 72% infant, and approximately 3% wound associated.

Botulism is not transmitted from person to person, and natural immunity to botulinum toxin does not develop, even after severe disease.

C. Rationale for passive immunotherapy. Patients with botulism may have free toxin circulating in serum, which is available for neutralization with antitoxins and hyperimmune globulins.

D. Passive immunotherapeutics. Two products are available in the United States:

- *Equine botulinum antitoxin, trivalent (types A, B, and E)*: This is a refined and concentrated preparation of horse globulins (taken from horses immunized with formaldehyde-inactivated botulinum toxin) that has been modified by enzymatic digestion. It is produced by Connaught Laboratories (Willowdale, Ontario) but is only available from the Centers for Disease Control and Prevention (CDC). The request for antitoxin must be initiated through state or local health departments (if this is not possible, the CDC Drug Service can be contacted at 404-639-3670 or 404-639-2888). The product is supplied as a liquid in 10-mL vials, each of which contains 7,500 IU (2,381 U.S. units) type A, 5,500 IU (1,839 U.S. units) type B, and 8,500 IU (8,500 U.S. units) type E antitoxin. It is licensed for treatment of suspected or proven cases of foodborne or wound botulinum toxin poisoning.

- *Human-derived botulinum antitoxin*: This product, formerly known as *human botulism immune globulin (BIG)*, is produced by the Massachusetts Public Health Biologic Laboratories and distributed under an investigational protocol by the Infant Botulism Treatment and Prevention Program of the California Department of Health Services. BIG consists of IgG derived from pooled human plasma from volunteers hyperimmunized with pentavalent botulinum toxoid; it is therefore polyclonal (it contains a variety of antibodies, including antibodies to other organisms). BIG is not licensed but is available as a treatment investigational new drug for infant botulism by calling 510-540-2646.

E. Storage, handling, and administration
- *Equine botulinum antitoxin*
  - Maintain temperature at 35° to 46°F (2° to 8°C)
  - Patients must first be tested for hypersensitivity under controlled conditions with availability of emergency equipment [see Chapter 3(V)]. Testing is performed in two stages: first a scratch, prick, or puncture test is performed; if this test is negative, an intradermal test is performed. Positive results are indicated by a wheal with surrounding erythema at least 3 mm larger than the negative control, read 15 to 20 minutes after application. A histamine control must be positive for valid interpretation. Testing should be performed when the patient has been off antihistamines for 24 to 48 hours, if possible.
    - *Scratch, prick, or puncture test*: Apply one drop of serum diluted 1:100 in 0.9% preservative-free saline to the site of a superficial scratch, prick, or puncture on the volar surface of the forearm. A positive control, consisting of histamine, and a negative control, consisting of saline, should also be applied at separate sites.
    - *Intradermal skin test*: Caution should be exercised because intradermal tests have resulted in fatalities. Inject intradermally 0.02 mL of a 1:1,000 dilution of serum in 0.9% preservative-free saline, raising a small wheal. Positive and negative controls should also be applied as

Table 11.8. Desensitization to animal-derived antitoxins

Dose number[a]	Dilution[b]	Volume of injection (mL)	Route	
			Preferred	Alternate
1	1:1,000	0.1	IV	ID
2	1:1,000	0.3	IV	ID
3	1:1,000	0.6	IV	SC
4	1:100	0.1	IV	SC
5	1:100	0.3	IV	SC
6	1:100	0.6	IV	SC
7	1:10	0.1	IV	SC
8	1:10	0.3	IV	SC
9	1:10	0.6	IV	SC
10	Undiluted	0.1	IV	SC
11	Undiluted	0.3	IV	SC
12	Undiluted	0.6	IV	IM
13	Undiluted	1.0	IV	IM

ID, intradermal.
[a]Successive doses are given at 15-minute intervals.
[b]Diluted in 0.9% sodium chloride.
Adapted from AAP. Antibodies of animal origin (animal antisera). In: Pickering LK, ed. *Red book: 2003 report of the Committee on Infectious Diseases*, 26th ed. Elk Grove Village, IL: American Academy of Pediatrics; 2003:60–63.

described for the scratch test. A negative initial intradermal test should be repeated with a 1:100 dilution of serum. For patients who have no history of animal allergy or exposure to animal serum, the 1:100 dilution may be used initially, provided that a negative scratch, prick, or puncture test is obtained first.
- If there is positive test for sensitivity or a history of previous administration of animal serum or allergy to animals, desensitization should be carried out by serial injections of diluted antitoxin as indicated in Table 11.8
- Should be administered with caution and emergency preparedness even in patients with negative tests for hypersensitivity
- Equine antitoxin can be administered intravenously or intramuscularly
- Dosing is variable and dependent on the clinical status of the patient; most adult patients receive between two and four vials
- Concurrent use of antihistamines with or without steroids may minimize reactions
- *Human-derived botulinum antitoxin*
  - Maintain temperature at 35° to 46°F (2° to 8°C)
  - The usual dose is 50 mg/kg
F. **Schedule.** Antitoxins should be administered as soon as botulism is suspected.

G. Efficacy
- *Equine botulinum antitoxin.* Onset of action is rapid, and there is no significant difference in circulating antitoxin levels whether the antitoxin is given intravenously or intramuscularly. The half-life is approximately 1 week. The sooner antitoxin is given, the better the prognosis. However, it may still be beneficial if administered as many as several days after onset, as circulating toxin may still be present several weeks after consumption of contaminated foods. Studies have shown reductions in mortality due to type E botulism from 49% to 3.5% and type A botulism from 46% to 27% when compared to untreated patients.
- *Human-derived botulinum antitoxin.* The half-life of BIG is approximately 21 days. A randomized, placebo-controlled trial of a single intravenous dose of BIG for infant botulism was completed in California under the sponsorship of the FDA's Orphan Drug Program. BIG recipients had a significant reduction in hospitalization—from 5.5 to 2.5 weeks—and a two-thirds reduction in the rate of intubation.

H. Official recommendations. Equine antitoxin is recommended for the treatment of foodborne and wound botulism. It is not used for infant botulism because there is no evidence of benefit, and there is the risk of inducing lifelong hypersensitivity to equine antigens. BIG is recommended for the treatment of infant botulism. Although no official recommendations exist, children receiving BIG can probably receive inactivated vaccines at any time, but live-attenuated vaccines should probably be deferred at least 9 months.

I. Safety. Approximately 20% of patients experience some degree of hypersensitivity to equine antitoxin. Anaphylactic reactions are IgE mediated and occur immediately. Acute febrile reactions can occur, and serum sickness, characterized by fever, rash, and arthritis, may occur as late as 3 weeks after administration. Certain safety issues common to all intravenous immune globulin products probably apply to BIG, including the possibility of renal failure, sensitization of IgA-deficient individuals, aseptic meningitis, and transmission of bloodborne pathogens [see Chapter 11(III)].

J. Contraindications
- *Equine botulinum antitoxin*: Anaphylactic reaction to horse serum
- *Human-derived botulinum antitoxin*
  - Anaphylactic reaction to a prior dose or to any immune globulin product
  - Selective IgA deficiency

K. Precautions. No specific precautions for these products have been published.

KEY CONCEPTS: BOTULISM ANTITOXINS
- Botulinum toxin is one of the most potent toxins known
- Infant disease is due to growth of *C. botulinum* in the gut
- Foodborne disease is due to preformed toxin
- Disease not transmitted from person to person
- Equine- and human-derived antitoxins available
- Testing for hypersensitivity is necessary before administering equine antitoxin
- Equine antitoxin not indicated for infant disease
- Human antitoxin is only available under an investigational protocol
- Antitoxin should be administered as soon as diagnosis is suspected

---

IX. Equine diphtheria antitoxin

Corynebacterium diphtheriae is an aerobic, pleomorphic gram-positive bacillus that produces a potent exotoxin.

The disease, epidemiology and transmission, and rationale for active vaccination are discussed in Chapter 5(I).

A. Rationale for passive immunotherapy. Because patients may deteriorate rapidly, passive immunization is indicated to neutralize toxin at the site of infection and in the circulation. Diphtheria antitoxin is not indicated for the prevention of diphtheria in exposed individuals; instead, surveillance, culture, and antibiotic prophylaxis should be initiated. Booster doses of vaccine may also be indicated [see Chapter 7(I)].

B. Passive immunotherapeutics. Equine diphtheria antitoxin is a refined and concentrated preparation of horse globulins (taken from horses immunized with diphtheria toxoid and toxin) that has been modified by enzymatic digestion. It is produced by Aventis Pasteur but is only available from the CDC. Physicians treating a suspected case of diphtheria should contact the diphtheria duty officer at 404-639-8255 (weekdays during business hours) or at 404-639-2889 (all other times). The product has a potency of 500 antitoxin units/mL or greater based on the U.S. Standard Diphtheria Antitoxin. It is supplied in 1,000 IU and 20,000 IU vials and is preserved with a cresol derivative. The original product was licensed for the prevention of diphtheria in nonimmunized individuals exposed to the disease and for the treatment of suspected or confirmed cases. However, since January 6, 1997, licensed diphtheria antitoxin with a valid expiration date has not been available in the United States. The CDC has a supply of European antitoxin that is comparable to the older U.S. product but is only available under a treatment investigational new drug protocol.

C. Storage, handling, and administration

- Maintain temperature at 35° to 46°F (2° to 8°C)
- Patients must first be tested for hypersensitivity under controlled conditions as described for equine botulinum antitoxin [see Chapter 11(VIII)]
- If there is positive test for sensitivity or a history of previous administration of animal serum or allergy to animals, desensitization should be carried out by serial injections of diluted antitoxin as indicated for equine botulinum antitoxin [see Chapter 11(VIII) and Table 11.8]
- Should be administered with caution and emergency preparedness even in patients with negative tests for hypersensitivity
- The dose is determined by the site and size of the diphtheritic membrane, the degree of toxicity, and the duration of the illness
  - Pharyngeal or laryngeal disease of 48 hours' duration or less: 20,000 to 40,000 units
  - Nasopharyngeal lesions: 40,000 to 60,000 units
  - Extensive disease of 3 days' duration or more or diffuse swelling of neck: 80,000 to 120,000 units
  - Consider 20,000 to 40,000 units for cutaneous disease
- Intravenous administration is preferred but should be done under the direction of the CDC
- Concurrent use of antihistamines with or without steroids may minimize reactions

D. Schedule. Equine diphtheria antitoxin should be administered as soon as the diagnosis is suspected, even before culture results are available.

E. Efficacy. Multiple studies have demonstrated that antitoxin is effective in reducing diphtheria mortality, primarily by preventing cardiovascular toxicity. There is a strong relationship between improved outcome and early administration of antitoxin. In a nonblinded trial, 8 of 242 patients (3.3%) treated with antitoxin died compared to 30 of 245 (12.2%) control patients. Other studies show that mortality ranges from 1.5% to 4.2% if antitoxin is given within the first 2 days of illness, compared to 6.9% to 20.2% if it is given on the third day or later.

F. Official recommendations. Equine diphtheria antitoxin is indicated for the treatment of suspected or confirmed cases of diphtheria. Use in unimmunized close contacts of a case is not recommended because there is no evidence that it provides benefit beyond antimicrobial prophylaxis and because of the risk of allergic reactions.

G. Safety. Approximately 20% of patients experience some degree of hypersensitivity reaction to equine antitoxin. Anaphylactic reactions are IgE mediated and occur immediately. Acute febrile reactions can occur, and serum sickness, characterized by fever, rash, and arthritis, may occur as late as 3 weeks after administration. A "thermal reaction" has been described, consisting of a chilly sensation,

slight difficulty breathing, and rapid rise in body temperature within 20 to 60 minutes of administration.
H. **Contraindications.** Anaphylactic reaction to horse
serum.
I. **Precautions.** No specific precautions for this product
have been published.

KEY CONCEPTS: EQUINE DIPHTHERIA ANTITOXIN

- Testing for hypersensitivity is necessary before administering
- Intravenous administration preferred
- Not recommended for postexposure prophylaxis
- Should be administered as soon as diagnosis is suspected

X. **Vaccinia immune globulin.** Vaccinia immune globulin
(VIG) was produced in the 1960s from the plasma of individuals who had recently received smallpox vaccination. It contained a high titer of neutralizing antibodies to vaccinia and
was available only for intramuscular injection. With the
reinstitution of smallpox vaccination in biodefense preparedness [see Chapter 9(I)], there is renewed interest in
the use of VIG to treat complications of vaccination. There is
currently enough VIG stored at the CDC to treat 600 to 800
adverse events, and the drug is available only under a treatment investigational new drug protocol. New lots of VIG are
being prepared for both IM and IV administration, but these
must undergo extensive testing before use. By 2004, there
should be approximately 30,000 doses available.

Historically, VIG was used approximately once for every
1 million primary vaccinees. Indications included extensive
inadvertent inoculation, eczema vaccinatum, severe generalized vaccinia, and vaccinia necrosum (progressive vaccinia). It was not recommended for mild complications,
erythema multiforme, or encephalitis, and it was contraindicated for vaccinia keratitis. Doses of 0.6 mL/kg were
used, but in severe cases, 1 to 10 mL/kg were given. For
assistance in managing complications of smallpox vaccination, clinicians should contact the CDC at 877-554-4625.

Vaccination in Special Circumstances

I. Impaired immunity. Vaccination of patients with impaired immunity requires special consideration for a number of reasons:

- *The risk-benefit ratio is complex*: Immunocompromised individuals are at greater risk for complications and death from vaccine-preventable diseases. At the same time, they may be at increased risk of complications from live vaccines, and the response to all vaccines may be suboptimal. Decisions regarding vaccination are therefore more complicated than they are in healthy individuals and must take into account the prevalence of disease and probability of exposure, the nature and degree of immunodeficiency, the type of vaccine and the likelihood of adverse effects, the efficacy of the vaccine when immunity is impaired, and the confounding effects of other interventions. Unfortunately, in many situations there are few data available to provide guidance.

- *Immunocompromised states differ qualitatively*: Qualitative differences dictate not only which vaccines are indicated but which vaccines represent a danger to the patient. Congenital immunodeficiencies may affect humoral immunity, cell-mediated immunity, phagocyte function, and complement function in different and interconnected ways. Humoral immune defects place patients at higher risk of invasive infection with encapsulated bacteria, demanding special consideration for vaccination against *Haemophilus influenzae* type b (Hib), pneumococcus, and meningococcus. Profound humoral defects increase the risk of serious enterovirus infection, making avoidance of oral poliovirus vaccine (OPV) of paramount importance. Alternatively, patients with isolated humoral defects are not at increased risk of complications from live varicella vaccine, because cellular responses are generally intact. In fact, varicella vaccine *is indicated* in these patients to prevent bacterial complications of chickenpox, for which they may be unusually susceptible. Complement deficiencies put patients at risk for bacterial infections but carry no implications for the safety of live or inactivated vaccines. Phagocyte dysfunction per se may not substantially weaken defenses against influenza virus, but it *does* increase the risk of bacterial superinfection. Thus, for example, patients with chronic granulomatous disease (whose neutrophils fail to undergo oxidative burst) should receive yearly inactivated influenza vaccine to prevent bacterial pneumonia. Secondary immune deficiency states, such as those resulting from immunosuppressive medications, nephrotic syndrome, malnutrition, splenectomy, or bone marrow transplantation, also differ qualitatively from one another.

- *Immunocompromised states differ quantitatively*: In general, patients with cell-mediated immune defects should not receive live vaccines because of the risk of dissemination. However, cellular defects may range from mild to profound, and these differences affect the risk-benefit ratio for vaccination. For example, although varicella vaccine should be avoided in human immunodeficiency virus (HIV)-infected individuals with low CD4 counts, poor T-cell function, and a history of opportunistic infections, it *should be given* to mildly symptomatic HIV-infected children with CD4 percentages of 25% or higher. In the former situation, the risk of vaccination is too great; in the latter, the risk of vaccination is small and is outweighed by the risk of natural disease. Along similar lines, DiGeorge syndrome, a quantitative T-cell deficiency resulting from thymic dysplasia, is quite variable in expression. Although those patients with low CD4 and CD8 counts and abnormal T-cell function *should not* receive live vaccines, live vaccines are probably safe in those patients with normal T-cell studies. Similarly, measles, mumps, and rubella vaccine (MMR) may be given to HIV-infected children *without profound immunosuppression* as determined by CD4 counts.
- *Immune responses may be suboptimal*: Data on the immunogenicity of many vaccines in immunocompromised individuals are lacking. Some patients would not be expected to respond at all. For example, there is no point in giving inactivated vaccines to patients with X-linked agammaglobulinemia because they do not make antibody. On the other hand, patients with common variable immunodeficiency may or may not respond, and such vaccines are worth giving with the hope of some benefit. Some patients who have normal concentrations of antibody may *still* not respond appropriately to certain vaccines. In fact, this constitutes an operational definition of "antibody deficiency with normal immunoglobulins" or "antibody dysfunction syndrome." In some cases, more intensive immunization regimens are necessary to achieve protective immunity. The polyclonal immune globulin for intravenous administration (IGIV) replacement therapy received by some patients with humoral defects protects them from disease but also limits the usefulness of live vaccines, which can be inactivated by passively acquired antibodies.
- *Immunization of close contacts is important but may carry risks*: Immunocompromised patients can be protected by ensuring that close contacts, especially other household members, are appropriately immunized. For example, acquired immunodeficiency syndrome (AIDS) patients may not respond well to influenza vaccine but can be protected from influenza by immunizing family members.

Certain vaccines, however, can be transmitted from vaccinees to immunocompromised contacts, resulting in complications. A classic example of this is vaccine-associated poliomyelitis resulting from transmission of OPV within the home. Although varicella vaccine *can* be transmitted horizontally, this probably only occurs if the vaccinee develops a rash after vaccination. Because natural varicella can be so devastating in immunocompromised hosts, many of whom cannot be vaccinated themselves, the risk-benefit ratio favors vaccinating household contacts. If a vaccinee develops a rash, he or she should avoid direct contact with the immunocompromised person until the lesions are crusted over. MMR vaccine is not horizontally transmitted and *should be given* to household contacts if indicated. Alternatively, smallpox vaccine should *not* be given to household contacts of immunocompromised persons because the risk of transmission is substantial, the complications are severe, and the risk of exposure to natural infection is (presumably) very low. Hepatitis A vaccine (Hep-A) should be given to contacts if the family resides in a high-incidence area.

- *Official recommendations may differ from product labeling*: Many package inserts list immunodeficiency states as contraindications to vaccination. This labeling reflects allowable claims and mandated precautions that derive from data presented to the U.S. Food and Drug Administration (FDA) at the time of licensure. Subsequent recommendations may be discordant with product labeling because of the availability of new data or reasoned reevaluations of the pertinent risks and benefits. Practitioners should be aware of these discrepancies. For example, the package insert for VARIVAX (varicella vaccine) states that the vaccine is contraindicated in individuals receiving immunosuppressive therapy and those with cellular or humoral immunodeficiencies. Official recommendations, however, allow for vaccination of certain individuals with these conditions.

The following sections give general guidelines for vaccination of persons with impaired immunity. Pre- and post-exposure passive immunoprophylaxis is discussed in Chapter 11.

A. Humoral deficiencies

- *Typical syndromes*: X-linked agammaglobulinemia, common variable immunodeficiency, IgA deficiency, IgG subclass deficiency, antibody deficiency with normal immunoglobulins (vaccine nonresponder state or antibody dysfunction syndrome), transient hypogammaglobulinemia of infancy
- *Contraindicated for safety reasons*: Live bacterial vaccines, vaccinia, and OPV are generally contraindicated. Varicella vaccine may be given, and MMR may be considered. Patients with selective IgA deficiency can probably receive all currently available vaccines safely because they have adequate serum IgG responses.

- *Special considerations*: Inactivated vaccines are not effective in patients with severe deficiencies of immune globulin synthesis. Because many of these patients receive monthly IGIV replacement therapy, live viral vaccines are unlikely to be effective, as they are neutralized by passively acquired antibodies. Less severely affected individuals who are not receiving IGIV may benefit from vaccination; in these cases, postimmunization antibody titers may be used to confirm responses.

B. Defects of cell-mediated immunity
  - *Typical syndromes* (humoral immunity is affected in most of these syndromes as well): severe combined immunodeficiency, DiGeorge syndrome, hyper-IgM syndrome, bare lymphocyte syndrome, autoimmune polyendocrinopathy-candidiasis-ectodermal dystrophy (chronic mucocutaneous candidiasis), Wiskott-Aldrich syndrome, ataxia-telangiectasia
  - *Contraindicated for safety reasons*: All live bacterial and viral vaccines are contraindicated.
  - *Special considerations*: Inactivated vaccines may be given, but effective responses are doubtful.

C. Phagocyte disorders
  - *Typical syndromes*: chronic granulomatous disease, leukocyte adhesion deficiency, Chédiak-Higashi syndrome, myeloperoxidase deficiency, hyperimmunoglobulinemia E/recurrent infection syndrome (Job syndrome), secondary granule deficiency
  - *Contraindicated for safety reasons*: All live bacterial vaccines are contraindicated.
  - *Special considerations*: Effective responses to all routine vaccines probably occur. Inactivated influenza vaccine is indicated to reduce the risk of secondary bacterial infection.

D. Complement deficiencies
  - *Typical syndromes*: deficiency of individual early (C1–C4) or late (C5–C9) components, properdin deficiency, factor I deficiency, secondary deficiency due to complement consumption
  - *Contraindicated for safety reasons*: No vaccines are contraindicated.
  - *Special considerations*: Patients with early component deficiencies are particularly susceptible to gram-positive organisms such as pneumococcus and should probably receive both pneumococcal and meningococcal vaccines. Those with late component deficiencies are uniquely susceptible to meningococcus and should be vaccinated against this pathogen. Inactivated influenza vaccine is indicated to reduce the risk of secondary bacterial infection.

E. Human immunodeficiency virus
  - *Perinatally exposed infants whose HIV status is indeterminate*: Infants born to HIV-infected mothers who are in the process of being evaluated for HIV infection should receive all routine inactivated vaccines. Inacti-

vated influenza vaccine should be given beginning at 6 months of age to the patient as well as to all household contacts, including the mother. OPV is contraindicated. Bacille Calmette-Guérin vaccine (BCG) may be given at birth in those parts of the world where it is routinely used.

- *Perinatally exposed infants who are not infected with HIV*: These are infants who have had at least two negative HIV polymerase chain reaction (PCR) tests, one at 1 month of age or older and one at 4 months of age or older, and have no other clinical or laboratory evidence of HIV infection. They should receive all routine vaccines, including MMR at 12 to 15 months of age and varicella vaccine at 12 to 18 months of age. Inactivated influenza vaccine should be given beginning at 6 months of age to the patient as well as to all household contacts, including the mother. OPV is contraindicated because of the possibility of spread to HIV-infected contacts.
- *HIV-infected infants and children*
  - OPV and BCG are contraindicated
  - The parenteral inactivated typhoid vaccine, rather than the live oral vaccine, should be given to persons at risk for typhoid fever
  - In general, live viral vaccines should be avoided, with the following exceptions:
    - *Yellow fever*: Travelers with asymptomatic HIV infection who cannot avoid exposure to yellow fever should be offered vaccination
    - *Measles, mumps, and rubella*: MMR may be given to HIV-infected patients with no or moderate immunosuppression (i.e., without *severe* immunosuppression as defined in Table 12.1) regardless of the presence or absence of symptoms. The second dose of MMR may be given any time 1 month or longer after the first dose. In fact, there is a strong rationale for giving the second dose early, as immune function may deteriorate before 4 to 6 years of age, when the second dose is usually recommended. Passive immunoprophylaxis for measles exposure is recommended by the American Academy of Pediatrics (AAP) for all HIV-infected children and adolescents, regardless of vaccination status, degree of symptoms, and level of immune suppression [the Advisory Committee on Immunization Practices (ACIP) recommendations specify only *symptomatic* HIV infection]. If the patient is already receiving IGIV and 2 weeks or more have elapsed since the last dose, consideration should be given to administering the next dose early.
    - *Varicella*: Asymptomatic or mildly symptomatic patients with no evidence of immunosuppression, as defined in Table 12.1, may receive varicella vaccine. The recommended schedule is two doses separated by 3 months. Patients who are already

Table 12.1.   CDC classification of HIV infection

Immuno-suppression	Age <12 mo		Age 1–5 yr		Age ≥6 yr	
	CD4 cells/μL	CD4 %	CD4 cells/μL	CD4 %	CD4 cells/μL	CD4 %
None	≥1,500	≥25	≥1,000	≥25	≥500	≥25
Moderate	750–1,499	15–24	500–999	15–24	200–499	15–24
Severe	<750	<15	<500	<15	<200	<15

Adapted from AAP. Human immunodeficiency virus infection. In: Pickering LK, ed. *Red book: 2003 report of the Committee on Infectious Diseases*, 26th ed. Elk Grove Village, IL: American Academy of Pediatrics, 2003:360–382.

receiving IGIV are assumed to be protected against varicella. Official guidelines for administration of human varicella-zoster immune globulin (VZIG) to HIV-infected individuals after exposure to chickenpox or shingles are incomplete because of a lack of data. The following guidelines seem reasonable:

- VZIG is indicated for *symptomatic and/or immunosuppressed* patients who are *susceptible* to varicella. "Susceptible" means no personal history of varicella or shingles and no history of immunization, or no detectable antibody despite a history of varicella and/or immunization. This definition is imperfect, because some individuals who lack antibody by commercial assays are still immune.

- Children with a personal history of varicella and/or adequate immunization (two doses given at a time when they were immunocompetent) may still be immune even if they have developed severe immunosuppression, and they are probably at more risk for reactivation of endogenous virus than reinfection with exogenous virus. Nevertheless, exposure of these children to chickenpox is a complex situation, and decisions regarding VZIG should be made with the assistance of an infectious disease specialist.

- Asymptomatic HIV-infected children without evidence of immunosuppression who have a personal history of varicella and/or adequate immunization do not need VZIG.

- It is difficult to know how to handle susceptible, asymptomatic children without evidence of immunosuppression. These children are probably at low risk for complicated varicella. One option is postexposure vaccination, which is recommended for children who do not have HIV [see Chapter 5(VII)]. However, data regarding efficacy in this situation are lacking, and the two doses recommended for HIV-infected children cannot be delivered in a postexposure time frame. Another option is to begin antiviral therapy at the first sign of illness. VZIG is probably not necessary.

- Adults who had varicella and/or adequate immunization before acquiring HIV probably do not need VZIG, regardless of the level of immunosuppression.
- VZIG should be considered for susceptible, asymptomatic adults without evidence of immunosuppression.

- HIV-infected patients may receive all routine inactivated vaccines and should receive yearly inactivated influenza vaccine beginning at 6 months of age (family members should receive this vaccine as well).
- For children who have completed the pneumococcal conjugate vaccine (PCV-7) series by 15 months of age, a dose of pneumococcal polysaccharide vaccine (Pne-PS) should be given at 24 months, and a single booster of Pne-PS should be considered 3 to 5 years later. For children 24 to 59 months of age who have not been immunized against pneumococcus, two doses of PCV-7 followed by a dose of Pne-PS should be given, each separated by 6 to 8 weeks; a booster dose of Pne-23 may be considered 3 to 5 years later. For unimmunized children 5 years of age or older, it would be reasonable to administer a dose of PCV-7 followed 6 to 8 weeks later by a dose of Pne-23, with a booster dose of Pne-23 3 to 5 years later.
- Meningococcal polysaccharide vaccine (Men-PS) is not routinely indicated for HIV-infected patients.
- *HIV-infected adolescents and adults*: Recommendations include yearly inactivated influenza vaccine and routine diphtheria and tetanus vaccine (Td) boosters. The hepatitis B vaccine (Hep-B) series should be given to patients who have not received it before. Pne-PS should be considered, as should Men-PS for college students.

F. Steroids. Because steroids may be immunosuppressive, they represent a potential problem in the use of live viral and bacterial vaccines. Any patient receiving steroids in any form who has clinical or laboratory evidence of immunosuppression should not receive live vaccines. In addition, patients whose underlying disease itself is immunosuppressive should not receive these vaccines, except under special circumstances. The following guidelines are offered for live vaccines in other situations:

- *Topical, inhaled, and compartmental depot injections*: Vaccination is acceptable
- *Physiologic replacement*: Vaccination is acceptable
- *Less than 2 mg/kg/day (less than 20 mg if over 10 kg; daily or alternating days) of prednisone or equivalent*: Vaccination is acceptable

- *Greater than 2 mg/kg/day (greater than 20 mg if over 10 kg; daily or alternating days) of prednisone or equivalent for less than 14 days*: Vaccinate right after stopping steroid therapy. Do not vaccinate if steroid therapy will extend to 14 days or more
- *Greater than 2 mg/kg/day (greater than 20 mg if over 10 kg; daily or alternating days) of prednisone or equivalent for 14 days or longer*: Vaccinate 1 month after stopping therapy

G. **Immunosuppressive chemotherapy.** Live-virus vaccines are usually withheld for 3 months or longer after immunosuppressive chemotherapy has been discontinued. This interval may vary with the type and intensity of immunosuppressive therapy, radiation therapy, underlying disease, and other factors. For children who are older than 12 months of age, previously immunized, and scheduled to undergo solid-organ transplantation, antibody titers against measles, mumps, rubella, and varicella should be obtained. Children who are susceptible should be given MMR vaccine, varicella vaccine, or both at least 1 month before transplantation. Antibody titers to measles, mumps, rubella, and varicella should be measured in all patients 1 year after transplantation. Although live-virus vaccines are usually contraindicated in these patients because they are receiving chronic immunosuppressive medications, those who are seronegative are candidates for passive immunization if exposed to disease. Solid-organ transplant patients should receive inactivated influenza vaccine 6 months or more after transplant and then annually for life. Hib vaccine and PCV-7 are only recommended in children and should be given before transplant. Men-PS is not routinely indicated. Inactivated vaccines should be given approximately 1 year after transplantation to ensure immunogenicity.

H. **Bone marrow transplantation.** Allogeneic bone marrow transplantation presents a complicated vaccination paradigm. The underlying disease itself may be immunosuppressive, the therapy used to prepare for transplantation ablates existing immunity, immunosuppressive therapy is given (sometimes for life) after the procedure, and graft-versus-host disease may further compromise immune function. Moreover, the adopted immune system of the donor provides unreliable immunity of uncertain duration; fortunately, immune memory can be recalled by immunization after engraftment (it is not clear whether lasting benefits accrue from immunization of the donor before transplant). Although graft-versus-host disease is not an issue with autologous transplantation and the conditioning regimens may be less severe, studies show that vaccine-induced immunity may be lost after transplantation.

Patients should be routinely revaccinated after bone marrow transplantation according to Table 12.2.

Table 12.2. Initial revaccination of bone marrow transplant patients

Disease	Vaccine/time after transplant		
	12 Mo	14 Mo	24 Mo
Diphtheria, tetanus, pertussis			
Age <7 yr	DTaP[a]	DTaP[a]	DTaP[a]
Age ≥7 yr	Td	Td	Td
Hepatitis A	Not routinely recommended[b]		
Hepatitis B	Hep-B[c]	Hep-B[c]	Hep-B[c]
Hib	Hib conjugate[d]	Hib conjugate[d]	Hib conjugate[d]
Inactivated influenza	Yearly beginning before transplant and resuming ≥6 mo after transplant (consider chemoprophylaxis as well)		
Measles, mumps, rubella	—	—	MMR if immunocompetent[e,f]
Meningococcus	Not routinely recommended		
Pneumococcus	Pne-PS[f]	—	Pne-PS[f]
Polio	IPV	IPV	IPV
Varicella	Contraindicated[g]		

[a]Diphtheria and tetanus vaccine for pediatric use (DT) if pertussis vaccine is contraindicated.

[b]Hep-A vaccine may be considered 12 months or more after transplantation for persons who have chronic liver disease or chronic graft-versus-host disease, persons living in endemic areas who otherwise qualify for routine vaccination, or persons living in areas experiencing outbreaks. Two doses should be given separated by 6 to 12 months. Polyclonal immune globulin for intramuscular administration (IGIM) is preferred for travel because data regarding immunogenicity of vaccine are lacking.

[c]Consider using the 40-μg dose (see Table 5.5). Test for anti-HBsAg antibody 1 to 3 months after the third dose; if negative, repeat the three-dose series one time.

[d]May be given regardless of age.

[e]A second dose should be given 6 to 12 months later. Patients with chronic graft-versus-host disease should not receive MMR.

[f]In children younger than 5 years of age, some clinicians would consider giving two doses of PCV-7 followed by one dose of Pne-PS, each separated by 6 to 8 weeks; one-time revaccination with Pne-PS in 3 to 5 years should be considered. In children 5 years of age or older, one dose of PCV-7 followed 6 to 8 weeks later by one dose of Pne-PS, with Pne-PS revaccination in 3 to 5 years, seems reasonable.

[g]Passive immunoprophylaxis should be given to all exposed patients regardless of personal history of disease or vaccination.

Adapted from CDC. Guidelines for preventing opportunistic infections among hematopoietic stem cell transplant recipients: Recommendations of CDC, the Infectious Disease Society of America, and the American Society of Blood and Marrow Transplantation. *MMWR* 2000;49(RR-10):1–128; AAP. Immunocompromised children. In: Pickering LK, ed. *Red book: 2003 report of the Committee on Infectious Diseases*, 26th ed. Elk Grove Village, IL: American Academy of Pediatrics, 2003:69–81.

I. Anatomic and functional asplenia. Patients with asplenia, whether anatomic (e.g., congenital, traumatic, or surgical) or functional (e.g., sickle cell disease, polysplenia syndrome), are at risk for life-threatening infection with encapsulated organisms, particularly pneumococcus. The basis for this risk lies in impaired clearance of opsonized bacteria, coordination of lymphocyte responses, and synthesis of IgM and phagocytosis-enhancing factors. The following guidelines are offered:

- *All asplenic individuals*: Yearly inactivated influenza vaccine should be given beginning at 6 months of age to prevent secondary bacterial infection. Family members should be immunized as well. Live vaccines may be given. Prophylactic antibiotics are indicated in certain individuals.
- *Children who are anatomically or functionally asplenic from birth (including sickle cell disease) or are splenectomized in the first 2 years of life*: PCV-7 and Hib conjugate should be given according to the routine schedule. At 2 years of age, Men-PS and Pne-PS should be given. A second dose of Pne-PS should be given 3 to 5 years later, and a second dose of Men-PS may be considered at that time. Children who were first vaccinated at less than 4 years of age should be considered for revaccination after 2 to 3 years. Revaccination for older children and adults 3 to 5 years after their first dose should also be considered. Only one revaccination with Pne-PS is indicated, and there are no clear-cut recommendations for repeated revaccination with Men-PS.
- *Elective splenectomy*: Under 2 years of age, a dose of PCV-7 and Hib conjugate should be given at least 2 weeks before surgery. Beyond 2 years of age, Hib, Pne-PS, and Men-PS should be given at least 2 weeks before the procedure. Consider one-time revaccination with Pne-PS and Men-PS 3 to 5 years later.
- *Traumatic splenectomy beyond 2 years of age*:
  - *Patient has already received the routine PCV-7 and Hib series*: The patient should receive one dose of Pne-PS and a booster dose of Hib.
  - *Patient never received PCV-7 or Hib (this includes adults)*: Children between 24 and 59 months of age should receive two doses of PCV-7 followed by one dose of Pne-PS, each separated by 6 to 8 weeks. They should also receive two doses of Hib vaccine, 2 months apart. Children 5 years of age or older should receive one dose of Hib and one dose of Pne-PS.
  - Men-PS may be considered beyond 2 years of age.

J. Chronic disease. Individuals with chronic underlying diseases may be unusually susceptible to infectious diseases, regardless of whether they have immune deficiency in the classic sense. As a general rule, all routine vaccines should be given unless they are specifically contraindicated. Additional vaccines are indicated as well. There is no reason (other than a true contraindication) not to give yearly inactivated influenza vaccine to any patient over 6 months of age who has a chronic underlying disease that might put him or her at risk for complications or secondary bacterial infection. This would include patients with chronic cardiac (e.g., congenital heart disease), respiratory (e.g., cystic fibrosis), allergic (e.g., asthma), hematologic (e.g., sickle cell disease), metabolic (e.g., diabetes), neuromuscular (e.g., muscular dystrophy), hepatic (e.g., cirrhosis), and renal (e.g., chronic renal failure) disorders. Patients who are particularly susceptible to pneumococcal infection, such as those with nephrotic syndrome, should receive pneumococcal vaccine as well. Patients with chronic liver disease are also at risk for severe hepatitis A and should receive Hep-A.

II. **Pregnancy and breast-feeding.** Although vaccination during pregnancy poses *theoretical* risks to the developing fetus, there is no evidence directly linking any vaccine (even live ones) to birth defects. Nevertheless, pregnant women should be vaccinated only when the vaccine is unlikely to cause harm, the risk for exposure to disease is high, and the infection would pose a significant risk to the mother or fetus. Delaying vaccination until the second or third trimester, when possible, is reasonable to minimize concerns about teratogenicity. In addition, thimerosal-free products should be used, if available.

In considering vaccines and pregnancy, clinicians should be aware of the following:

- Approximately 2% of all newborns have a congenital malformation; it follows that some women who are vaccinated during pregnancy have infants with birth defects. Although a causal relationship with the vaccine may be lacking, there may be a tendency to attribute the birth defect to the vaccine. Pregnant women should be counseled about this before being vaccinated.
- Very few vaccines have been tested for safety and efficacy in large numbers of pregnant women. For this reason, most vaccines are classified as Pregnancy Category C by the FDA, meaning that although there are no adequate and well-controlled studies in humans (regardless of whether animal studies have been done or show fetal harm), the benefits in pregnant women may be acceptable despite the potential risks. Even vaccines that *are indicated* in pregnancy, such as inactivated influenza vaccine, carry this labeling.
- Live vaccines are generally contraindicated during pregnancy. However, inadvertent receipt of live vaccines is not a reason to terminate the pregnancy because there is no definitive evidence of maternal-fetal transmission or fetal harm. Women who have received MMR or varicella vaccines should wait at least 1 month before becoming pregnant. There is no contraindication to giving either of these vaccines to household contacts. In the case of varicella vaccine, if the pregnant woman is known to be sus-

ceptible to varicella and a close contact develops a rash after vaccination, exposure should be avoided until the vaccinee's lesions are crusted over. One situation in which a live vaccine might be given during pregnancy is when a women is traveling to an area where she will be at substantial risk of exposure to yellow fever. Another example in which the benefits of live-virus vaccination outweigh the risks is exposure of a pregnant woman to smallpox.

- There are no known risks of passive immunization during pregnancy. In fact, VZIG *is recommended* for susceptible pregnant women who are exposed to varicella, because the risk of complicated disease in the mother is high (it is not know whether VZIG protects the fetus).
- Breast-feeding per se is not a contraindication to the use of any vaccines, including live-attenuated ones, except for preevent use of smallpox vaccine.

Td and inactivated influenza are routinely recommended for pregnant women in the United States. Those who have not received a tetanus booster in the last 10 years should be given a dose of Td, and those who are unimmunized or partially immunized should receive a primary series. Inactivated influenza vaccine should be administered to all women who will be at or beyond 14 weeks of pregnancy during the influenza season. Vaccines that should be considered if the benefits outweigh the risks include Pne-PS, Hep-A, Hep-B, and inactivated poliovirus vaccine (IPV).

III. **International adoptees, refugees, and immigrants.** Since 1996, the Immigration and Naturalization Act has required all immigrant children entering the United States to show proof of having received all ACIP-recommended vaccines before an immigration visa is granted. International adoptees are exempted from this requirement, but the adoptive parents must sign a waiver indicating their intention to comply with immunization requirements after the child arrives. Refugees are also exempted from immunization requirements at the time of entry, but they must show proof of immunization at the time at which they apply for permanent residency, usually within 3 years of arrival.

The following issues are relevant in the immunization management of individuals from other countries, particularly international adoptees:

- Vaccination records are considered valid only if in written form and containing the vaccines, dates of administration, intervals between doses, and age at the time of immunization
- Written records must be translated and interpreted correctly, and even then may be inaccurate or fraudulent
- The immunization schedule in many countries differs from that in the United States
- Vaccines in some countries may have inadequate potency, especially because of handling issues
- Serologic correlates of protection exist for some diseases but not for others. Testing may be expensive, and results require interpretation.

- There is no harm in revaccinating individuals who have already been vaccinated, although reactogenicity to diphtheria, tetanus, and acellular pertussis vaccine (DTaP) and Pne-PS may increase with successive doses

It is desirable for all individuals entering the United States permanently to receive all routinely recommended vaccines. For reasons mentioned above, the simplest approach is to start over and revaccinate. Young infants can be vaccinated according to the routine childhood schedule (see Table 1.9); older children can be vaccinated according to catch-up schedules (see Table 1.12). Individuals from hepatitis B–endemic areas should be screened for hepatitis B virus surface antigen (HBsAg); if positive, vaccination is unnecessary. For older children, an alternative—although somewhat less practical—approach is to test for antibodies to the major vaccine antigens and administer those vaccines to which the child has no immunity. For adults who immigrate to the United States, consideration should be given to vaccination with MMR, Td, Hep-B, and varicella.

IV. **Health care personnel.** Health care workers, as well as individuals who work in residential institutions, may be exposed to vaccine-preventable diseases and may transmit them to patients or residents. Individuals who fit into this category include staff, physicians, nurses, students, and ancillary personnel—in essence, anyone who might have contact with patients. The risks of infection might be particularly high for people working in emergency departments or ambulatory care settings, especially if the facility serves underimmunized populations. The consequences of transmission to patients might be particularly high wherever there are vulnerable patients, such as intensive care units, newborn nurseries, obstetric wards, chronic care facilities, and oncology or transplant units. Health care workers should be up-to-date on all routinely recommended vaccines, including, for example, tetanus boosters. Diseases that deserve particular attention include the following:

- *Rubella*: Individuals born before 1957 are considered immune to rubella regardless of whether they recall having had the disease. However, health care facilities should recommend MMR vaccine to unimmunized workers born before 1957 who lack rubella antibodies (workers with direct patient contact should be tested). Persons should be considered immune only on the basis of serologic tests or documented proof of immunization at 12 months of age or older. A personal history of rubella is unreliable and should not be used to judge immune status, because so many rash illnesses can mimic the disease. All susceptible persons should be immunized with MMR or monocomponent rubella vaccine (if immunity to measles and mumps has been documented).
- *Measles*: Individuals born before 1957 are considered immune to measles regardless of whether they recall having had the disease. Health care personnel born in

1957 or later should have evidence of immunity as established by physician-documented measles, a positive serologic test, or receipt of two doses of a live measles vaccine (such as MMR) at 12 months of age or older. Health care facilities should consider offering at least one dose of a measles-containing vaccine to workers born before 1957 who lack proof of immunity (workers with direct patient contact should be tested), particularly in communities with ongoing measles transmission.

- *Hepatitis B*: Hep-B is recommended for all health care workers who are likely to be exposed to blood or blood-containing body fluids. Those who are at ongoing risk for sharps injuries should be tested for antibodies to HBsAg after the three-dose series, and those who test negative should receive another three-dose series one time only. If they remain seronegative, they should be tested for HBsAg, as chronic carriage could explain failure to respond to the vaccine.

- *Mumps*: Adults born before 1957 are considered to be immune to mumps regardless of whether they recall having had the disease. Those born in 1957 or later are considered immune if they have had a single dose of mumps vaccine at 12 months of age or older, or if they have mumps antibody.

- *Varicella*: Varicella immunity is strongly recommended for all health care personnel. Proof of immunity is constituted by a reliable personal history of chickenpox or physician-documented disease, a positive antibody test, or prior receipt of two doses of vaccine separated by at least 1 month. Vaccinated individuals can return to work immediately, but if a rash develops (for example, vesicles at the inoculation site), the worker should not have contact with immunocompromised patients; he or she can continue to work with patients who are not immunosuppressed as long as the lesions are kept covered. Workers who develop generalized rash should be furloughed until the rash is resolved. Vaccinated workers who are exposed should be tested immediately for antibody, as vaccination does not always result in seroconversion. If seronegative, they may be retested 5 to 6 days later. If antibody is present at that time, disease is unlikely to develop; if antibody is not present, the worker should be furloughed or monitored closely for disease.

- *Influenza*: Influenza immunization programs for health care workers should be organized in the fall of each year.

Hospitals and other facilities may develop policies that require documentation of immunization or immunity. Documentation of immunization or immunity of all health care workers against vaccine-preventable diseases should be included as part of a comprehensive occupational health program at health care facilities. Immunizations should be provided at no cost to the worker. Studies have shown that this preventative strategy is more cost-effective than treating patients and their contacts for vaccine-preventable diseases. The extent to which these recommendations are carried out varies considerably from institution to institution. Vaccination cannot be forced on a health care worker who is reluctant to be vaccinated. In these situations, it should be emphasized that exposure to a vaccine-preventable disease could result in leave without pay during the period of potential communicability, and workers' compensation benefits would not apply unless the disease actually developed.

V. **Travel.** Travelers going to Canada, Western Europe, Australia, and New Zealand are probably at no higher risk of illness than those traveling within the United States. For other destinations, however, consideration may need to be given to other vaccines or to accelerated schedules for routine vaccines, depending to some extent on what circumstances the traveler will encounter. Travel to certain areas may require other considerations, including malaria chemoprophylaxis, insect avoidance, food hygiene, and the availability of emergency medical services. Moreover, certain individuals may be at higher risk than others for particular diseases.

Travel medicine clinics, which may be available at local health departments, academic medical centers, or in private practice settings, maintain up-to-date information and provide vaccination services for travelers. Primary care physicians who choose to provide travel vaccines to their patients should be aware of the following:

- *Planning*: Consultation should take place 4 to 6 weeks before departure to allow for the development of protective immunity after vaccination. More time may be required if certain vaccines must be ordered.
- *Itinerary*: It is not enough to know to what country the person is traveling. The duration of stay and the particular activities in which the person will be engaged can help determine risk. For example, a 2-day stay in a sophisticated urban hotel carries different risks than extended field work in rural areas.
- *Routine vaccines*: All travelers should be up-to-date on routinely recommended vaccines. Some special considerations are listed below:
  - *Childhood vaccination schedule*: The routine childhood schedule (see Table 1.9) provides some flexibility in the timing of doses. For example, the third dose of Hep-B and IPV can be given as early as 6 months of age, and the fourth dose of Hib and PCV-7 can be given as early as 12 months of age. The fourth dose of DTaP can be given as early as 12 months of age, provided that 6 months or more have elapsed since the third dose. Varicella vaccine can be given as early as 12 months of age. The first dose of MMR can be given as early as 6 months of age if travel to an endemic area is expected (reimmunization with two doses after the first birthday is necessary). For infants immunized after the first birthday, the second dose of MMR can be

given as early as 4 weeks after the first dose. Physicians should be aware of flexibility in the schedule and administer all eligible vaccines before the anticipated date of travel.

- *Td*: Although boosters are recommended only every 10 years in adults, consideration should be given to a dose if more than 5 years have elapsed and the person will be working in situations in which dirty wounds might be incurred or traveling to regions where diphtheria outbreaks have occurred.
- *Polio*: Previously immunized adults traveling to endemic areas should receive one dose of IPV (this does not need to be given again for subsequent travel). If travel of an infant to an endemic area is imminent, three doses of IPV can be given at 4-week intervals.
- *Influenza*: Inactivated influenza vaccine may be given to anyone 6 months of age or older who is traveling to areas with influenza activity. This should especially be considered for children 6 to 23 months of age and is recommended for adults 50 years of age or older. Live-attenuated influenza vaccine can be used in healthy individuals 5 to 49 years of age.
- *Pne-PS*: All adults 65 years of age or older should be immunized.
- *Hep-B*: For those individuals who might have missed universal immunization, Hep-B vaccine should be given if such travelers might be exposed to blood, have sexual contact with the local population, stay longer than 6 months, or be exposed through medical treatment.

- *Mandatory vaccines*: The only vaccine covered by international health regulations at the present time is yellow fever, for which travelers to certain countries must have a valid International Certificate of Vaccination [see Chapter 8(XI)]. However, some countries have their own regulations. For example, Saudi Arabia requires meningococcal vaccine for pilgrims visiting Mecca for the Hajj, and some countries may require the vaccine for individuals returning from the Hajj.
- *Recommended vaccines*: Table 12.3 gives some general guidelines regarding vaccines for travel to certain parts of the world. Specific information about the vaccines is contained in the referenced sections of this book. Because disease outbreaks are always occurring and guidelines frequently change, the best advice is to check updated resources (see below) before traveling.
- *Resources*: Excellent online travel health resources are available to physicians, some of which are listed in Table 12.4. Of particular note are two publications by the Centers for Disease Control and Prevention (CDC), both of which are available online:
  - *Health Information for International Travel* (www.cdc.gov/travel/yb/index.htm): The "Yellow Book" is published every 2 years and serves as a reference for those who advise international travelers of health risks

Table 12.3.   General travel recommendations

Region	Diphtheria [5(I), 7(I)]	Hepatitis A [8(IV)]	Polio [5(IV)]	Japanese encephalitis virus [8(V)]	Meningococcus [8(VII)]	Rabies[a] [8(VIII)]	Typhoid[b] [8(IX)]	Yellow fever[c] [8(X)]
Central Africa		✓	✓		✓	✓	✓	✓
East Africa		✓	✓		✓	✓	✓	✓
North Africa		✓	✓			✓	✓	
Southern Africa		✓	✓			✓	✓	
West Africa		✓	✓		✓	✓	✓	✓
East Asia		✓		✓		✓	✓	
South Asia		✓		✓		✓	✓	
Southeast Asia		✓[d]		✓		✓	✓	
Australia and the South Pacific		✓				✓	✓	
Caribbean		✓				✓	✓	✓
Central America and Mexico		✓				✓	✓	✓
Eastern Europe	✓					✓	✓	
Western Europe								
Indian Subcontinent		✓		✓		✓	✓	
Middle East		✓			✓	✓	✓	

Vaccine-preventable diseases of particular interest [chapter]

(continued)

Table 12.3. *Continued*

Region	Vaccine-preventable diseases of particular interest [chapter]							
	Diphtheria [5(I), 7(I)]	Hepatitis A [8(IV)]	Polio [5(IV)]	Japanese encephalitis virus [8(V)]	Meningococcus [8(VII)]	Rabies[a] [8(VIII)]	Typhoid[b] [8(IX)]	Yellow fever[c] [8(X)]
Former Soviet Union	✓	✓	—	—	—	✓	✓	—[e]
Temperate South America	—	✓	—	—	—	✓	✓	✓
Tropical South America	—	✓	—	—	—	✓	✓	✓

[a] If exposure to wild or domestic animals is expected.
[b] If visiting developing countries in the region.
[c] Vaccinees should receive a valid International Certificate of Vaccination. Some countries require a certificate from travelers arriving from infected areas. Others require vaccination of all entering travelers; still others may waive the requirements for travelers coming from noninfected areas and staying less than 2 weeks. Vaccination is also recommended for travel outside of urban areas of countries in endemic areas that do not officially report the disease. Some countries require a traveler who has been in any country thought to harbor the disease to have a valid certificate, even if only in transit.
[d] Except Australia and New Zealand.
[e] Outside urban areas in Argentina.
Adapted from CDC, National Center for Infectious Diseases: Travelers' Health: www.cdc.gov/travel/index.htm (accessed 01/21/03).

Table 12.4.   Travel medicine resources

Organization	URL
Centers for Disease Control and Prevention: National Center for Infectious Diseases	www.cdc.gov/travel
World Health Organization: International Travel and Health	www.who.int/ith
International Society of Travel Medicine	www.istm.org
MDtravelhealth.com	www.mdtravelhealth.com
Travel Medicine, Inc.	www.travmed.com

- *Summary of Health Information for International Travel* (www.cdc.gov/travel/blusheet.htm): The "Blue Sheet" is continuously updated and contains information that supplements the Yellow Book, including notices about recent disease outbreaks or changes in vaccination requirements
- **VI. Other special situations.** Table 12.5 summarizes other situations and groups that deserve special attention for certain vaccines.

Table 12.5.   Vaccination in special circumstances[a]

Condition or circumstance	Particular risks and special considerations
Animal workers and veterinarians	Anthrax, rabies, plague
Bleeding diathesis	Use intramuscular vaccines with caution
	Hep-A and Hep-B for patients receiving clotting factors
Children and adolescents on long-term aspirin therapy	Inactivated influenza
College students living in dormitories	Meningococcus, influenza
Field personnel (e.g., Peace Corps workers)	Rabies, plague, typhoid fever
Food handlers	Hepatitis A (based on local epidemiology)
Foresters	Rabies, plague
Injecting illegal drug users	Hepatitis A, hepatitis B
Laboratory workers	Any pathogen used for which a vaccine is available
Men who have sex with men	Hepatitis A, hepatitis B
Military personnel	Children receive routine vaccines
	Meningococcus, adenovirus, influenza
	Vaccines for bioterrorism
	Travel vaccines

(continued)

Table 12.5.   *Continued*

Condition or circumstance	Particular risks and special considerations
Morticians	Hepatitis B
Native Americans and Alaskans	Pneumococcus, Hib
Patients with cochlear implants or cerebrospinal fluid leaks	Pneumococcus
Premature infants	Follow routine schedule at appropriate chronologic age Do not reduce doses Hep-B: see Chapters 5(III) and 11(II) Consider Synagis (Palivizumab; RSV-mAb) or RespiGam (RSV-IGIV)
Providers of essential community services	Influenza
Public safety workers	Hepatitis B
Residents of long-term care facilities	Influenza
Sewage workers	Typhoid, hepatitis A,[b] hepatitis B
Spelunkers	Rabies
Staff of correctional facilities	Influenza, hepatitis B
Staff of day care centers	Hepatitis A[b]
Staff of institutions for developmentally disabled	Influenza, hepatitis A,[b] hepatitis B

[a]These considerations assume that all routinely recommended series and boosters have been given.

[b]The ACIP states that there is no occupationally related increased risk of hepatitis A for these workers.

Vaccine Regulation, Policy, and Safety

I. Licensure and monitoring of vaccines in the United States. A tremendous amount of effort is involved in developing vaccine candidates. The biology of the agent and pathogenesis of the disease must be elucidated. Correlates of immunity, and the laboratory tools to measure them, must be developed. Animal models of efficacy must be investigated. Issues such as immunopotentiation, formulation, and delivery must be worked out, and consistent test lots must be produced. At that point, candidate vaccines are ready for field-testing in humans, a process that is rigorously overseen and strictly regulated. The principal agency involved in regulating this process and ensuring public safety in the United States is the U.S. Food and Drug Administration (FDA), an operating division of the Public Health Service (PHS) of the Department of Health and Human Services (DHHS). After licensure, other agencies and advisory bodies are involved in making recommendations for use and, along with the FDA, monitoring safety. Finally, overall direction for the country's vaccine program is provided by coordinating offices with input from a variety of academic organizations. The big picture of this sometimes-confusing process is given in Figure 13.1, which is useful to refer to in the discussion that follows. Chapter 14 gives contact information for many of these agencies.

Vaccines are produced under standards that ensure purity and consistency in a process regulated by the Centers for Biologics Evaluation and Research (CBER), a center within the FDA that acts under the authority of statutes in the Code of Federal Regulations. The World Health Organization (WHO) provides guidance for products that are used internationally. Laboratory testing of vaccine purity and consistency is required before and after licensure. An intensive search is performed for known viral, bacterial, and fungal agents that may contaminate vaccines, and potency tests are applied. Manufacturers are required to conform to Good Manufacturing Practices, a vast collection of rules and guidances maintained by the FDA that covers everything from raw materials quality assurance to record keeping, cleanliness standards, personnel qualifications, in-house testing, process controls, warehousing, and distribution. At least six large lots of vaccine (each containing tens of thousands of doses) with identical potencies must be produced in a manner that is demonstrated to be consistent and reliable. In addition, manufacturers are required to provide information regarding appropriate vaccine storage, handling, and safe injection practices. Fulfilling the requirements of CBER

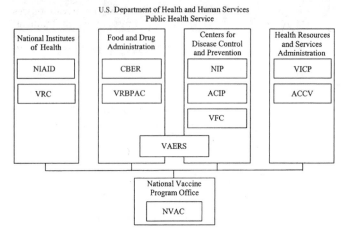

Figure 13.1.   Governmental agencies involved in vaccine research, policy, and implementation. ACCV, Advisory Commission on Childhood Vaccines; ACIP, Advisory Committee on Immunization Practices; CBER, Center for Biologics Evaluation and Research; NIAID, National Institutes of Allergy and Infectious Diseases; NIP, National Immunization Program; NVAC, National Vaccine Advisory Committee; VAERS, Vaccine Adverse Event Reporting System; VFC, Vaccines For Children program; VICP, Vaccine Injury Compensation Program; VRBPAC, Vaccines and Related Biological Products Advisory Committee; VRC, Vaccine Research Center

often takes between 5 and 10 years and is extraordinarily expensive. The average cost to develop a vaccine before licensure is between $500 and $700 million. This is one of several reasons why most vaccines can only be manufactured by large corporations.

The FDA receives advice on vaccine issues from the Vaccines and Related Biological Products Advisory Committee (VRBPAC), which consists of 15 members appointed by the FDA Commissioner. Although most members have recognized expertise in fields related to vaccinology, one member who is identified with consumer interests may be appointed. In addition, a nonvoting representative of the pharmaceutical industry may be invited. This ensures that all interested parties have input into which vaccines are tested and licensed.

Once a candidate vaccine has undergone extensive laboratory testing and is approved as an investigational new drug for use in clinical trials, studies of safety, immunogenicity, and efficacy are performed. Some of these studies are conducted by the National Institutes of Health (NIH) through the Vaccine Clinical Trials Units (VCTUs), whereas others are conducted at academic centers or private offices by pharmaceutical companies or clinical research organizations using local principal investigators. Either way, strict federal guidelines apply regarding the protection of human subjects and the management of potential conflicts of interest. Clinical trials generally proceed in three stages or phases:

- *Phase 1*: These trials usually involve only 20 to 80 volunteers and are intended to provide basic information on safety and tolerability. Because of their small size, they can detect only extremely common adverse events. Subjects are often not drawn from the intended vaccine target population. For example, pediatric vaccine candidates might undergo initial testing in adults until basic safety is assured.
- *Phase 2*: These trials enroll 100 to 200 subjects and give information about the vaccine's immunogenicity, dosage, and common side effects. These studies are performed in the proposed target group and may also provide some information on efficacy.
- *Phase 3*: These studies enroll thousands to tens of thousands of subjects, using sample sizes large enough to ensure that questions about safety and efficacy will be answered. Subjects are carefully followed for adverse events in the immediate postvaccination period (usually a maximum of 42 days). Longer periods of observation allow for determination of protection from disease and longevity of immune responses. Large trials also evaluate the consistency of responses and look at concomitant use with other vaccines. Because phase 3 trials include placebo recipients, it is relatively simple to determine whether a particular adverse event is related to the vaccine. However, prelicensure trials cannot detect rare side effects, adverse events with delayed onset, or potential reactions in culturally or ethnically diverse subpopulations.

The FDA grants licensure based on data from these studies filed by the company. It also approves a package insert, which contains official indications and statements on efficacy, contraindications, warnings, precautions, and adverse events. Unfortunately, because of litigation concerns, the package insert often lists adverse events not proved to be caused by the vaccine.

Unpredictable adverse events, which may occur as infrequently as once in every 10,000 to 100,000 doses administered, must by necessity be detected through continuing and comprehensive vaccine safety assessment after licensure.

II. **Vaccine policy and recommendations.** The Centers for Disease Control and Prevention (CDC), also an operating division of the PHS, houses the National Immunization Program (NIP), which provides leadership in the planning, coordination, and conduct of immunization activities throughout the country. The NIP assists health departments in implementing immunization programs, supports the establishment of vaccine supply contracts for state and local programs through the Vaccines For Children (VFC) Program, assists in the development of information management systems, administers research and operational programs, and supports surveillance for vaccine-preventable diseases.

The CDC is the principal body that makes recommendations for use after a vaccine is licensed by the FDA. In this role, the CDC receives advice from the following bodies:

- *Advisory Committee on Immunization Practices (ACIP)*— The ACIP provides advice and guidance to the Secretary of Health and Human Services, the Assistant Secretary, and the CDC regarding the most appropriate application of vaccines to control communicable diseases in the civilian population. It is the only entity in the federal government to function in this capacity. The 15-member committee meets three times each year and issues written recommendations that include periodicity, dosage, and contraindications. In collaboration with the other two agencies listed below, the ACIP establishes the routine childhood immunization schedule and, therefore, controls which vaccines are in the VFC program. Members with financial conflicts of interest concerning particular vaccines cannot vote on recommendations that pertain to those products.

- *American Academy of Pediatrics (AAP)*—The AAP is an organization of pediatricians and pediatric medical and surgical subspecialists that advocates for the health of children and their families and supports practitioners in their educational development and service. The Committee on Infectious Diseases (COID) develops policy recommendations on the use of vaccines and publishes the *Red Book*. The academy also partners with the CDC in implementing the Childhood Immunization Support Program, with goals to improve delivery practices, enable effective communication, and establish a network of providers promoting implementation of the best immunization practices within a medical home.

- *American Association of Family Physicians (AAFP)*— The AAFP promotes high quality standards for family doctors who provide comprehensive care to the public.

These three bodies work together to create a harmonized routine childhood immunization schedule, which is published in *Pediatrics* and *MMWR: Morbidity and Mortality Weekly Report* in January of every year. Supplemental recommendations are periodically published throughout the year. All ACIP statements are now released as joint statements with AAP and AAFP.

The National Vaccine Program Office (NVPO) was created in 1986 to coordinate the activities of all federal agencies by developing and implementing the National Vaccine Plan, which calls for the development of new and improved vaccines, ensuring optimal safety and effectiveness, better education of the medical and lay communities, and more effective use of existing vaccines. Collaboration with the commercial vaccine industry, global organizations, consumer groups, and academic institutions is also sought. The National Vaccine Advisory Committee (NVAC) makes recommendations to the NVPO regarding the supply of safe and effective vaccines, research priorities, areas of cooperation, and ways to achieve optimal prevention of infectious diseases through vaccine development while minimizing adverse reactions. The 15 members include physicians and individuals involved in research, manufacturing, parent organizations, and public health.

III. **The vaccine safety net.** The inherent limitations of assessing vaccine safety before licensure necessitate vigilance once a vaccine is brought to market. The safety net in the United States includes the following:

A. **Vaccine Adverse Event Reporting System (VAERS).** VAERS is a postmarketing surveillance system created by the National Childhood Vaccine Injury Act (NCVIA) of 1986 (Public Law 99-660) described in more detail in Chapter 2(IV). Information from VAERS reports is entered into a database, and selected serious events and deaths are compiled and analyzed. Approximately 200,000 forms are distributed, and approximately 10,000 reports are received annually. A significant limitation of VAERS is that it only receives information regarding vaccinated persons in whom an adverse event occurs. Because it does not receive information about the number of vaccine doses administered or the occurrence of adverse events in unvaccinated persons, causal relationships between vaccines and particular adverse events cannot be established. In addition, underreporting, poor data quality, incomplete reports, differences between public and private sector reporting rates, lack of consistent diagnostic criteria for disease, and simultaneous administration of multiple vaccines limit the information that can be derived from VAERS. Moreover, significant reporting biases exist. For example, increased reporting is seen immediately after licensure and when particular vaccines are "in the news."

Despite these limitations, VAERS is the only surveillance system that covers the entire U.S. population, and it includes the largest number of case reports temporally associated with vaccination. It serves to generate the signal that triggers further investigation and can provide early warning of potential problems, including new, rare, or unusual adverse events. A good example of the use of VAERS data was in prompting investigation of the relationship between rotavirus vaccine and intussusception. Unfortunately, VAERS data have also been misunderstood by the media and misused by antivaccine activists, who have made the erroneous supposition that temporal association means causation.

B. **Vaccine Safety Datalink.** The Vaccine Safety Datalink (VSD) is an active surveillance system using large linked databases that was created by the CDC in 1990.

Information regarding vaccine history and medical outcome is collected prospectively from the computerized clinical databases of four health maintenance organizations in Seattle, WA; Portland, OR; Oakland, CA; and Los Angeles, CA. Approximately 6 million people of all ages are studied through this process, amounting to 2% of the entire U.S. population. Given these numbers, relatively rare adverse events can be detected. Other strengths of the VSD include improved reporting, reduced recall bias, and the ability to study unvaccinated control subjects. For these reasons, the VSD is an excellent way to determine whether the relationship between a vaccine and an adverse event is causal or coincidental.

Formal postlicensure assessments of vaccine safety (phase 4 studies) are often required of vaccine manufacturers. These studies usually rely on large linked databases and enhance the ability to detect adverse events not apparent in prelicensure trials.

C. **Clinical Immunization Safety Assessment (CISA) centers.** Before the creation of the first CISA centers in 2001, there was no coordinated effort to evaluate and treat vaccine adverse events in individual patients. These centers, essentially partnerships between academic medical institutions and the CDC, now serve to systematically evaluate patients who experience adverse events as reported in the VAERS. In addition, health care providers can refer patients to CISA centers for consultation. The major goals of this program are to develop standard protocols for evaluation and management of adverse events, elucidate the mechanisms of these events, and provide guidelines regarding continuation of the particular vaccine series in these patients. Current CISA centers are located at Johns Hopkins University (Baltimore, MD), Northern California Kaiser Permanente (San Francisco, CA), Vanderbilt University (Nashville, TN), Boston University (Boston, MA), and Columbia Presbyterian Hospital (New York, NY).

D. **Immunization Safety Review Committee.** The Institute of Medicine (IOM) was established in 1970 by the National Academy of Sciences, a private, nonprofit, nongovernmental organization of distinguished scholars operating under a charter granted by Congress in 1863. Its purpose is to provide independent, objective, timely, authoritative information and advice to the federal government on health and science policy. On January 11, 2001, the IOM convened the Immunization Safety Review Committee, consisting of 15 members with expertise in pediatrics, internal medicine, infectious diseases, immunology, epidemiology and biostatistics, public health, nursing, ethics, and risk communication, among other disciplines. Committee members were subject to strict selection criteria to avoid real or perceived conflicts of interest. The committee was charged with reviewing,

Table 13.1. Immunization Safety Review Committee activity to date[a]

Meeting date	Issue addressed
March 8, 2001	MMR vaccine and autism
July 16, 2001	Thimerosal-containing vaccines and neurodevelopmental disorders
November 12, 2001	Multiple immunizations and immune dysfunction
March 11, 2002	Hep-B vaccine and demyelinating neurologic disorders
July 11, 2002	SV40 contamination of polio vaccine and cancer
October 28, 2002	Vaccinations and sudden unexpected death in infancy
March 13, 2003	Influenza vaccine and possible neurologic complications

[a]Reports available at www.iom.edu/IOM/IOMHome.nsf/Pages/immunization+safety+review.

over a 3-year period, nine different vaccine safety hypotheses selected by the Interagency Vaccine Group representing the NVPO, NIP, NIH, Department of Defense, FDA, National Vaccine Injury Compensation Program (VICP), Health Care Financing Administration (HCFA), and the Agency for International Development. Each review was to assess (a) scientific plausibility based on epidemiologic and clinical evidence of causality and experimental evidence for biologic mechanisms and (b) the significance of the issue in a broader societal context. Before release, the committee's reports are reviewed and critiqued by an independent panel of experts overseen by the National Research Council's Report Review Committee. Table 13.1 summarizes the issues addressed by the committee to date.

E. Task Force on Safer Childhood Vaccines. The NCVIA of 1986 mandated the establishment of the Task Force on Safer Childhood Vaccines, comprising representatives of several PHS agencies. The charge to the Task Force was to make recommendations promoting the development of safer vaccines and assuring improvement in licensing, manufacturing, processing, testing, labeling, warning, use instructions, distribution, storage, administration, field surveillance, adverse reaction reporting, recall of reactogenic lots, and research. Their report, released in 1998, emphasized the need to assess and address public concerns about the risks and benefits of vaccines, conduct research on the biologic basis for vaccine reactions, foster partnership between stakeholders, enhance the ability to detect adverse events, and improve the coordination of efforts between agencies.

F. **The safety net in action.** The release of rhesus-human reassortant rotavirus vaccine, tetravalent (RRV-TV; Rota-Shield) in the United States and its rapid withdrawal illustrate how well the safety net works. The vaccine was licensed based on demonstrated safety and efficacy in clinical trials wherein nearly 11,000 children received the vaccine in its final formulation. With universal use, the vaccine was expected to prevent 55,000 hospitalizations and 25 deaths each year. Before licensure, an ACIP Working Group, the NIH, and the AAP considered the possibility of an association between the vaccine and intussusception but rejected a causal relationship based on the following:

- Intussusception occurred in 5 of 10,054 vaccinees and 1 of 4,633 controls, a difference that was not statistically significant
- Natural rotavirus infection was not linked to intussusception
- Cases occurred at an age when one normally finds intussusception in the general population
- No cases occurred after the first dose

Nevertheless, the package insert listed intussusception as a possible adverse reaction, and postlicensure surveillance was mandated. The subsequent timeline is given in Table 13.2.

It is now estimated that intussusception attributable to RRV-TV occurred once for every 11,000 children vaccinated. This level of risk is so small that it could not have been detected in the prelicensure trials, given the number of children enrolled. However, the machinery in place to detect serious adverse events and protect the public performed remarkably well. Current trials of candidate rotavirus vaccines [see Chapter 10(XIII)] will involve tens of thousands of children to detect even a weak association with intussusception. Ultimately, the decision to use new rotavirus vaccines, or any new vaccine for that matter, must necessarily balance the known risks, however small, with the known complications of disease.

IV. **Current public concerns about vaccines.** What do we mean when we say that vaccines are *safe*? One definition of the word *safe* is "harmless." This definition would imply that any negative consequence of vaccines would make them unsafe. However, all vaccines have side effects. For example, parenterally administered vaccines can cause pain, redness, swelling, and tenderness at the site of injection. Some vaccines cause more severe side effects. For example, pertussis vaccine can very rarely cause persistent, inconsolable crying; high fever; hypotonic-hyporesponsive syndrome; and seizures with or without fever. Although none of these severe symptoms results in permanent damage, they can be quite frightening to parents. There are historic examples of serious side effects as well. For example, Guillain-Barré syndrome was seen after immunization with A/New Jersey/76 influenza (swine flu)

Table 13.2. Timeline of rotavirus vaccine experience in the United States

Date	Event
August 31, 1998	FDA grants licensure
October 22, 1998	AAP recommends universal use
March 19, 1999	ACIP publishes recommendation for universal use
July 7, 1999	VAERS contains 15 reports of intussusception
	13 cases after the first dose
	Most occurred within 1 wk
	Surveillance data from California and Minnesota suggest a causal association
July 16, 1999	CDC recommends postponing vaccination, and manufacturer voluntarily ceases further distribution
September 1999	AAP publishes recommendation to postpone vaccination
October 15, 1999	Manufacturer voluntarily withdraws product from market
October 22, 1999	ACIP withdraws recommendation
January 21, 2000	Workshop convened by the NIH and the NVPO to focus research on pathogenesis and enable progress toward safer rotavirus vaccines
Final analysis (approximate)	1.8 million doses distributed
	1.5 million doses administered
	1.0 million children received vaccine
	15,000 hospitalizations prevented
	10 deaths from dehydration prevented
	100 excess intussusceptions
	1 death from vaccine

vaccine, but there were only 8.6 to 9.7 cases per million vaccinees. Similarly, oral poliovirus vaccine (OPV) caused paralytic polio, but only one case for every 2.3 million doses distributed. The recommendation to change to inactivated poliovirus vaccine (IPV) in the year 2000 was based on recognition of this extremely rare side effect, which had by then become more of a risk than natural polio itself.

Few things in life meet the definition of "harmless." Even everyday activities contain hidden dangers. For example, each year in the United States, 350 people are killed in bath- or shower-related accidents, and 200 people are killed when food lodges in their trachea. Just being outdoors can be dangerous; for example, each year, 100 people are killed by lightning. Therefore, by the "harmless" criterion, even routine daily activities could be considered unsafe.

Another definition of the word *safe* is "having been preserved from a real danger." Using this definition, the danger (the disease) must be significantly greater than the means of protecting against the danger (the vaccine). Or, said another way, a vaccine's benefits must clearly and definitively outweigh its risks. For all routinely recommended vaccines, the benefits clearly outweigh the risks.

What follows is a series of questions that parents (and patients) may ask regarding vaccines. The answers may serve as a basis for effective communication of the true risks and benefits. Some of the issues have been addressed by the IOM Immunization Safety Review Committee (Table 13.1).

A. **Are vaccines still necessary?** Because many diseases that vaccines prevent are rare, it can be hard for parents to understand why it is still important to protect against them. Vaccines are still necessary for three reasons:

- *To prevent common infections*—For example, varicella, pertussis, hepatitis B, and pneumococcal disease are common enough that the choice not to vaccinate is the choice to take a significant risk of getting the disease.
- *To prevent infections that could easily reemerge*— Some diseases in this country continue to occur at very low levels [e.g., *Haemophilus influenzae* type b (Hib), measles, mumps, and rubella]. If immunization rates in our schools or communities are low, outbreaks of these diseases are likely to occur. This is exactly what happened between 1989 and 1991 in the United States, when there were approximately 55,000 reported cases of measles, 11,000 hospitalizations, and 123 deaths from the disease.
- *To prevent infections that could easily be imported from other parts of the world*—Although some diseases have been completely eliminated (polio) or virtually eliminated (diphtheria) from this country, they still occur in other parts of the world. Children still get polio in India, and diphtheria outbreaks have occurred in Russia. Because the United States has a high rate of tourist, immigrant, and international business travel, outbreaks of these diseases are only a plane ride away.

B. **Do children get too many vaccines at one time?** One hundred years ago, children received one vaccine (the smallpox vaccine). Forty years ago, children received five vaccines routinely (diphtheria, pertussis, tetanus, polio, and smallpox) and as many as eight shots by two years of age. Today, children receive 11 or 12 vaccines routinely and as many as 20 shots by two years of age. Some parents wonder whether we have gone too far.

However, vaccines are just a small part of what babies encounter in an immunologic sense every day. Within a matter of hours, the gastrointestinal tract of the newborn, initially relatively free of microbes, is heavily colonized with bacteria. The most common of these colonizing bacteria include facultative anaerobes such as *E. coli* and streptococci and strict anaerobes such as *Bacteroides* and *Clostridium*. Specific secretory IgA responses directed against these potentially harmful bacteria are produced by the neonate's intestinal lymphocytes during the first week of life. The vast

Table 13.3. Number of separate antigens contained in routinely administered vaccines

Vaccine	Year 1960	Year 1980	Year 2000
Smallpox	200	—	—
Diphtheria	1	1	1
Tetanus	1	1	1
Pertussis	~3,000[a]	~3,000[a]	2–5[b]
Polio	15	15	15
Measles	—	10	10
Mumps	—	9	9
Rubella	—	5	5
Hib	—	—	2
Varicella	—	—	69
PCV-7	—	—	8
Hep-B	—	—	1
Total	~3,217	~3,041	123–126

[a]Whole-cell vaccine.
[b]Acellular vaccine.
Adapted from Offit PA, Quarles J, Gerber MA, et al. Addressing parents' concerns: do multiple vaccines overwhelm or weaken the infant's immune system? *Pediatrics* 2002;109:124–129.

majority of infants meet these microbial challenges very effectively.

Even though children receive more vaccines today than they did 40 years ago, the number of separate immunologic challenges (i.e., bacterial and viral proteins and bacterial polysaccharides) has actually *decreased* dramatically (Table 13.3). The main reason for this is the elimination of smallpox vaccine, containing approximately 200 proteins, and the whole-cell pertussis vaccine, containing approximately 3,000 antigens.

C. **Do vaccines weaken the immune system?** Some parents are concerned that vaccines might weaken the immune system and cause a child to be more susceptible to infections with viruses or bacteria not contained in the vaccines (so-called *heterologous infections*). Vaccines may cause temporary suppression of delayed-type hypersensitivity skin reactions or alter certain lymphocyte function tests *in vitro*. In addition, the measles vaccine may decrease immunogenicity of the varicella vaccine if the latter is administered within 30 days. However, the short-lived immunosuppression caused by certain vaccines does not result in an increased risk of heterologous infections. Vaccinated children are not at increased risk of subsequent infection with other pathogens when compared to unvaccinated children. On the contrary, a study of 496 vaccinated and unvaccinated children in Germany found that children who received the diphtheria, pertussis, tetanus, Hib, and polio vaccines in the first 3 months of life actually had *fewer* infections with vaccine-related and vaccine-unrelated pathogens.

Bacterial and viral *infections*, on the other hand, often predispose children and adults to severe, invasive infections with other pathogens. For example, influenza infection clearly predisposes patients to pneumococcal pneumonia. Similarly, varicella infection increases susceptibility to group A beta-hemolytic streptococcal infections including necrotizing fasciitis, toxic shock syndrome, and bacteremia. Thus, if susceptibility to heterologous infection is the concern, vaccination makes more sense than no vaccination.

D. Do vaccines cause autism? In 1998, Wakefield and his coworkers in London described 12 children with regressive developmental disorders and chronic enterocolitis; ten of these children had autism. In eight children, the onset of regressive neurologic symptoms was temporally linked by the child's parent or physician to receipt of measles, mumps, and rubella vaccine (MMR). The average length of time between receipt of MMR and onset of neurologic symptoms was 6.3 days (range, 1–14 days). Nine of these children also had lymphoid nodular hyperplasia in the terminal ileum determined by endoscopy. The authors concluded that a unique disease process characterized by intestinal inflammation and regressive autism might be caused by MMR, and they have subsequently advocated monovalent measles, mumps, and rubella vaccines rather than the combination. However, because this report did not include control groups who did not receive the vaccine, a causal relationship between MMR and autism could not be determined.

Subsequent to Wakefield's publication, several investigators studied the hypothesis that MMR causes autism. Taylor and colleagues performed a population-based study of children in eight health districts in the North Thames region of the United Kingdom. Children with autistic spectrum disorder (ASD) born after 1979 were identified from computerized registries and school records. The authors identified 498 children with ASD that included typical autism, atypical autism, and Asperger's syndrome. Three statistical analyses were performed. First, in a time-series analysis, an increase in cases of ASD was not seen after introduction of MMR to the United Kingdom, which occurred in 1988. Second, among children with ASD born after 1987, the proportion that had received MMR was similar to that for children in the general population. Third, there was no significant clustering of cases of ASD at various intervals up to 1 year after receipt of MMR vaccine. A second study by this group expanded these observations to include one and two doses of MMR and longer intervals after receipt of vaccine, again finding no evidence for a causal association.

Two additional studies supported the findings of Taylor and coworkers. One examined trends in autism and MMR immunization rates in California between 1980 and 1994. Although there was an increase in the number of autism cases during that period (possibly caused by increased recognition of the syndrome or demographic changes in the state), immunization rates remained steady and did not parallel the autism rates. Very similar results were seen in a population-based study from the United Kingdom covering the years 1988 to 1993.

To evaluate whether MMR vaccine was associated with a new form of autism that included intestinal symptoms, two large, well-controlled, retrospective studies were performed. One found that the proportion of children with developmental regression (25%) or bowel symptoms (17%) did not change significantly between 1979 and 1998, a period that included the introduction of MMR. Similarly, a study of 262 patients with autism found no evidence for the emergence of a new form of the disease that included intestinal symptoms after widespread use of MMR. Finally, a recent population-based study from Denmark examined a cohort of children born between 1991 and 1998, representing a total of 2,129,864 person years. The relative risk of autistic disorder in vaccinated children compared to unvaccinated children was 0.92. [For reference, a relative risk of 1.0 means no relationship, a value significantly greater than 1.0 implies a causal association (as long as there are no confounding variables), and a value significantly less than 1.0 means the vaccine actually may protect against the outcome.] There was also no association between autistic disorder and age at vaccination, the interval since vaccination, or the date of vaccination.

Taken together, the above studies convincingly refute the notion that MMR causes autism, and there remains no reason to give the monovalent components in lieu of the combination.

E. Did the whole-cell pertussis vaccine cause permanent brain damage? In 1974, Kulenkampff and coworkers published an uncontrolled case series of children who allegedly developed mental retardation and epilepsy after receipt of the whole-cell pertussis vaccine. Over the next several years, fear of the pertussis vaccine generated by media coverage of this report caused a decrease in pertussis immunization rates in British children from 81% to 31% and resulted in more than 100,000 cases and 36 deaths from pertussis. Media coverage of the Kulenkampff report also caused decreased immunization rates and increased pertussis deaths in Japan, Sweden, and Wales. However, many excellent, well-controlled studies have found that whole-cell pertussis vaccine is not a cause of chronic neurologic disease.

F. Does natural infection induce better immunity than immunization? It is true that natural infection almost always induces stronger and longer-lasting immunity than vaccines. Whereas immunity from disease often follows a single natural infection, immunity from vaccines usually occurs only after several doses. However, the difference between vaccination and natural infection is the price paid for immunity, which, in the latter case, might be pneumonitis and respiratory failure from chickenpox, mental retardation from Hib meningitis, empyema from pneumococcus, deafness from congenital rubella, liver cancer from hepatitis B, or encephalitis and death from measles.

G. Are vaccines made from fetal tissues? Rubella, hepatitis A (Hep-A), rabies, and varicella vaccines are grown in cultured human embryo fibroblasts (MRC-5 or WI-38) because these are the only cells that replicate the viruses in high enough titer for mass production. Each cell line was first obtained from an aborted fetus in the early 1960s. These same embryonic cells have been passaged in tissue culture in the laboratory since then, and no new fetal material has ever been involved. Nevertheless, this situation represents a moral dilemma for some individuals. In helping parents work through this, it may help to emphasize that the original abortion was not done specifically with the intent to produce vaccines, that the vaccine producers never intended to abort fetuses, and that the moral imperative to save lives through vaccination might outweigh their objection to what they consider to be a singular, distant moral transgression.

H. Do vaccines cause allergies? Developed countries have seen an increase in the incidence of allergic diseases during the same time that many new vaccines have been introduced, leading some to believe there is a relationship. The theoretical basis for this belief has to do with the "hygiene hypothesis," which holds that "clean living" brought on in part by the elimination of vaccine-preventable diseases creates an immunologic environment during ontogeny that is replete with type 2 helper T cells and deficient in T-regulator cells, an environment that promotes allergy and autoimmunity. However, several large epidemiologic studies favor rejection of this hypothesis. One well-controlled study identified 18,407 children with asthma who were born between 1991 and 1997 and compared them to a control group without asthma. Relative risks of asthma in vaccinated compared to unvaccinated children were 0.92 for diphtheria, tetanus, and whole-cell pertussis vaccine (DTP), 1.09 for OPV, and 0.97 for MMR. In children who had at least two medical encounters during their first year of life, the relative risk for asthma was 1.07 after receipt of the Hib vaccine and 1.09 after receipt of the hepatitis B vaccine (Hep-B). All of these relative risks imply no association.

Another large well-controlled study of 669 children prospectively evaluated the risk of allergies after receipt of the pertussis vaccine. Infants were randomized to receive a two-component diphtheria, tetanus, and acellular pertussis vaccine (DTaP2); a five-component DTaP (DTaP5); DTP; or diphtheria and tetanus vaccine for pediatric use (DT) beginning at 2 months of age. Children were followed for more than 2 years, and the risk of allergies was determined by parent questionnaires and examination of medical records. Allergic disorders studied included asthma, atopic dermatitis, allergic rhinoconjunctivitis, urticaria, and food allergies. No difference in the incidence of allergic diseases was observed in children who did or did not receive pertussis vaccine. Of interest, children with natural pertussis infections were more likely to develop allergic diseases than children not infected with pertussis. Taken together, these studies and others argue strongly that vaccines do not cause allergic diseases.

I. **Do vaccines cause diabetes mellitus?** Several uncontrolled observational studies claimed that the introduction of vaccines, particularly Hib, into certain populations caused an increase in the incidence of type 1 diabetes. The purported link is vaccine-induced enhancement of preexisting subclinical islet cell autoimmunity. Perhaps the best study evaluating the relationship between vaccines and type 1 diabetes was performed using data from the VSD. Two hundred fifty-two cases of type 1 diabetes were compared with 768 matched controls without diabetes. The odds ratio was 0.28 for the association between diabetes and the whole-cell pertussis vaccine, 1.36 for MMR, 1.14 for Hib, 0.81 for Hep-B, 1.16 for varicella vaccine, and 0.92 for acellular pertussis (the odds ratio is an approximation to the relative risk). For children vaccinated at birth with Hep-B, the odds ratio for diabetes was 0.51; for those vaccinated at 2 months of age or later, the odds ratio was 0.86.

In addition, 21,421 children who received the Hib conjugate vaccine between 1988 and 1990 in the United States were followed for 10 years, and the risk of type 1 diabetes was 0.78 compared to a group of 22,557 children who did not receive the vaccine. Several other well-controlled retrospective studies also found that immunizations were not associated with an increased risk of developing type 1 diabetes.

J. **Do vaccines cause multiple sclerosis?** The hypothesis that vaccines might cause multiple sclerosis (MS) was fueled by anecdotal reports of MS after Hep-B immunization and two case-control studies showing an increase in the incidence of MS in vaccinated individuals that was not statistically significant. However, two large case-control studies evaluated whether Hep-B causes MS or whether Hep-B, tetanus, or influenza vaccines exacerbate symptoms of MS. The first study used a cohort of nurses followed since 1976 to identify 192 women with

MS and 645 matched controls. The relative risk of multiple sclerosis associated with exposure to Hep-B was 0.9, and the relative risk within 2 years before the onset of disease was 0.7. There was also no association between the number of doses of Hep-B and the risk of multiple sclerosis. The second study included 643 patients in Europe with MS relapse occurring between 1993 and 1997. Exposure to vaccination in the 2-month period before relapse was compared with the four previous 2-month control periods to determine relative risks. The relative risk of relapse associated with the use of any vaccine was 0.71 and was 0.67, 0.75, and 1.08 with Hep-B, tetanus, and influenza vaccines, respectively.

Other well-controlled studies also found that influenza vaccine did not exacerbate symptoms of MS. In a retrospective study of 180 patients with relapsing MS, infection with influenza virus was more likely than immunization with influenza vaccine to cause an exacerbation of symptoms, suggesting that influenza vaccine is actually likely to prevent exacerbations of MS.

K. Did the thimerosal in some vaccines cause harm? In 1997, the FDA was required by the FDA Modernization Act to compile a list of drugs and foods that contained mercury because of the observation that high levels of mercury can damage the nervous system and kidneys. Studies in the Faroe Islands, the Seychelles, and Iraq found that fetuses could be harmed when pregnant women ingested large quantities of mercury contained in contaminated fish or fumigated (disinfected) grain. Because some vaccines used thimerosal as a preservative, which contains an organic form of mercury, they were included in the list generated by the FDA. Preservatives prevent vaccines from becoming contaminated with bacteria or fungi and are especially important for multidose vials.

The amount of mercury contained in vaccines was within the acceptable range published by the FDA, the Agency for Toxic Substance and Disease Registry, and the WHO. However, the cumulative levels of mercury represented by multiple vaccine doses slightly exceeded those considered to be safe by the Environmental Protection Agency (EPA). To determine "safe" levels of mercury, the EPA evaluated a study performed in Iraq in which pregnant women were accidentally exposed to large quantities of methylmercury (a more toxic organic compound than the ethylmercury contained in thimerosal) that had been used to fumigate grain. The EPA then estimated the lowest dose of mercury that was found to cause neurodevelopmental delay in infants as a result of fetal exposure. From these data, the EPA calculated the lowest dose of methylmercury that could possibly harm an unborn child and divided this dose by ten to determine the lowest acceptable dose of mercury.

There are many problems with using the study in Iraq to determine levels of thimerosal in vaccines that would be safe in children:

- The mercury contained in thimerosal is in the form of ethylmercury, which is quickly excreted in the stool and is less likely to accumulate in the body
- Vaccines are administered to children after, not before, they are born, when the nervous system is more mature and, therefore, much less likely to be susceptible to the harmful effects of mercury
- By including a safety factor of ten, the EPA estimate was very conservative

At this point in time, thimerosal has been removed from childhood vaccines as a precaution. However, there was never convincing evidence directly linking thimerosal to harm in any child, and a recent study demonstrated that administration of thimerosal-containing vaccines to infants does not raise blood levels of mercury beyond safe values. Furthermore, preliminary (unpublished) studies show no relationship between the level of mercury contained in vaccines and neurologic problems.

L. **Do vaccines contain the agent associated with "mad cow disease"?** By July of 2000 approximately 175,000 cows in the United Kingdom had developed a disease called *mad cow disease* (MCD)—a progressive deterioration of the nervous system. At the same time, more than 70 people in the United Kingdom had developed a progressive neurologic disease termed *variant Creutzfeldt-Jakob disease* (vCJD) that likely resulted from eating meat prepared from cows with MCD. Both MCD and vCJD are caused by prions, which are proteinaceous, self-replicating infectious particles. On July 27, 2000, CBER convened a meeting to discuss the possibility that some vaccines were made using serum or gelatin derived from cows in countries in which MCD had been found, including England. Although the risk of transmission of vCJD to humans from such vaccines was considered theoretical and remote, CBER recommended that vaccines use bovine materials originating from countries without endogenous MCD. This recommendation was published as a Notice to Readers in the *MMWR: Morbidity and Mortality Weekly Report* on December 22, 2000, and was followed by a New York Times article published on February 8, 2001 entitled "Five Drug Makers Use Material with Possible Mad Cow Link."

Prions are found in the brains of cows with MCD and in the brains of humans with vCJD. They can also be found in the spinal cord and retina. However, blood from infected animals and infected people has never been shown to be a source of infection for humans. The likely source of prions for people in England was hamburger, not steak, and hamburger may be prepared in a manner that includes the spinal cord. Steak, on the other hand, represents only the muscles of cows and, therefore, does not contain prions.

Vaccines may contain trace amounts of animal products used during the manufacturing process. For example, vaccines are grown in laboratory cells that require many growth factors for maintenance. An excellent source of these growth factors is fetal bovine serum, which is naturally filtered by the six-layered bovine placenta. Many proteins are excluded from the bovine fetal circulation by these layers (for example, bovine fetal blood contains 1/500th of the antibodies found in bovine maternal blood). Maternal-fetal transmission of prions has never been documented in animals, and fetal blood is not known to contain prions. Moreover, the fetal bovine serum used in vaccine manufacture is highly diluted and eventually removed from cells during purification of vaccine viruses. It should be pointed out as well that prions propagate in mammalian brain but not cell culture.

Another product from cows and pigs that may be used in vaccines is gelatin, a protein formed by boiling skin or connective tissue such as hooves. Gelatin is used to stabilize vaccines so that they remain effective after distribution. Because prions are not detected in the skin or connective tissue of animals, gelatin does not represent a risk to patients.

Final reassurance comes from the fact that transmission of prions occurs from eating the brains of infected animals or from directly inoculating preparations of brains of infected animals into the brains of experimental animals. Transmission of prions has not been documented after inoculation into the muscles or under the skin, which are the routes used for vaccination. Taken together, the chances that currently licensed vaccines contain prions and represent a risk to humans are essentially zero.

M. Do vaccines cause cancer? The polio vaccine used in the late 1950s and early 1960s was contaminated with a monkey virus called simian virus 40 (SV40), present in the monkey kidney cells used to grow the vaccine. Recently, investigators found SV40 DNA in biopsy specimens obtained from patients with mesothelioma, osteosarcoma, and non-Hodgkin's lymphoma. However, several facts should be noted:

- SV40 was present in the cancers of people who had or had not received the polio vaccine that was contaminated with SV40
- People with cancer who were born after 1963, when SV40 was no longer a contaminant of the polio vaccine, were found to have evidence of SV40 in their cancerous cells
- Using current techniques, it is difficult to distinguish SV40 from other common and related agents such as JC and BK viruses

- Epidemiologic studies do not show an increased risk of cancers in those who received polio vaccine between 1955 and 1963

Taken together, these findings argue against the hypothesis that SV40 contained in polio vaccines caused cancers. The data further suggest that SV40 is likely be transmitted to people by a mechanism other than vaccines.

N. Did the polio vaccine start the AIDS epidemic? In 1999, Edward Hooper published a book entitled *The River: A Journey to the Source of HIV and AIDS*. The central hypothesis was that the origin of AIDS could be traced to poliovirus vaccines that were administered orally in the Belgian Congo between 1957 and 1960. This assertion was based on the following assumptions: (a) all poliovirus vaccines were grown in monkey kidney cells; (b) those cells were contaminated with simian immunodeficiency virus (SIV), which is closely related to HIV; and (c) people were inadvertently infected with SIV that then mutated to HIV and caused the AIDS epidemic.

The following facts, however, exonerate polio vaccines as a cause of AIDS:

- SIV is found in chimpanzees, not monkeys, and chimpanzee cells were never used to grow polio vaccine
- SIV and HIV are not very close genetically, and mutation from SIV to HIV would have required centuries, not years
- Both SIV and HIV are enveloped viruses that are easily disrupted by extremes of pH. If given by mouth (as was OPV), both of these viruses would likely be destroyed in the acidic environment of the stomach
- Original lots of the polio vaccine (including those used in Africa for the polio vaccine trials) did not contain HIV, SIV, or chimpanzee genetic sequences when analyzed by molecular amplification techniques

Unfortunately, fears of polio vaccine based on this unfounded theory might have adversely affected vaccine use where it is needed most—in the developing world, where the last vestiges of wild-type poliovirus reside.

O. Do vaccines cause sudden infant death syndrome? In 1999, the ABC news program *20/20* aired a story claiming that Hep-B caused sudden infant death syndrome (SIDS). The story included a picture of a 1-month-old girl who died of SIDS only 16 hours after receiving the second dose of Hep-B. In 1999, when routine use of Hep-B was recommended for all infants, approximately 5,000 children died every year from SIDS. Within 10 years of the introduction of universal Hep-B immunization, vaccine uptake had increased to approximately 90%, and the incidence of SIDS had decreased dramatically to approximately 1,600 cases per year. This decrease was due to the introduction of the "Back to Sleep" program, in which parents were encouraged to place infants on their backs or sides to sleep. The lack of an ecologic correlation between SIDS and Hep-B is supported by VAERS data that show very few neonatal deaths after Hep-B vaccination after approximately 86 million doses were given. Several studies actually show *lower* SIDS rates among infants who receive vaccines compared to those who do not. Although this may reflect a bias wherein healthier or better-cared-for infants are the ones who are immunized, the data clearly do not indicate vaccines as a risk factor for SIDS. Temporal associations arise because some vaccines happen to be given just at the time of the peak age incidence of SIDS.

Sources of Information about Vaccines*

I. National and international policy agencies

Name:	National Immunization Program (NIP)
	Centers for Disease Control and Prevention
Address:	Mail Stop E-05
	1600 Clifton Rd., N.E.
	Atlanta, GA 30333
Phone number:	800-232-2522
Web site:	www.cdc.gov/nip

Name:	National Vaccine Program Office (NVPO)
	Centers for Disease Control and Prevention
Address:	Mail Stop D-66
	1600 Clifton Rd., N.E.
	Atlanta, GA 30333
Phone number:	404-687-6672
Web site:	www.cdc.gov/od/nvpo

Name:	National Institute of Allergy and Infectious Diseases (NIAID)
Address:	Building 31, Room 7A-50
	31 Center Dr., MSC 2520
	Bethesda, MD 20892
Phone number:	301-496-5717
Web site:	www.niaid.nih.gov

Name:	Food and Drug Administration (FDA)
Address:	5600 Fishers Ln.
	Rockville, MD 20857
Phone number:	888-463-6332
Web site:	www.fda.gov

Name:	World Health Organization (WHO)
	Department of Vaccines and Biologicals
Address:	Avenue Appia 20
	1211 Geneva 27, Switzerland
Phone number:	+41-22-791-21-11
Web site:	www.who.int/vaccines

Name:	Pan American Health Organization (PAHO)
	Division of Vaccines and Immunization
Address:	525 23rd St., N.W.
	Washington, DC 20037
Phone number:	202-974-3000
Web site:	www.paho.org

*Web sites in Chapter 14 accessed 1/27/03.

II. Advisory boards and committees

Name:	Advisory Committee on Immunization Practices (ACIP)
	Centers for Disease Control and Prevention
Address:	Mail Stop E-16
	1600 Clifton Rd., N.E.
	Atlanta, GA 30333
Phone number:	404-639-8096
Web site:	www.cdc.gov/nip/acip

Name:	National Vaccine Advisory Committee (NVAC)
	Centers for Disease Control and Prevention
Address:	Mail Stop D-66
	1600 Clifton Rd., N.E.
	Atlanta, GA 30333
Phone number:	404-687-6672
Web site:	www.cdc.gov/od/nvpo/comittee.htm#nvac

III. Professional associations

Name:	American Academy of Pediatrics (AAP)
Address:	141 Northwest Point Blvd.
	Elk Grove Village, IL 60007
Phone number:	800-433-9016
Web site:	www.aap.org

Name:	American Academy of Family Physicians (AAFP)
Address:	11400 Tomahawk Creek Pkwy.
	Leawood, KS 66211
Phone number:	800-274-2237
Web site:	www.aafp.org

Name:	American Nurses Association (ANA)
Address:	600 Maryland Ave., S.W.
	Suite 100 West
	Washington, DC 20024
Phone number:	800-274-4262
Web site:	www.ana.org

Name:	Infectious Diseases Society of America (IDSA)
Address:	66 Canal Center Plaza
	Suite 600
	Alexandria, VA 22314
Phone number:	703-299-0200
Web site:	www.idsociety.org

Name:	American Public Health Association (APHA)
Address:	800 I St., N.W.
	Washington, DC 20001
Phone number:	202-777-2742
Web site:	www.apha.org

Name:	Association of Teachers of Preventive Medicine (ATPM)
Address:	1660 L St., N.W. Suite 208 Washington, DC 20036
Phone number:	866-474-2876
Web site:	www.atpm.org

Name:	American College Health Association (ACHA)
Address:	P.O. Box 28937 Baltimore, MD 21240
Phone number:	410-859-1500
Web site:	www.acha.org

Name:	American Pharmaceutical Association (APhA)
Address:	2215 Constitution Ave., N.W. Washington, DC 20037
Phone number:	202-628-4410
Web site:	www.aphanet.org

IV. Vaccine safety

Name:	Vaccine Adverse Event Reporting System (VAERS)
Address:	8401 Colesville Rd. Suite 200 Silver Spring, MD 20910
Phone number:	800-822-7967
Web site:	www.vaers.org

Name:	National Vaccine Injury Compensation Program (VICP)
Address:	Parklawn Building, Room 8A-46 5600 Fishers Ln. Rockville, MD 20857
Phone number:	800-338-2382
Web site:	www.hrsa.gov/osp/vicp

Name:	Advisory Commission on Childhood Vaccines (ACCV)
Address:	Parklawn Building, Room 8A-46 5600 Fishers Ln. Rockville, MD 20857
Phone number:	301-443-2124
Web site:	www.hrsa.gov/osp/vicp/accv.htm

Name:	Immunization Safety Review (ISR) Committee Institute of Medicine (IOM)
Address:	500 5th St., N.W. Suite 868 Washington, DC 20001
Phone number:	202-334-1342
Web site:	www.iom.edu/IOM/IOMHome.nsf/Pages/immunization+safety+review

Name:	Institute for Vaccine Safety Johns Hopkins Bloomberg School of Public Health
Address:	615 N. Wolfe St. Room W5041 Baltimore, MD 21205
Phone number:	Not available
Web site:	www.vaccinesafety.edu

Name:	Clinical Immunization Safety Assessment Centers
Phone number:	404-639-8256
Web site:	www.cdc.gov/nip/home-hcp.htm

V. Advocacy and implementation

Name:	Vaccines for Children (VFC) program Centers for Disease Control and Prevention
Address:	Mail Stop E-61 1600 Clifton Rd., N.E. Atlanta, GA 30333
Phone number:	800-232-2522
Web site:	www.cdc.gov/nip/vfc

Name:	Immunization Action Coalition (IAC)
Address:	1573 Selby Ave. Suite 234 St. Paul, MN 55104
Phone number:	651-647-9009
Web site:	www.immunize.org

Name:	National Coalition for Adult Immunization
Address:	4733 Bethesda Ave. Suite 750 Bethesda, MD 20814
Phone number:	301-656-0003
Web site:	www.nfid.org/ncai

Name:	Vaccine Education Center Children's Hospital of Philadelphia
Address:	34th and Civic Center Blvd. Philadelphia, PA 19104
Phone number:	215-590-9990
Web site:	www.vaccine.chop.edu

Name:	Albert B. Sabin Vaccine Institute
Address:	58 Pine St. New Canaan, CT 06840
Phone number:	203-972-7907
Web site:	www.sabin.org

Name:	Children's Vaccine Program at Program for Appropriate Technology in Health (PATH) Bill and Melinda Gates Foundation
Address:	4 Nickerson St. Seattle, WA 98109
Phone number:	206-285-3500
Web site:	www.childrensvaccine.org

Name:	National Network for Immunization Information (NNii)
Address:	66 Canal Center Plaza Suite 600 Alexandria, VA 22314
Phone number:	877-341-6644
Web site:	www.immunizationinfo.org

Name:	Every Child by Two
Address:	666 11th St., N.W. Suite 202 Washington, DC 20001
Phone number:	202-783-7034
Web site:	www.ecbt.org

Name:	Global Alliance for Vaccines and Immunization
Address:	Palais des Nations 1211 Geneva 10, Switzerland
Phone number:	+41-22-909-50-19
Web site:	www.vaccinealliance.org

Name:	National Partnership for Immunization
Address:	4733 Bethesda Avenue Suite 750 Bethesda, MD 20814
Phone number:	301-656-0003
Web site:	www.partnersforimmunization.org

Name:	Parents of Kids with Infectious Diseases
Address:	P.O. Box 5666 Vancouver, WA 98668
Phone number:	360-695-0293
Web site:	www.pkids.org

Name:	All Kids Count
Address:	750 Commerce Dr. Suite 400 Decatur, GA 30030
Phone number:	800-874-4338
Web site:	www.allkidscount.org

VI. Immunization coverage

Name:	National Notifiable Disease Surveillance System (NNDSS)
Address:	Division of Public Health Surveillance and Informatics Epidemiology Program Office Centers for Disease Control and Prevention 4770 Buford Highway, Mail Stop K74 Atlanta, GA 30341
Phone number:	770-488-8359
Web site:	www.cdc.gov/epo/dphsi/phs.htm

Name:	National Immunization Survey (NIS)
Address:	Abt Associates, Inc. 55 Wheeler St. Cambridge, MA 02138
Phone number:	617-492-7100
Web site:	www.nisabt.org

Name:	National Health Interview Survey (NIHS)
Address:	National Center for Health Statistics Centers for Disease Control and Prevention 6525 Belcrest Rd. Hyattsville, MD 20782
Phone number:	301-458-4636
Web site:	www.cdc.gov/nchs

Name:	Clinic Assessment Software Application (CASA)
Address:	Systems Development Team Attn: CASA National Immunization Program Centers for Disease Control and Prevention CDC Mail Stop E-62 1600 Clifton Road Atlanta, GA 30333
Phone number:	404-639-8921
Web site:	www.cdc.gov/nip/casa

Name:	Behavioral Risk Factor Surveillance System (BRFSS)
Address:	National Center for Chronic Disease Prevention and Health Promotion Centers for Disease Control and Prevention Mail Stop K-47 4770 Buford Highway, N.E. Atlanta, GA 30341
Phone number:	770-488-2455
Web site:	www.cdc.gov/brfss

Name:	Health Plan Employer Data and Information Set (HEDIS)
Address:	National Committee for Quality Assurance 2000 L Street, N.W. Suite 500 Washington, DC 20036
Phone number:	202-955-3500
Web site:	www.ncqa.org/programs/hedis

VII. State health departments
See Table 14.1.

VIII. U.S. manufacturers and distributors
See Table 14.2.

IX. Other Web sites

Name:	Immunofacts: The Immunization Gateway—Your Vaccine Fact-Finder
Web site:	www.immunofacts.com
Sponsor:	Facts and Comparisons, a Wolters Kluwer Company

Name:	The Vaccine Page
Web site:	www.vaccines.com
Sponsor:	Children's Vaccine Program at Program for Appropriate Technology in Health (PATH)

Name:	Allied Vaccine Group
Web site:	www.vaccine.org

Table 14.1. State health department immunization programs

State	Phone number	Web site
Alabama	334-206-5023	www.adph.org/immunization
Alaska	907-269-8088	www.epi.hss.state.ak.us/programs/infect/immune.stm
Arizona	602-230-5852	www.hs.state.az.us/phs/immun
Arkansas	501-661-2169	www.healthyarkansas.com
California	510-540-2067	www.dhs.ca.gov/ps/dcdc/izgroup
Colorado	303-692-2650	www.cdphe.state.co.us/ps/mch/imm/immhom.asp
Connecticut	860-509-7929	www.dph.state.ct.us/bch/infectious-dise/immuniza.htm
Delaware	302-739-4746	www.state.de.us/dhss/dph/imm-home.html
District of Columbia	202-576-7130	www.dchealth.dc.gov/services/administration_offices/phsa/immunization/index.shtm
Florida	850-245-4342	www9.myflorida.com/disease_ctrl/immune
Georgia	404-657-3158	www.ph.dhr.state.ga.us/programs/immunization
Hawaii	808-586-8300	www.state.hi.us/doh/immunization
Idaho	800-554-2922	www2.state.id.us/dhw/immun/immun.htm
Illinois	217-782-4977	www.idph.state.il.us/about/shots.htm
Indiana	317-233-7704	www.in.gov/isdh/programs/immuni-zation.htm
Iowa	515-281-4917	idph.state.ia.us/ch/immunization.asp
Kansas	785-296-5591	www.kdhe.state.ks.us/immunize
Kentucky	502-564-4478	chs.state.ky.us/publichealth/index-immunization_programs.htm
Louisiana	504-483-1900	oph.dhh.state.la.us/immunization
Maine	207-287-3746	www.state.me.us/dhs/boh/mip
Maryland	410-767-6679	mdpublichealth.org/edcp/html/immpg.html
Massachusetts	617-624-6000	www.state.ma.us/dph/cdc/epii/imm/imm.htm
Michigan	517-335-8159	www.michigan.gov/mdch
Minnesota	612-676-5237	www.health.state.mn.us/divs/dpc/adps/immprov.htm
Mississippi	601-576-7751	www.mdhs.state.ms.us/ocy.html
Missouri	573-751-6133	www.dhss.state.mo.us/Immuniza-tions

(continued)

Table 14.1. *Continued*

State	Phone number	Web site
Montana	406-444-5580	www.dphhs.state.mt.us
Nebraska	402-471-3727	www.hhs.state.ne.us/imm/immin-dex.htm
Nevada	775-684-5939	health2k.state.nv.us/immune/index.htm
New Hamp-shire	603-271-4482	www.dhhs.state.nh.us/DHHS/IMMU-NIZATION/default.htm
New Jersey	609-588-7512	www.state.nj.us/health/cd/vpd-phome.htm
New Mexico	505-827-2366	www.health.state.nm.us
New York	518-473-4437	www.health.state.ny.us/nysdoh/immun/immunization.htm
North Caro-lina	919-733-7752	wch.dhhs.state.nc.us/imm.htm
North Dakota	701-328-2378	www.ehs.health.state.nd.us/disease/immune
Ohio	614-466-4643	www.immunize-ohio.org
Oklahoma	405-271-4073	www.health.state.ok.us/program/imm/index.html
Oregon	503-731-4020	www.ohd.hr.state.or.us/imm
Pennsylvania	717-787-5681	webserver.health.state.pa.us/health/cwp/view.asp?a=178&Q=199020
Rhode Island	401-222-2312	www.healthri.org/family/immuniza-tion/home.htm
South Caro-lina	803-898-0159	www.scdhec.net/hs/diseasecont/immunization/child_vacc.htm
South Dakota	605-773-3737	www.state.sd.us/doh/Disease/immun.htm
Tennessee	615-741-7343	www2.state.tn.us/health/CEDS/immunization.htm
Texas	512-458-7284	www.tdh.state.tx.us/immunize/default.htm
Utah	801-538-9450	www.immunize-utah.org/default.htm
Vermont	802-863-7333	www.healthyvermonters.info
Virginia	804-786-6246	www.vdh.state.va.us/imm/index.htm
Washington	360-236-3595	www.doh.wa.gov/cfh/Immunize/default.htm
West Virginia	304-558-2188	www.wvdhhr.org/immunizations
Wisconsin	608-267-9959	www.dhfs.state.wi.us/immunization/index.htm
Wyoming	307-777-7652	wdhfs.state.wy.us/immunization

Table 14.2. U.S. manufacturers, distributors, and product information

Alpha Therapeutic Corporation 2410 Lillyvale Ave. Los Angeles, CA 90032 Venoglobulin-S	**Phone: 323-225-2221** **Web site: www.alphather.com** Immune globulin intravenous, human (IGIV)
American Red Cross Plasma Services Division 1300 Wilson Blvd. Arlington, VA 22209 Panglobulin (manufactured by ZLB Bioplasma) Polygam (manufactured by Baxter)	**Phone: 800-261-5772** **Web site: plasmaservices.redcross.org** Immune globulin intravenous, human (IGIV) Immune globulin intravenous, human (IGIV)
Aventis Behring L.L.C. (formerly Centeon) 1020 First Ave. P.O. Box 61501 King of Prussia, PA 19406 Gammar-P I.V.	**Phone: 800-504-5434** **Web site: www.aventisbehring.com** Immune globulin intravenous, human (IGIV)
Aventis Pasteur, Inc. (AP) (formerly Pasteur **Mérieux Connaught and Rhône-Poulenc S.A.)** Discovery Dr. Swiftwater, PA 18370 ActHIB, OmniHIB (distributed by GlaxoSmithKline) DAPTACEL Diphtheria and Tetanus Toxoids Adsorbed USP (Pediatric) Fluzone Imogam Rabies-HT IMOVAX RABIES IPOL	**Phone: 800-822-2463** **Web site: www.us.aventispasteur.com** *Haemophilus influenzae* polyribosylribotol phosphate–tetanus toxoid conjugate (PRP-T) Diphtheria and tetanus toxoids, 5-component acellular pertussis (DTaP5) Diphtheria and tetanus toxoids (DT) Inactivated influenza, trivalent, subvirion Rabies immune globulin, human (RIG) Rabies, human diploid cell, inactivated (HDCV) Poliovirus, inactivated (IPV)

(continued)

Table 14.2.   Continued

JE-VAX	Japanese encephalitis, inactivated (JEV)
Menomune–A/C/Y/W-135	Meningococcal polysaccharide, groups A, C, Y, and W-135 (Men-PS)
Mycobax	Bacille Calmette-Guérin, live (BCG)
TriHIBit	*Haemophilus influenzae* polyribosylribitol phosphate–tetanus toxoid conjugate (ActHIB); reconstituted with diphtheria and tetanus toxoids, 2-component acellular pertussis (Tripedia) (PRP-T/DTaP2)
Tetanus and Diphtheria Toxoids Adsorbed (Adult)	Diphtheria and tetanus toxoids (Td)
Tetanus Toxoid Adsorbed USP	Tetanus toxoid (TT)
Tetanus Toxoid USP	Tetanus toxoid for booster only (TT)
Tripedia (preservative free)	Diphtheria and tetanus toxoids, 2-component acellular pertussis (DTaP2)
Typhim Vi	Typhoid Vi polysaccharide (Ty-ViPS)
YF-VAX	Yellow fever; live-attenuated (YF)
Baxter Healthcare Corporation	**Phone: 800-422-9837**
One Baxter Pkwy.	**Web site: www.baxter.com**
Deerfield, IL 60015	
GAMMAGARD S/D	Immune globulin intravenous, human (IGIV)
Iveegam EN	Immune globulin intravenous, human (IGIV)
Bayer Corporation	**Phone: 203-812-2000**
400 Morgan Ln.	**Web site: www.ubayerus.com**
West Haven, CT 06516	
BayGam	Immune globulin intramuscular, human (IGIM)
BayHep B	Hepatitis B immune globulin, human (HBIG)
BayRab	Rabies immune globulin, human (RIG)
BayTet	Tetanus immune globulin, human (TIG)
Gamimune N 10%	Immune globulin intravenous, human (IGIV)
Polygam (distributed by American Red Cross)	Immune globulin intravenous, human (IGIV)

Berna Products Corporation(North American subsidiary of Swiss Serum and Vaccine Institute, Berne) **4216 Ponce de Leon Blvd.** **Coral Gables, FL 33146** Vivotif Berna	**Phone: 800-533-5899** **Web site: www.bernaproducts.com** Typhoid, live-attenuated (Ty21a)
BioPort Corporation **3500 North Martin Luther King, #J** **Lansing, MI 48906** BioThrax	**Phone: 517-327-5540** **Web site: www.bioport.com** Anthrax vaccine adsorbed, cell free
Chiron Corporation **4560 Horton St.** **Emeryville, CA 94608** RabAvert	**Phone: 510-655-8730** **Web site: www.chiron.com** Rabies, purified chick embryo cell, inactivated (PCEC)
Evans Vaccines, Ltd. (a subsidiary of PowderJect Pharmaceuticals, Plc.; in May 2003, Chiron announced its intention to acquire PowderJect) **Gaskill Rd., Speke, Merseyside** **L24 9GR, United Kingdom** Fluvirin	**Phone: +44-01-51-705-50-51** **Web site: www.evansvaccines.com** Inactivated influenza, trivalent, subvirion
FFF Enterprises **41093 County Center Dr.** **Temecula, CA 92591** Immune Globulin (Human) USP (manufactured by MPHBL) Varicella-Zoster Immune Globulin (manufactured by MPHBL)	**Phone: 909-296-2500** **Web site: www.fffenterprises.com** Immune globulin intramuscular, human (IGIM) Varicella-zoster immune globulin, human (VZIG)

(continued)

Table 14.2. *Continued*

General Injectables & Vaccines (GIV) P.O. Box 9 **Bastian, VA 24314**	**Phone: 800-521-7468** **Web site: www.giv.com**	
		Tetanus and Diphtheria Toxoids Adsorbed for Adult Use (manufactured by MPHBL) — Diphtheria and tetanus toxoids (Td)
GlaxoSmithKline (GSK) (formerly GlaxoWellcome and SmithKline Beecham) 1 Franklin Plaza P.O. Box 7929 **Philadelphia, PA 19101**	**Phone: 888-825-5249** **Web site: www.gsk.com**	
Engerix-B		Hepatitis B, recombinant (Hep-B)
Havrix		Hepatitis A, inactivated (Hep-A)
Infanrix		Diphtheria and tetanus toxoids, 3-component acellular pertussis (DTaP3)
LYMErix		Lyme disease, recombinant outer surface protein A (rOspA)
Pediarix		Diphtheria and tetanus toxoids, 3-component acellular pertussis; hepatitis B, recombinant; poliovirus, inactivated (DTaP3/Hep-B/IPV)
Twinrix		Hepatitis A, inactivated; hepatitis B, recombinant (Hep-A/Hep-B)
Massachusetts Public Health Biologic Laboratories (MPHBL) 305 South St. **Boston, MA 02130** **(Products are distributed by MPHBL within Massachusetts but by other companies outside the state)**	**Phone: 617-983-6400** **Web site: Not available**	
Human-Derived Botulinum Antitoxin (available under investigational protocol from the California Department of Health)		Botulism immune globulin, human (BIG)
Immune Globulin (Human) USP (distributed by FFF Enterprises)		Immune globulin intramuscular, human (IGIM)

Tetanus and Diphtheria Toxoids Adsorbed for Adult Use (distributed by General Injectables & Vaccines, Inc.)

Varicella-Zoster Immune Globulin (distributed by FFF Enterprises)

Diphtheria and tetanus toxoids (Td)

Varicella-zoster immune globulin, human (VZIG)

MedImmune, Inc.
35 W. Watkins Mill Rd.
P.O. Box 7929
Gaithersburg, MD 20878
CytoGam (manufactured by MPHBL)
Flumist (marketed by Wyeth)
Synagis
RespiGam (manufactured by MPHBL)

Phone: 301-417-0770
Web site: www.medimmune.com

Cytomegalovirus immune globulin intravenous, human (CMV-IGIV)
Live-attenuated influenza vaccine, intranasal (LAIV)
Palivizumab (humanized murine monoclonal antibody to RSV; RSV-mAb)
RSV immune globulin intravenous, human (RSV-IGIV)

Merck & Co., Inc.
P.O. Box 4
West Point, PA 19486
COMVAX

Phone: 800-672-6372
Web site: www.merckvaccines.com

Haemophilus influenzae polyribosylribotol phosphate–meningococcal outer membrane protein conjugate; hepatitis B, recombinant (PRP-OMP/Hep-B)

MERUVAX_{II}
M-M-R_{II}
PedvaxHIB

Rubella, live-attenuated
Measles, mumps and rubella, live-attenuated (MMR)
Haemophilus influenzae polyribosylribotol phosphate–meningococcal outer membrane protein conjugate (PRP-OMP)

PNEUMOVAX 23
RECOMBIVAX HB
VAQTA
VARIVAX

Pneumococcal polysaccharide, 23-valent (Pne-PS)
Hepatitis B, recombinant (Hep-B)
Hepatitis A, inactivated (Hep-A)
Varicella, live-attenuated

Nabi (North American Biologicals, Inc.)
5800 Park of Commerce Blvd. N.W.
Boca Raton, FL 33487
Nabi-HB

Phone: 561-989-5800
Web site: www.nabi.com

Hepatitis B immune globulin, human (HBIG)

(continued)

Table 14.2. *Continued*

Novartis Pharmaceuticals Corporation **One Health Plaza** **East Hanover, NJ 07936**	**Phone: 973-781-8300** **Web site: www.novartis.com**
Sandoglobulin (manufactured by ZLB Bioplasma AG, Swiss Red Cross; no longer available in the United States)	Immune globulin intravenous, human (IGIV)
Organon, Inc. **375 Mt. Pleasant Ave.** **West Orange, NJ 07052**	**Phone: 800-241-8812** **Web site: www.organoninc.com**
BCG VACCINE U.S.P.	Bacille Calmette-Guérin, live (BCG)
Wyeth (formerly American Home Products, includes former companies Ayerst, McKenna & Harrison Ltd; A.H. Robins; and Lederle Laboratories) **5 Giralda Farms** **Madison, NJ 07940**	**Phone: 800-934-5556** **Web site: www.wyeth.com**
Dryvax	Smallpox vaccine, dried, calf-lymph type
FluShield (no longer available)	Inactivated influenza, trivalent, subvirion
HibTITER	*Haemophilus influenzae* polyribosylribotol phosphate–mutant diphtheria protein (CRM_{197}) conjugate (HbOC)
Pnu-Imune 23 (no longer available)	Pneumococcal polysaccharide, 23-valent (Pne-PS)
Prevnar	Pneumococcal polysaccharide–mutant diphtheria protein (CRM_{197}) conjugate, 7-valent (PCV-7)
ZLB Bioplasma, Inc. [U.S. distributor for ZLB (Zentrallaboratorium Blutspendedienst) Bioplasma AG, now a subsidiary of ACSL Limited] **801 N. Brand Blvd.** **Suite 1150** **Glendale, CA 91203**	**Phone: 866-244-2952Web site: www.zlbusa.com**
Carimune	Immune globulin intravenous, human (IGIV)
Panglobulin (distributed by American Red Cross)	Immune globulin intravenous, human (IGIV)

X. Books and monographs

Title:	Vaccines (3rd ed.)
Author:	Stanley A. Plotkin, Walter A. Orenstein
Publisher:	WB Saunders
Year:	1999 (new edition due in 2003)
ISBN number:	0721674437

Title:	Vaccinating Your Child: Questions and Answers for the Concerned Parent
Author:	Sharon G. Humiston, Cynthia Good
Publisher:	Peachtree
Year:	2000
ISBN number:	1561451770

Title:	Epidemiology and Prevention of Vaccine-Preventable Diseases (Pink Book)
Author:	William Atkinson, Charles Wolfe
Publisher:	Public Health Foundation
Year:	2002
ISBN number:	None (available through CDC)

Title:	Your Child's Best Shot: A Parent's Guide to Vaccination
Author:	Ronald Gold
Publisher:	Canadian Paediatric Society
Year:	2002
ISBN number:	0968240968

Title:	Red Book: 2003 Report of the Committee on Infectious Diseases
Author:	Larry K. Pickering, American Academy of Pediatrics
Publisher:	American Academy of Pediatrics
Year:	2003
ISBN number:	1581100957

Title:	Vaccines: What You Should Know
Author:	Paul A. Offit, Louis M. Bell
Publisher:	John Wiley and Sons
Year:	2003
ISBN number:	0471420042

XI. Videotapes and multimedia

Title:	A Paralyzing Fear: The Story of Polio in America
Type:	Videotape
Author:	Nina Gilden Seavey, Paul Wagner, Olympia Dukakis, Catherine Shields
Publisher:	Center for History in the Media, George Washington University and Paul Wagner Productions
Year:	2000

Title:	Vaccines: Separating Fact From Fear
Type:	Videotape
Author:	Vaccine Education Center

Publisher:	Vaccine Education Center at the Children's Hospital of Philadelphia
Year:	2001

Title:	Increasing Adult Vaccination Rates: What Works
Type:	CD-ROM
Author:	Association of Teachers of Preventive Medicine, Centers for Disease Control and Prevention
Publisher:	Association of Teachers of Preventive Medicine, Centers for Disease Control and Prevention
Year:	2001

Title:	The Immunization Encounter
Type:	Videotape
Author:	William Atkinson, Judy V. Schmidt, Donna L. Weaver
Publisher:	Public Health Training Network, CDC
Year:	2002

Title:	Vaccines and Your Baby
Type:	Videotape
Author:	Vaccine Education Center
Publisher:	Vaccine Education Center at the Children's Hospital of Philadelphia
Year:	2002

XII. Vaccine protest organizations

Vaccines are now safer than at any time in history. Despite this, new challenges to the safety, efficacy, and necessity of vaccines arise daily, many brought forward by activists and popularized in the lay press and on the Internet. Although very few (if any) of the claims made hold up to scientific scrutiny, well-meaning parents may nevertheless be heavily influenced by the negative things they hear and read. The resultant fear of vaccination can translate directly into personal and public harm.

A simple Internet search using terms like "vaccines" or "immunization" yields a multitude of Web sites that contain non–peer-reviewed data, frightening anecdotes, and pseudoscientific arguments intermingled with legitimate concerns such as fever and local reactogenicity; parents may have trouble filtering the information from the misinformation. Many of these Web sites are sponsored by organizations that claim authority, credibility, and scientific rigor; offer strong emotive or political appeals; make explicit claims about vaccines that are unsupported or even contradicted by published data; and call parents to action in opposing vaccine policy. Table 14.3 lists some Web sites that have a vaccine protest orientation. Providers should remain informed about the content of these sites to be better prepared to address issues that parents may raise.

Table 14.3. Web sites with vaccine protest orientation

Web site	Sponsor
avn.org.au	Australian Vaccination Network
www.empiricaltherapies.com	Center for Empirical Medicine
www.unc.edu/~aphillip/www/chf	Citizens for Healthcare Freedom
home.sprynet.com/%7Egyrene	Concerned Parents for Vaccine Safety
www.ctanet.fr/vaccination-information	French National League for Liberty in Vaccination
www.gval.com	Global Vaccine Awareness League
www.ias.org.nz	Immunization Awareness Society
members.aol.com/_ht_a/mccfhc	Missouri Citizens Coalition for Freedom in Health Care
www.909shot.com	National Vaccine Information Center
www.nyvic.org	New Yorkers for Vaccination Information and Choice
www.vaccineinfo.net	Parents Requesting Open Vaccine Education
www.vaccines.bizland.com	People Advocating Vaccine Education
www.thinktwice.com	Thinktwice Global Vaccine Institute
home.san.rr.com/via	Vaccine Information & Awareness
www.van.org.uk	Vaccine Information Service
vaccines.net	Classen Immunotherapies, Inc.

Adapted from Davies P, Chapman S, Leask J. Antivaccination activists on the World Wide Web. *Arch Dis Child* 2002;87:22–25; Poland GA, Jacobson RM, Understanding those who do not understand: a brief review of the anti-vaccine movement. *Vaccine* 2001;19:2440–2445; and Wolfe RM, Sharp LK, Lipsky MS. Content and design attributes of antivaccination Web sites. *JAMA* 2002;287:3245–3248.

Suggested Readings

Chapter 1: General considerations
Section IV: Contraindications and precautions

AAP. Active immunizations. In: Pickering LK, ed. *Red book: 2003 report of the Committee on Infectious Diseases*, 26th ed. Elk Grove Village, IL: American Academy of Pediatrics; 2003:7–53, 798–801.

CDC. General recommendations on immunization. In: Atkinson W, Wolfe C, eds. *Epidemiology and prevention of vaccine-preventable diseases*, 7th ed. Atlanta, GA: Public Health Foundation; 2002:7–22.

Section VI: Effective vaccine delivery

CDC. Impact of missed opportunities to vaccinate preschool-aged children on vaccination coverage levels—Selected U.S. sites, 1991–1992. *MMWR* 1994;43:709–711;717–718.

Rappo PD, Cox EO, Green JL, et al. Policy on the development of immunization tracking systems. *Pediatrics* 1996;97:927.

Szilagyi PG, Rodewald LE, Humiston SG, et al. Effect of two urban emergency department immunization programs on childhood immunization rates. *Arch Pediatr Adolesc Med* 1997;151:999–1006.

Szilagyi PG, Bordley C, Vann JC, et al. Effect of patient reminder/recall interventions on immunization rates: a review. *JAMA* 2000;284:1820–1827.

CDC. Development of community- and state-based immunization registries: CDC response to a report from the National Vaccine Advisory Committee. *MMWR* 2001;50 (RR-17).

CDC. Immunization registry progress—United States, 2002. *MMWR* 2002;51:760–762.

Section VII: Monitoring immunization coverage and effectiveness

CDC. Surveillance for vaccination coverage among children and adults—United States. *MMWR* 2000;49:SS-9.

CDC. National, state, and urban area vaccination coverage levels among children aged 19–35 months—United States, 2001. *MMWR* 2002;51:664–666.

Luman ET, Barker LE, McCauley MM, et al. A measure of success: findings from the National Immunization Survey. *Am J Prev Med* 2001;20(4S):1–154.

Luman ET, McCauley MM, Stokley S, et al. Timeliness of childhood immunizations. *Pediatrics* 2002;110:935–939.

National Immunization Program. Immunization coverage in the U.S. www.cdc.gov/nip/coverage (accessed 01/26/03).

CDC. Standards for pediatric immunization practices. *MMWR* 1993;42(No. RR-5):1–13.

Gardner P, Pickering LK, Orenstein WA, et al. Guidelines for quality standards for immunization. *Clin Infect Dis* 2002;35:503–511.

National Vaccine Program Office. The standards for pediatric immunization practice. www.cdc.gov/od/nvpo/standar.htm (accessed 01/24/03).

Section V: Occupational Safety and Health Administration (OSHA)

OSHA. Occupational exposure to bloodborne pathogens; needlestick and other sharps injuries; final rule. *Federal Register* 2001;66:5318–5325.

OSHA. Bloodborne pathogens. www.osha.gov/SLTC/bloodbornepathogens/index.html (accessed 01/25/03).

Section VI: School mandates and state legislation

AAP. Religious objections to medical care. *Pediatrics* 1997;99:279–281.

Feikin DR, Lezotte DC, Hamman RF, et al. Individual and community risks of measles and pertussis associated with personal exemptions to immunization. *JAMA* 2000;284:3145–3150.

Orenstein WA, Hinman AR. The immunization system in the United States—the role of school immunization laws. *Vaccine* 1999;17:S19–S24.

Salmon DA, Haber M, Gangarosa EJ, et al. Health consequences of religious and philosophical exemptions from immunization laws: individual and societal risks. *JAMA* 1999;282:47–53.

Chapter 3: The vaccine encounter
Section I: Communicating about vaccines

Ball LK, Evans G, Bostrom A. Risky business: challenges in vaccine risk communication. *Pediatrics* 1998;101:453–458.

Davis TC, Frederickson DD, Arnold CL, et al. Childhood vaccine risk/benefit communication in private practice office settings: a national survey. *Pediatrics* 2001;107:e17.

Davis TC, Fredrickson DD, Bocchini C, et al. Improving vaccine risk/benefit communication with an immunization education package: a pilot study. *Ambul Pediatr* 2002;2:193–200.

Evans G, Bostrom A, Johnston RB, et al. *Risk communication and vaccination: summary of a workshop*. Washington, DC: National Academy Press, 1997.

Fredrickson DD, Davis TC, Bocchini JA. Explaining the risks and benefits of vaccines to parents. *Pediatr Ann* 2001;30:400–406.

LeBaron CW, Rodewald L, Humiston S. How much time is spent on well-child care and vaccinations? *Arch Pediatr Adolesc Med* 1999;153:1154–1159.

Marshall GS. Vaccines under fire: the importance of perspective. *Pediatr Ann* 2001;30:379–380, 390.

Marshall GS. Truths about vaccines. In: *An ounce of prevention: communicating the benefits and risks of vaccines to parents*. CME monograph distributed as a supplement to *Infectious Diseases in Children* (Brunell PA, ed.): January, 2003.

Chapter 4: The business of vaccines in practice
Section I: Coding and billing

American Medical Association. *Current procedural terminology: CPT 2003*. Chicago, IL: AMA Press, 2002.

Hart AC, Hopkins CA, eds. *International classification of diseases: 9th revision: clinical modification*, 6th ed. Salt Lake City, UT: Ingenix, Inc., 2002.

Section III: Funding vaccine services

Freed GL, Clark SJ, Pathman D, et al. Impact of North Carolina's universal vaccine purchase program by children's insurance status. *Arch Pediatr Adolesc Med* 1999;153:748–754.

Zimmerman RK, Mieczkowski TA, Mainzer HM, et al. Effect of the Vaccines for Children Program on physician referral of children to public vaccine clinics: a pre-post comparison. *Pediatrics* 2001;108:297–304.

Section IV: Vaccine shortages

Cohen J. U.S. vaccine supply falls seriously short. *Science* 2002;295:1998–2001.

National Vaccine Advisory Committee. Strengthening the supply of routinely recommended vaccines in the United States. www.cdc.gov/od/nvpo/nvac-vsr.htm (accessed 03/17/03).

Orenstein WA. Protecting our kids: What is causing the current shortage in childhood vaccines? Testimony before the Committee on Governmental Affairs, U.S. Senate. www.cdc.gov/nip/news/testimonies/vac-shortages-walt-6-12-2002.htm (accessed 01/24/03).

Chapter 5: Universal vaccines for children and adolescents
Section I: Diphtheria, tetanus, and pertussis

AAP. Diphtheria. In: Pickering LK, ed. *Red book: 2003 report of the Committee on Infectious Diseases*, 26th ed. Elk Grove Village, IL: American Academy of Pediatrics; 2003:263–266.

AAP. Pertussis. In: Pickering LK, ed. *Red book: 2003 report of the Committee on Infectious Diseases*, 26th ed. Elk Grove Village, IL: American Academy of Pediatrics; 2003:472–486.

AAP. Tetanus. In: Pickering LK, ed. *Red book: 2003 report of the Committee on Infectious Diseases*, 26th ed. Elk Grove Village, IL: American Academy of Pediatrics; 2003:611–616.

CDC. Pertussis vaccination: use of acellular pertussis vaccines among infants and young children: recommendations of the Advisory Committee on Immunization Practices (ACIP). *MMWR* 1997;46(RR-7):1–25.

CDC. Use of diphtheria toxoid-tetanus toxoid-acellular pertussis vaccine as a five-dose series: supplemental recommendations of the Advisory Committee on Immunization Practices (ACIP). *MMWR* 2000;49(RR-13):1–8.

CDC. Pertussis—United States, 1997–2000. *MMWR* 2002;51:73–76.

Decker MD, Edwards KM. Acellular pertussis vaccines. *Pediatr Clin North Am* 2000;47:309–335.

Section II: *Haemophilus influenzae* type b

AAP. *Haemophilus influenzae* infections. In: Pickering LK, ed. *Red book: 2003 report of the Committee on Infectious Diseases*, 26th ed. Elk Grove Village, IL: American Academy of Pediatrics; 2003:293–301.

CDC. *Haemophilus* b conjugate vaccines for prevention of *Haemophilus influenzae* type b disease among infants and children two months of age and older: recommendations of the Immunization Practices Advisory Committee (ACIP). *MMWR* 1991;40(RR-1):1–7.

CDC. *Haemophilus influenzae* invasive disease among children aged <5 years—California. *MMWR* 1998;47: 737–740.

CDC. Progress toward elimination of *Haemophilus influenzae* type b disease among infants and children—United States, 1998–2000. *MMWR* 2002;51: 234–237.

Decker MD, Edwards KM. *Haemophilus influenzae* type b vaccines: history, choice and comparisons. *Pediatr Infect Dis J* 1998;17:S113–116.

Section III: Hepatitis B

AAP. Universal hepatitis B immunization. *Pediatrics* 1992;89:795–800.

AAP. Hepatitis B. In: Pickering LK, ed. *Red book: 2003 report of the Committee on Infectious Diseases*, 26th ed. Elk Grove Village, IL: American Academy of Pediatrics; 2003:318–336.

CDC. A comprehensive strategy for the elimination of hepatitis B transmission in the United States through universal childhood immunization. *MMWR* 1991;40(RR-13):1–25.

CDC. Update: Recommendations to prevent hepatitis B transmission—United States. *MMWR* 1995;44:574–575.

CDC. Update: Recommendations to prevent hepatitis B transmission—United States. *MMWR* 1999;48:574–575.

CDC. Achievements in public health: hepatitis B vaccination—U.S., 1982–2002. *MMWR* 2002;51:549–552, 563.

Lee WM. Hepatitis B virus infection. *N Engl J Med* 1997;337:1733–1745.

Yusuf HR, Daniels D, Smith P, et al. Association between administration of hepatitis B vaccine at birth and completion of the hepatitis B and 4:3:1:3 vaccine series. *JAMA* 2000;284:978–983.

Section IV: Polio

AAP. Prevention of poliomyelitis: recommendations for use of only inactivated poliovirus vaccine for routine immunization. *Pediatrics* 1999;104:1404–1406.

AAP. Poliovirus infections. In: Pickering LK, ed. *Red book: 2003 report of the Committee on Infectious Diseases*, 26th ed. Elk Grove Village, IL: American Academy of Pediatrics; 2003:505–509.

CDC. Poliomyelitis prevention in the United States: introduction of a sequential vaccination schedule of inactivated poliovirus vaccine followed by oral poliovirus vaccine. *MMWR* 1997;46(RR-3):1–25.

CDC. Revised recommendations for routine poliomyelitis vaccination. *MMWR* 1999;48:590.

CDC. Poliomyelitis prevention in the United States: updated recommendations of the Advisory Committee on Immunization Practices (ACIP). *MMWR* 2000;49(RR-5):1–22.

Hull HF. The future of polio eradication. *Lancet* 2001;1:299–303.

Strebel PM, Sutter RW, Cochi SL, et al. Epidemiology of poliomyelitis in the United States one decade after the last reported case of indigenous wild virus–associated disease. *Clin Infect Dis* 1992;14:568–579.

Section V: Measles, mumps, and rubella

AAP. Age for routine administration of the second dose of measles-mumps-rubella vaccine. *Pediatrics* 1998; 101:129–133.

AAP. Measles. In: Pickering LK, ed. *Red book: 2003 report of the Committee on Infectious Diseases*, 26th ed. Elk Grove Village, IL: American Academy of Pediatrics; 2003:419–429.

AAP. Mumps. In: Pickering LK, ed. *Red book: 2003 report of the Committee on Infectious Diseases*, 26th ed. Elk Grove Village, IL: American Academy of Pediatrics; 2003:439–443.

AAP. Rubella. In: Pickering LK, ed. *Red book: 2003 report of the Committee on Infectious Diseases*, 26th ed. Elk Grove Village, IL: American Academy of Pediatrics; 2003:536–541.

CDC. Measles, mumps, and rubella—Vaccine use and strategies for elimination of measles, rubella, and congenital rubella syndrome and control of mumps. *MMWR* 1998;47(RR-8):1–58.

National Vaccine Advisory Committee. The measles epidemic: the problems, barriers, and recommendations. *JAMA* 1991;266:1547–1552.

Cochi SL, Preblud SR, Orenstein WA. Perspectives on the relative resurgence of mumps in the United States. *Am J Dis Child* 1988;142:499–507.

Reef SE, Plotkin S, Cordero JF, et al. Preparing for elimination of congenital rubella syndrome (CRS): summary of a workshop on CRS elimination in the United States. *Clin Infect Dis* 2000;31:85–95.

Section VI: Pneumococcal conjugate

AAP. Policy statement: recommendations for the prevention of pneumococcal infections, including the use of pneumococcal conjugate vaccine (Prevnar), pneumococcal polysaccharide vaccine, and antibiotic prophylaxis. *Pediatrics* 2000;106:362–366.

AAP. Technical report: prevention of pneumococcal infections, including the use of pneumococcal conjugate and polysaccharide vaccines and antibiotic prophylaxis. *Pediatrics* 2000;106:367–376.

AAP. Pneumococcal infections. In: Pickering LK, ed. *Red book: 2003 report of the Committee on Infectious Diseases*, 26th ed. Elk Grove Village, IL: American Academy of Pediatrics; 2003:490–500.

CDC. Preventing pneumococcal disease among infants and young children: recommendations of the Advisory Committee on Immunization Practices (ACIP). *MMWR* 2000;49(RR-9):1–38.

Giebink GS. The prevention of pneumococcal disease in children. *N Engl J Med* 2001;345:1177–1183.

Pelton SI, Klein JO. The future of pneumococcal conjugate vaccines for prevention of pneumococcal diseases in infants and children. *Pediatrics* 2002;110:805–814.

Section VII: Varicella

AAP. Varicella vaccine update. *Pediatrics* 2000;105:136–141.

AAP. Varicella-zoster infections. In: Pickering LK, ed. *Red book: 2003 report of the Committee on Infectious Diseases*, 26th ed. Elk Grove Village, IL: American Academy of Pediatrics; 2003:672–686.

CDC. Prevention of varicella: update recommendations of the Advisory Committee on Immunization Practices (ACIP). *MMWR* 1999;48(RR-6):1–5.

CDC. Simultaneous administration of varicella vaccine and other recommended childhood vaccines—United States, 1995–1999. *MMWR* 2001;50:1058–1061.

Clements DA, Zaref JI, Bland CL, et al. Partial uptake of varicella vaccine and the epidemiological effect on varicella disease in 11 day-care centers in North Carolina. *Arch Pediatr Adolesc Med* 2001;155:455–461.

Izurieta HS, Strebel PM, Blake PA, et al. Postlicensure effectiveness of varicella vaccine during an outbreak in a child care center. *JAMA* 1997;278:1495–1499.

Meyer PA, Seward JF, Jumaan AO, et al. Varicella mortality: trends before vaccine licensure in the United States, 1970–1994. *J Infect Dis* 2000;182:383–390.

Seward JF, Watson BM, Peterson CL, et al. Varicella disease after introduction of varicella vaccine in the United States, 1995–2000. *JAMA* 2002;287:606–611.

Vazquez M, LaRussa PS, Gershon AA, et al. The effectiveness of the varicella vaccine in clinical practice. *N Engl J Med* 2001;344:955–960.

Chapter 6: Combination vaccines
Section I: General considerations

AAP. Combination vaccines for childhood immunization: recommendations of the Advisory Committee on Immunization Practices (ACIP), the American Academy of Pediatrics (AAP), and the American Academy of Family Physicians (AAFP). *Pediatrics* 1999;103:1064–1077.

Breiman R, Goldenthal K, eds. International symposium on combination vaccines. *Clin Infect Dis* 2001;33(Suppl 4):S261–S375.

Greenberg DP, ed. Recent developments in combination vaccines: clinical implications. *Pediatr Infect Dis J* 2001;20(Suppl):S5–S62.

Insel RA. Potential alterations in immunogenicity by combining or simultaneously administering vaccine components. *Ann N Y Acad Sci* 1995;754:35–47.

Section II: Diphtheria, tetanus, pertussis, and *Haemophilus influenzae*

CDC. Notice to readers: FDA approval of a *Haemophilus influenzae* b conjugate vaccine combined with an acellular pertussis vaccine. *MMWR* 1996;45:993–995.

Section III: *Haemophilus influenzae* type b and hepatitis

CDC. Notice to readers: FDA approval for infants of a *Haemophilus* b conjugate and hepatitis B (recombinant) combined vaccine. *MMWR* 1997;46:107–109.

Section IV: Hepatitis A and hepatitis B

CDC. Notice to readers: FDA approval for a combined hepatitis A and B vaccine. *MMWR* 2001;50:806–807.

Section V: Diphtheria, tetanus, pertussis, hepatitis B, and polio

Blatter MM, Reisinger K, Bottenfield GW, et al. Evaluation of the reactogenicity and immunogenicity of a new combined DTPa-HBV-IPV vaccine co-administered with Hib vaccine at 2, 4, and 6 months of age (abstract 648). In: *Infectious Diseases Society of America. Program and Abstracts of the 37th Annual Meeting of the Infectious Diseases Society of America.* Alexandria, VA: IDSA, 1999:152.

CDC. FDA licensure of diphtheria and tetanus toxoids and acellular pertussis adsorbed, hepatitis B (recombinant), and poliovirus vaccine combined (Pediarix), for use in infants. *MMWR* 2003;52:203–204.

Greenberg DP, Wong VK, Partridge S, et al. Safety and immunogenicity of a combination diphtheria–tetanus toxoids–acellular pertussis–hepatitis B vaccine administered at two, four and six months of age compared with monovalent hepatitis B vaccine administered at birth, one month and six months of age. *Pediatr Infect Dis J* 2002;21:769–777.

Gylca R, Gylca V, Benes O, et al. A new DTPa-HBV-IPV vaccine co-administered with Hib, compared to a commercially available DTPw-IPV/Hib vaccine co-administered with HBV, given at 6, 10 and 14 weeks following HBV at birth. *Vaccine* 2001;19:825–833.

Pichichero ME, Blatter MM, Reisinger KS, et al. Impact of a birth dose of hepatitis B vaccine on the reactogenicity and immunogenicity of diphtheria-tetanus–acellular pertussis–hepatitis B–inactivated poliovirus–*Haemophilus influenzae* type b combination vaccination. *Pediatr Infect Dis J* 2002;21:854–859.

Yeh SH, Ward JI, Partridge S, et al. Safety and immunogenicity of a pentavalent diphtheria, tetanus, pertussis, hepatitis B and polio combination vaccine in infants. *Pediatr Infect Dis J* 2001;20:973–980.

Zepp F, Schuind A, Meyer C, et al. Safety and reactogenicity of a novel DTPa-HBV-IPV combined vaccine given along with commercial Hib vaccines in comparison with separate concomitant administration of DTPa, Hib, and OPV vaccines in infants. *Pediatrics* 2002;109:e58.

Chapter 7: Vaccines for adults and selected children
Section I: Tetanus and diphtheria [see also Chapter 5(I)]

CDC. Diphtheria, tetanus, and pertussis: recommendations for vaccine use and other preventive measures: recommendations of the Immunization Practices Advisory Committee (ACIP). *MMWR* 1991;40(RR-10):1–28.

CDC. Update on adult immunization: recommendations of the Immunization Practices Advisory Committee (ACIP). *MMWR* 1991;40(RR-12):1–77.

Section II: Pneumococcal polysaccharide

CDC. Prevention of pneumococcal disease: recommendations of the Advisory Committee on Immunization Practices (ACIP). *MMWR* 1997;46(RR-8):1–24.

Robinson KA, Baughman W, Rothrock G, et al. Epidemiology of invasive *Streptococcus pneumoniae* infections in the United States, 1995–1998: opportunities for prevention in the conjugate vaccine era. *JAMA* 2001;285:1729–1735.

Whitney CG, Farley MM, Hadler J, et al. Increasing prevalence of multidrug-resistant *Streptococcus pneumoniae* in the United States. *N Engl J Med* 2000;343:1917–1924.

Section III: Influenza

Bridges CB, Thompson WW, Meltzer MI, et al. Effectiveness and cost-benefit of influenza vaccination of healthy working adults: a randomized controlled trial. *JAMA* 2000;284:1655–1663.

CDC. Immunization of health-care workers: recommendations of the Advisory Committee on Immunization Practices (ACIP) and the Hospital Infection Control Practices Advisory Committee (HICPAC). *MMWR* 1997;46(RR-18):1–42.

CDC. Prevention and control of influenza: recommendations of the Advisory Committee on Immunization Practices (ACIP). *MMWR* 2002;51(RR-3):1–31 (Note: these recommendations are revised annually.)

Couch RB. Prevention and treatment of influenza. *N Engl J Med* 2000;343:1778–1787.

Izurieta HS, Thompson WW, Kramarz P, et al. Influenza and the rates of hospitalization for respiratory disease among infants and young children. *N Engl J Med* 2000;342:232–239.

Neuzil KM, Zhu Y, Griffin MR, et al. Burden of interpandemic influenza in children younger than 5 years: a 25-year prospective study. *J Infect Dis* 2002;185:147–152.

Nichol KL, Lind A, Margolis KL, et al. The effectiveness of vaccination against influenza in healthy, working adults. *N Engl J Med* 1995;333:889–893.

Thompson WW, Shay DK, Weintraub E, et al. Mortality associated with influenza and respiratory syncytial virus in the United States. *JAMA* 2003;289:179–186.

Chapter 8: Vaccines for specialized use
Section I: Adenovirus

Brandt CD, Kim HW, Vargosko AJ, et al. Infections in 18,000 infants and children in a controlled study of respiratory tract diseases. I. Adenovirus pathogenicity in relation to serologic type and illness syndrome. *Am J Epidemiol* 1969;90:484–500.

D'Angelo LJ, Hierholzer JC, Holman RC, et al. Epidemic keratoconjunctivitis caused by adenovirus type 8: epidemiologic and laboratory aspects of a large outbreak. *Am J Epidemiol* 1981;113:44–49.

Dingle JH, Langmuir AD. Epidemiology of acute respiratory diseases in military recruits. *Am Rev Respir Dis* 1968;97:1–65.

Edwards KM, Thompson J, Paolini J, et al. Adenovirus infections in young children. *Pediatrics* 1985;76:420–424.

Kolavic-Gray SA, Binn LN, Sanchez JL, et al. Large epidemic of adenovirus type 4 infection among military trainees: epidemiological, clinical, and laboratory studies. *Clin Infect Dis* 2002;35:808–818.

Peckinpaugh RO, Pierce WE, Rosenbaum MJ, et al. Mass enteric live adenovirus vaccination during epidemic acute respiratory disease. *JAMA* 1968;205:75–80.

Ruuskanen O, Meurman O, Sarkkinen H. Adenoviral diseases in children: a study of 105 hospital cases. *Pediatrics* 1985;76:79–83.

Sherwood RW, Buescher EL, Nitz RE. Effect of adenovirus vaccine on acute respiratory disease in U.S. Army recruits. *JAMA* 1961;178:1115–1127.

Top FH, Grossman RA, Bartelloni PJ. Immunization with live types 7 and 4 adenovirus vaccines: antibody response and protective effect against acute respiratory disease due to adenovirus type 7. *J Infect Dis* 1971;124:155–160.

Section II: Bacille Calmette-Guérin

AAP. Tuberculosis. In: Pickering LK, ed. *Red book: 2003 report of the Committee on Infectious Diseases*, 26th ed. Elk Grove Village, IL: American Academy of Pediatrics; 2003:642–660.

Brewer TF, Colditz GA. Relationship between bacilli Calmette-Guérin (BCG) strains and the efficacy of BCG vaccine in the prevention of tuberculosis. *Clin Infect Dis* 1995;20:126–135.

CDC. The role of BCG vaccine in the prevention and control of tuberculosis in the United States: a joint statement by the Advisory Council for the Elimination of Tuberculosis and the Advisory Committee on Immunization Practices. *MMWR* 1996;45(RR-4):1–18.

Colditz GA, Brewer TF, Berkey CS, et al. Efficacy of BCG vaccine in the prevention of tuberculosis: meta-analysis of the published literature. *JAMA* 1994;271:698–702.

Filho VW, de Castilho EA, Rodrigues LC, et al. Effectiveness of BCG vaccination against tuberculous meningitis: a case-control study in Sao Paulo, Brazil. *Bull World Health Org* 1990;68:69–74.

Khan MA, Kovnat DM, Bachus B, et al. Clinical and roentgenographic spectrum of pulmonary tuberculosis in the adult. *Am J Med* 1977;62:31–38.

Lotte A, Wasz-Hockert O, Poisson N, et al. BCG complications: estimates of the risks among vaccinated subjects and statistical analysis of their main characteristics. *Adv Tuberc Res* 1984;21:107–193.

Raviglione MC, Snider DE, Kochi A. Global epidemiology of tuberculosis: morbidity and mortality of a worldwide epidemic. *JAMA* 1995;273:220–226.

Sirinavin S, Chotpitayasunondh T, Suwanjutha S, et al. Protective efficacy of neonatal bacillus Calmette-Guérin vaccination against tuberculosis. *Pediatr Infect Dis J* 1991;10:359–365.

Starke JR. Bacille Calmette-Guérin vaccine. *Semin Pediatr Infect Dis* 1991;2:153–158.

Ussery XT, Valway SE, McKenna M, et al. Epidemiology of tuberculosis among children in the United States: 1985 to 1994. *Pediatr Infect Dis J* 1996;15:697–704.

Section III: Cholera

AAP. Cholera. In: Pickering LK, ed. *Red book: 2003 report of the Committee on Infectious Diseases*, 26th ed. Elk Grove Village, IL: American Academy of Pediatrics; 2003:686–688.

Blake PA. Epidemiology of cholera in the Americas. *Gastroenterol Clin North Am* 1993;22:639–660.

CDC. Recommendations of the Immunization Practices Advisory Committee: cholera vaccine. *MMWR* 1988; 37:617–624.

Clemens JD, Sack DA, Harris JR, et al. Field trial of oral cholera vaccines in Bangladesh: results from three-year follow-up. *Lancet* 1990;335:270–273.

Committee to Advise on Tropical Medicine and Travel. Statement on oral cholera vaccination. *Can Commun Dis Rep* 1998;24(ACS-5):1–5.

Cyrz SJ, Levine MM, Kaper JB, et al. Randomized double-blind placebo controlled trial to evaluate the safety and immunogenicity of the live oral cholera vaccine strain CVD 103-HgR in Swiss adults. *Vaccine* 1990;8:577–580.

Guthmann JP. Epidemic cholera in Latin America: spread and routes of transmission. *J Trop Med Hyg* 1995;98:419–427.

Mosley WH, Aziz KM, Mizanur Rahman AS, et al. Report of the 1966–67 cholera vaccine trial in rural East Pakistan. *Bull World Health Org* 1972;47:229–238.

Philippines Cholera Committee. A controlled field trial of the effectiveness of the intradermal and subcutaneous administration of cholera vaccine in the Philippines. *Bull World Health Org* 1973;49:389–394.

Ryan ET, Calderwood SB. Cholera vaccines. *Clin Infect Dis* 2000;31:561–565.

Sommer A, Mosley WH. Ineffectiveness of cholera vaccination as an epidemic control measure. *Lancet* 1973; 1:1232–1235.

WHO. Cholera vaccines. *World Epidemiol Record* 2001; 76:117–124.

Section IV: Hepatitis A

AAP. Hepatitis A. In: Pickering LK, ed. *Red book: 2003 report of the Committee on Infectious Diseases*, 26th ed. Elk Grove Village, IL: American Academy of Pediatrics; 2003:309–318.

Averhoff F, Shapiro CN, Bell BP, et al. Control of hepatitis A through routine vaccination of children. *JAMA* 2001;286:2968–2973.

CDC. Prevention of hepatitis A through active or passive immunization: recommendations of the Advisory Committee on Immunization Practices (ACIP). *MMWR* 1999;48(RR-12):1–37.

Hollinger FB, ed. An overview of the clinical development of hepatitis A vaccine. *J Infect Dis* 1995;171(Suppl 1):S1–S77.

Innis BL, Snitbhan R, Kunasol P, et al. Protection against hepatitis A by an inactivated vaccine. *JAMA* 1994;271:1328–1334.

Koff RS. Clinical manifestations and diagnosis of hepatitis A virus infection. *Vaccine* 1992;10(Suppl 1):S15–S17.

McMahon BJ, Beller M, Williams J, et al. A program to control an outbreak of hepatitis A in Alaska by using an inactivated hepatitis A vaccine. *Arch Pediatr Adolesc Med* 1996;150:733–739.

Shapiro CN, Coleman PJ, McQuillan GM, et al. Epidemiology of hepatitis A: seroepidemiology and risk groups in the U.S.A. *Vaccine* 1992;10(Suppl 1):S59–S62.

Shapiro CN, Margolis HS. Worldwide epidemiology of hepatitis A virus infection. *J Hepatol* 1993;18(Suppl 2):S11–S14.

Werzberger A, Mensch B, Kuter B, et al. A controlled trial of formalin-inactivated hepatitis A vaccine in healthy children. *N Engl J Med* 1992;327:453–457.

Section V: Japanese encephalitis

CDC. Inactivated Japanese encephalitis virus vaccine: recommendations of the Advisory Committee on Immunization Practices (ACIP). *MMWR* 1993;42(RR-1):1–15.

Chambers TJ, Tsai TF, Pervivkov Y, et al. Vaccine development against dengue and Japanese encephalitis: report of a World Health Organization meeting. *Vaccine* 1997;15:1494–1502.

Hoke CH, Nisalak A, Sangawhipa N, et al. Protection against Japanese encephalitis by inactivated vaccines. *N Engl J Med* 1988;319:609–614.

Robinson HC, Russell ML, Csokonay WM. Japanese encephalitis vaccine and adverse effects among travelers. *Can Dis Weekly Report* 1991;17;173–174,177.

Ruff TA, Eisen D, Fuller A, et al. Adverse reactions to Japanese encephalitis vaccine. *Lancet* 1991;338:881–882.

Thongcharoen P. Japanese encephalitis virus encephalitis: an overview. *Southeast Asian J Trop Med Public Health* 1989;20:559–573.

Section VI: Lyme disease

AAP. Lyme disease. In: Pickering LK, ed. *Red book: 2003 report of the Committee on Infectious Diseases*, 26th ed. Elk Grove Village, IL: American Academy of Pediatrics; 2003:407–411.

CDC. Recommendations for the use of Lyme disease vaccine: recommendations of the Advisory Committee on Immunization Practices (ACIP). *MMWR* 1999;48(RR-7):1–25.

Gerber MA, Shapiro ED, Burke GS, et al. Lyme disease in children in Southeastern Connecticut. *N Engl J Med* 1996;335:1270–1274.

Keller D, Koster FT, Marks DH, et al. Safety and immunogenicity of a recombinant outer surface protein A Lyme vaccine. *JAMA* 1994;271:1764–1768.

Sigal LH, Zahradnik JM, Lavin P, et al. A vaccine consisting of recombinant *Borrelia burgdorferi* outersurface protein A to prevent Lyme disease. *N Engl J Med* 1998;339:216–222.

Steere AC, Sikand VK, Meurice F, et al. Vaccination against Lyme disease with recombinant *Borrelia burgdorferi* outer-surface protein A vaccine. *J Infect Dis* 1996;174:739–746.

Steere AC, Sikand VK, Meurice F, et al. Vaccination against Lyme disease with recombinant *Borrelia burgdorferi* outer-surface lipoprotein A with adjuvant. *N Engl J Med* 1998;339:209–216.

Steere AC. Lyme disease. *N Engl J Med* 2001;345:115–125.

Younus F, Luft BJ. Vaccines for Lyme disease. *Curr Clin Top Infect Dis* 2001;21:349–365.

Section VII: Meningococcus

AAP. Meningococcal infections. In: Pickering LK, ed. *Red book: 2003 report of the Committee on Infectious Diseases*, 26th ed. Elk Grove Village, IL: American Academy of Pediatrics; 2003:430–436.

Armand J, Arminjon F, Mynard MC, et al. Tetravalent meningococcal polysaccharide vaccine groups A, C, Y, W-135: clinical and serological evaluation. *J Biol Stand* 1982;10:335–339.

Bruce MG, Rosenstein NE, Capparella JM, et al. Risk factors for meningococcal disease in college students. *JAMA* 2001;286:688–693.

CDC. Control and prevention of serogroup C meningococcal disease: evaluation and management of suspected outbreaks: recommendations of the Advisory Committee on Immunization Practices (ACIP). *MMWR* 1997;46(RR-5):13–21.

CDC. Prevention and control of meningococcal disease: recommendations of the Advisory Committee on Immunization Practices (ACIP). *MMWR* 2000;49(RR-7):1–10.

CDC. Meningococcal disease and college students: recommendations of the Advisory Committee on Immunization Practices (ACIP). *MMWR* 2000;49(RR-7):11–20.

De Wals P, De Serres G, Niyonsenga T. Effectiveness of a mass immunization campaign against serogroup C meningococcal disease in Quebec. *JAMA* 2001;285:177–181.

Lennon D, Gellin B, Hood D, Voss L. Successful intervention in a group A meningococcal outbreak in Auckland, New Zealand. *Pediatr Infect Dis J* 1992;11:617–623.

Lieberman JM, Chiu SS, Wong VK, et al. Safety and immunogenicity of a serogroups A/C *Neisseria meningitidis* oligosaccharide–protein conjugate vaccine in young children. *JAMA* 1996;275:1499–1503.

Peltola H, Makela PH, Kayhty H, et al. Clinical efficacy of meningococcus group A capsular polysaccharide vaccine in children three months to five years of age. *N Engl J Med* 1977;297:686–691.

Rosenstein NE, Perkins BA, Stephens DS, et al. The changing epidemiology of meningococcal disease in the United States, 1992–1996. *J Infect Dis* 1999;180: 1894–1901.

Rosenstein NE, Perkins BA, Stephens DS, et al. Meningococcal disease. *N Engl J Med* 2001;344:1378–1388.

Section VIII: Rabies

AAP. Rabies. In: Pickering LK, ed. *Red book: 2003 report of the Committee on Infectious Diseases*, 26th ed. Elk Grove Village, IL: American Academy of Pediatrics; 2003:514–521.

CDC. Human rabies prevention—United States, 1999: recommendations of the Advisory Committee on Immunization Practices (ACIP). *MMWR* 1999;48(RR-1):1–21.

Dreesen DW, Fishbein DB, Kemp DT, et al. Two-year comparative trial on the immunogenicity and adverse effects of purified chick embryo cell rabies vaccine for pre-exposure immunization. *Vaccine* 1989;7:397–400.

Moran GJ, Talan DA, Mower W, et al. Appropriateness of rabies postexposure prophylaxis treatment for animal exposures. *JAMA* 2000;284:1001–1007.

Morimoto K, Patel M, Corisdeo S, et al. Characterization of a unique variant of bat rabies virus responsible for newly emerging human cases in North America. *Proc Natl Acad Sci U S A* 1996;93:5653–5658.

Plotkin SA. Rabies vaccine prepared in human cell cultures: progress and perspectives. *Rev Infect Dis* 1980;2:433–447.

Plotkin SA. Rabies. *Clin Infect Dis* 2000;30:4–12.

Remington PL, Shope T, Andrews J. A recommended approach to the evaluation of human rabies exposure in an acute-care hospital. *JAMA* 1985;254:67–69.

Section IX: Typhoid

AAP. *Salmonella* infections. In: Pickering LK, ed. *Red book: 2003 report of the Committee on Infectious Diseases*, 26th ed. Elk Grove Village, IL: American Academy of Pediatrics; 2003:541–547.

Acharya VI, Lowe CU, Thapa R, et al. Prevention of typhoid fever in Nepal with the Vi capsular polysaccharide of *Salmonella typhi*: a preliminary report. *N Engl J Med* 1987;317:1101–1104.

CDC. Typhoid immunization: recommendations of the Advisory Committee on Immunization Practices (ACIP). *MMWR* 1994;43(RR-14):1–7.

Ferreccio C, Levine MM, Rodriguez H, et al. Comparative efficacy of two, three, or four doses of Ty21a live oral typhoid vaccine enteric-coated capsules: a field trial in an endemic area. *J Infect Dis* 1989;159:766–769.

Levine MM, Ferreccio C, Black RE, et al. Large-scale field trial of Ty21a live oral typhoid vaccine in enteric-coated capsule formulation. *Lancet* 1987;1: 1049–1052.

Levine MM, Ferreccio C, Black RE, et al. Progress in vaccines against typhoid fever. *Rev Infect Dis* 1989;11(Suppl 3):S552–S567.

Lin FY, Ho VA, Khiem HB, et al. The efficacy of a *Salmonella typhi* Vi conjugate vaccine in two-to-five-year-old children. *N Engl J Med* 2001;344:1263–1269.

Mahle WT, Levine MM. *Salmonella typhi* infection in children younger than five years of age. *Pediatr Infect Dis J* 1993;12:627–631.

Parry CM, Hien TT, Dougan G, et al. Typhoid fever. *N Engl J Med* 2002;347:1770–1782.

Taylor DN, Pollard RA, Blake PA. Typhoid in the United States and risk to the international traveler. *J Infect Dis* 1980;142:934–938.

Section X: Yellow fever

AAP. Arboviruses. In: Pickering LK, ed. *Red book: 2003 report of the Committee on Infectious Diseases*, 26th ed. Elk Grove Village, IL: American Academy of Pediatrics; 2003:199–205.

CDC. Fever, jaundice, and multiple organ system failure associated with 17D-derived yellow fever vaccination, 1996–2001. *MMWR* 2001;50:643–645.

CDC. Adverse events associated with 17D-derived yellow fever vaccination—United States, 2001–2002. *MMWR* 2002;51:989–993.

CDC. Yellow fever vaccine: recommendations of the Advisory Committee on Immunization Practices (ACIP). *MMWR* 2002;51(RR-17):1–10.

Monath TP, Nichols R, Archambault WT, et al. Comparative safety and immunogenicity of two yellow fever 17D vaccines (ARILVAX and YF-VAX) in a phase III multicenter, double-blind clinic trial. *Am J Trop Med Hyg* 2002;66:533–541.

Poland JD, Calisher CH, Monath TP, et al. Persistence of neutralizing antibody 30–35 years after immunization with 17D yellow fever vaccine. *Bull World Health Organ* 1981;59:895–900.

Vianio J, Cutts F. Yellow fever. World Health Organization Global Program for Vaccines and Immunization, 1998. Publication No. (WHO/EPI/GEN) 98.11. www.who.int/emc-documents/yellow_fever/whoepigen9811c.html (accessed 12/03/02).

Chapter 9: Bioterrorism
Section I: Smallpox

Behbehani AM. The smallpox story: historical perspective. *ASM News* 1991;57:571–576.

Bozzette SA, Boer R, Bhatnagar V, et al. A model for a smallpox-vaccination policy. *N Engl J Med* 2003;348:416–425.

CDC. Vaccinia (amallpox) vaccine: recommendations of the Advisory Committee on Immunization Practices (ACIP), 2001. *MMWR* 2001:50(RR-10):1–25.

CDC. Summary of October 2002 ACIP smallpox vaccination recommendations. www.bt.cdc.gov/agent/smallpox/vaccination/acip-recs-oct2002.asp (accessed 02/01/03).

CDC. Recommendations for using smallpox vaccine in a pre-event vaccination program: supplemental recommendations of the Advisory Committee on Immunization Practices (ACIP) and the Healthcare Infection Control Practices Advisory Committee (HICPAC). *MMWR* 2003;52(RR-7):1–16.

CDC. Smallpox vaccination and adverse reactions: guidance for clinicians. *MMWR* 2003;52:1–29.

CDC. Interim Centers for Disease Control and Prevention (CDC) guidance for use of smallpox vaccine, cidofovir, and vaccinia immune globulin (VIG) for prevention and treatment in the setting of an outbreak of monkeypox infections. www.phppo.cdc.gov/han/Documents/AlertDocs/146.asp (accessed 06/23/03).

CDC. Multistate outbreak of monkeypox—Illinois, Indiana, and Wisconsin, 2003. *MMWR* 2003;52:537–540.

Frey SE, Couch RB, Tacket CO, et al. Clinical responses to undiluted and diluted smallpox vaccine. *N Engl J Med* 2002;346:1265–1274.

Frey SE, Newman FK, Cruz J, et al. Dose-related effects of smallpox vaccine. *N Engl J Med* 2002;346:1275–1280.

Henderson DA, Inglesby TV, Bartlett JG, et al. Smallpox as a biological weapon: medical and public health management. *JAMA* 1999;281:2127–2137.

Holloran ME, Longini IM, Nizam A, et al. Containing bioterrorist smallpox. *Science* 2002;298:1428–1431.

Section II: Anthrax

CDC. Use of anthrax vaccine in the United States: recommendations of the Advisory Committee on Immunization Practices. *MMWR* 2000;49(RR-15):1–20.

CDC. Occupational health guidelines for remediation workers at *Bacillus anthracis*–contaminated sites—United States, 2001–2002. *MMWR* 2002;51:786–789.

CDC. Use of anthrax vaccine in response to terrorism: supplemental recommendations of the Advisory Committee on Immunization Practices. *MMWR* 2002;51:1024–1026.

Dixon TC, Meselson M, Guillemin J, et al. Anthrax. *N Engl J Med* 1999;341:815–826.

Inglesby TV, O'Toole T, Henderson DA, et al. Anthrax as a biological weapon, 2002: updated recommendations for management. *JAMA* 2002;287:2236–2252.

Swartz MN. Recognition and management of anthrax: an update. *N Engl J Med* 2001;345:1621–1626.

Section III: Other category A agents

Arnon SS, Schechter R, Inglesby TV, et al. Botulinum toxin as a biological weapon: medical and public health management. *JAMA* 2001;285:1059–1070.

Borio L, Inglesby T, Peters CJ, et al. Hemorrhagic fever viruses as biological weapons: medical and public health management. *JAMA* 2002;287:2391–2405.

Dennis DT, Inglesby TV, Henderson DA, et al. Tularemia as a biological weapon: medical and public health management. *JAMA* 2001;285:2763–2773.

Inglesby TV, Dennis DT, Henderson DA, et al. Plague as a biological weapon: medical and public health management. *JAMA* 2000;283:2281–2290.

Chapter 10: Vaccines in development for general use
Section II.A: New combinations: DTaP5/Hib/IPV

Lee CY, Thipphawong J, Huang LM, et al. An evaluation of the safety and immunogenicity of a five-component acellular pertussis, diphtheria, and tetanus toxoid vaccine (DTaP) when combined with a *Haemophilus influenzae* type b–tetanus toxoid conjugate vaccine (PRP-T) in Taiwanese infants. *Pediatrics* 1999;103:25–30.

Mills E, Gold R, Thipphawong J, et al. Safety and immunogenicity of a combined five-component pertussis-diphtheria-tetanus–inactivated poliomyelitis–*Haemophilus* b conjugate vaccine administered to infants at two, four and six months of age. *Vaccine* 1998;16:576–585.

Section II.B: New combinations: MMRV

Arbeter AM, Baker L, Starr SE, et al. Combination measles, mumps, rubella and varicella vaccine. *Pediatrics* 1986;78:742–747.

Berger R, Just M. Interference between strains in live virus vaccines. II: Combined vaccination with varicella and measles-mumps-rubella vaccine. *J Biol Stand* 1988;16:275–279.

Brunell PA, Novelli VM, Lipton SV, et al. Combined vaccine against measles, mumps, rubella and varicella. *Pediatrics* 1988;81:779–784.

Just M, Berger R, Just V. Evaluation of a combined measles-mumps-rubella-chickenpox vaccine. *Dev Biol Stand* 1986;65:85–88.

Reuman PD, Sawyer MH, Kuter BJ, et al. Safety and immunogenicity of concurrent administration of measles-mumps-rubella-varicella vaccine and PedvaxHIB vaccines in healthy children twelve to eighteen months old. *Pediatr Infect Dis J* 1997;16:662–667.

Vesikari T, Ohrling A, Baer M, et al. Evaluation of live attenuated varicella vaccine (Oka-RIT strain) and combined varicella and MMR vaccination in 13–17-month-old children. *Acta Paediatr Scand* 1991;80: 1051–1057.

Watson BM, Laufer DS, Kuter BJ, et al. Safety and immunogenicity of a combined live attenuated measles, mumps, rubella, and varicella vaccine (MMR$_{II}$V) in healthy children. *J Infect Dis* 1996;173:731–734.

White CJ, Stinson D, Staehle B, et al. Measles, mumps, rubella, and varicella combination vaccine: safety and immunogenicity alone and in combination with other vaccines given to children. *Clin Infect Dis* 1997;24:925–931.

Section II.C: New combinations: other combinations

Liese JG, Stojanov S, Berut F, et al. Large scale safety study of a liquid hexavalent vaccine (D-T-acP-IPV-PRP-T-HBs) administered at 2, 4, 6 and 12–14 months of age. *Vaccine* 2001;20:448–454.

Mallet E, Fabre P, Pines E, et al. Immunogenicity and safety of a new liquid hexavalent combined vaccine compared with separate administration of reference licensed vaccines in infants. *Pediatr Infect Dis J* 2000;19:1119–1127.

Rennels M, Reisinger K, Rathore M, et al. Safety and immunogenicity of combined conjugate 9-valent *S pneumoniae*–meningococcal group C (9vPnC-MnCC) and *H influenzae* b-9vPnC-MnCC (HbOC-9vPnC-MnCC) vaccine. Abstracts of the 41st Interscience Conference on Antimicrobial Agents and Chemotherapy, December, 2001, p. 283, Abstract G-2039.

Section III: Cytomegalovirus

Adler SP, Starr SE, Plotkin SA, et al. Immunity induced by primary human cytomegalovirus infection protects against secondary infection among women of child-bearing age. *J Infect Dis* 1995;171:26–32.

Adler SP, Plotkin SA, Gönczöl E, et al. A canarypox vector expressing cytomegalovirus (CMV) glycoprotein B primes for antibody responses to a live attenuated CMV vaccine (Towne). *J Infect Dis* 1999;180:843–846.

Balfour HH, Welo PK, Sachs GW. Cytomegalovirus vaccine trial in 400 renal transplant candidates. *Transplant Proc* 1985;17:81–83.

Fowler KB, Stagno S, Pass RF, et al. The outcome of congenital cytomegalovirus infection in relation to maternal antibody status. *N Engl J Med* 1992;326: 663–667.

Mitchell DK, Holmes SJ, Burke RL, et al. Immunogenicity of a recombinant human cytomegalovirus gB vaccine in seronegative toddlers. *Pediatr Infect Dis J* 2002;21:133–138.

Plotkin SA, Starr SE, Friedman HM, et al. Effect of Towne live virus vaccine on cytomegalovirus disease after renal transplant: a controlled trial. *Ann Intern Med* 1991;114:525–531.

Plotkin SA. Vaccination against cytomegalovirus. *Arch Virol* 2001;17:121–134.

Section IV: Epstein-Barr virus

Cohen JI. Epstein-Barr virus infection. *N Engl J Med* 2000;343:481–492.

Khanna R, Moss DJ, Burrows SR. Vaccine strategies against Epstein-Barr virus-associated diseases: lessons from studies on cytotoxic T-cell–mediated immune regulation. *Immunol Rev* 1999;170:49–64.

Khanna R, Sherritt M, Burrows SR. EBV structural antigens, gp350 and gp85, as targets for ex vivo virus-specific CTL during acute infectious mononucleosis: potential use of gp350/gp85 CTL epitopes for vaccine design. *J Immunol* 1999;162:3063–3069.

Macsween KF, Crawford DH. Epstein-Barr virus—Recent advances. *Lancet Infect Dis* 2003;3:131–140.

Morgan AJ. Epstein-Barr virus vaccines. *Vaccine* 1992; 10:563–571.

Ranieri E, Herr W, Gambotto A, et al. Dendritic cells transduced with an adenovirus vector encoding Epstein-Barr virus latent membrane protein 2B: a new modality for vaccination. *J Virol* 1999;73:10416–10425.

Spring SB, Hascall G, Gruber J. Issues related to development of Epstein-Barr virus vaccines. *J Natl Cancer Inst* 1996;88:1436–1441.

Section V: Herpes simplex virus

Corey L, Langenberg AGM, Ashley R, et al. Recombinant glycoprotein vaccine for the prevention of genital HSV-2 infection: two randomized controlled trials. *JAMA* 1999;282:331–340.

Fleming DT, McQuillan GM, Johnson RE, et al. Herpes simplex virus type 2 in the United States, 1976 to 1994. *N Engl J Med* 1997;337:1105–1111.

Stanberry LR, Cunningham AL, Mindel A, et al. Prospects for control of herpes simplex virus disease through immunization. *Clin Infect Dis* 2000;30:549–566.

Stanberry LR, Spruance SL, Cunningham AL, et al. Glycoprotein-D-adjuvant vaccine to prevent genital herpes. *N Engl J Med* 2002;347:1652–1661.

Whitley RJ, Kimberlin DW, Roizman B. Herpes simplex viruses. *Clin Infect Dis* 1998;26:541–553.

Whitley RJ, Roizman B. Herpes simplex viruses: is a vaccine tenable? *J Clin Invest* 2002;110:145–151.

Section VI: Human immunodeficiency virus

Dolin R. HIV vaccines for prevention of infection and disease in humans. *Infect Dis Clin North Am* 2000;14: 1001–1016.

Graham BS. Clinical trials of HIV vaccines. *Ann Rev Med* 2002;53:207–221.

Letvin NL, Barough DH, Montefiore DC. Prospects for vaccine protection against HIV-1 infection and AIDS. *Ann Rev Immunol* 2002;20:73–99.

Nathanson N, Mathieson BJ. Biological considerations in the development of a human immunodeficiency virus vaccine. *J Infect Dis* 2000;182:579–589.

Section VII: Human papillomavirus

Adams M, Borysiewicz L, Fiander A, et al. Clinical studies of human papilloma vaccines in pre-invasive and invasive cancer. *Vaccine* 2001;19:2549–2556.

Breitburd F, Coursaget P. Human papillomavirus vaccines. *Semin Cancer Biol* 1999;9:431–445.

Cornelison T. Human papillomavirus genotype 16 vaccines for cervical cancer prophylaxis and treatment. *Curr Opin Oncology* 2000;12:466–473.

Kaufman RH, Adam E, Vladimir V. Human papillomavirus infection and cervical carcinoma. *Clin Obstet Gynecol* 2000;43:363–380.

Koutsky LA, Ault KA, Wheeler CM, et al. A controlled trial of a human papillomavirus type 16 vaccine. *N Engl J Med* 2002;347:1645–1651.

Section VIII: Live cold-adapted influenza [see also Chapter 7(III)]

Belshe RB, Mendelman PM, Treanor J, et al. The efficacy of live attenuated, cold-adapted, trivalent, intranasal influenzavirus vaccine in children. *N Engl J Med* 1998;338:1405–1412.

Belshe RB, Gruber WC, Mendelman PM, et al. Efficacy of vaccination with live attenuated, cold-adapted, trivalent, intranasal influenza virus vaccine against a variant (A/Sydney) not contained in the vaccine. *J Pediatr* 2000;136:168–175.

Bradshaw J, Wright PF. Cold-adapted influenza vaccines. *Curr Opin Pediatr* 2002;14:95–98.

Jacobson RM, Poland GA. Universal vaccination of healthy children against influenza. *Pediatr Drugs* 2002;4:65–71.

Neuzil KM, Dupont WD, Wright PF, et al. Efficacy of inactivated and cold-adapted vaccines against influenza A infection, 1985 to 1990: the pediatric experience. *Pediatr Infect Dis J* 2001;20:733–740.

Neuzil KM, Edward KM. Influenza vaccines in children. *Semin Pediatr Infect Dis* 2002;13:174–181.

Piedra PA. Safety of the trivalent, cold-adapted influenza vaccine (CAIV-T) in children. *Semin Pediatr Infect Dis* 2002;13:90–96.

Rennels MB, Meissner HC, AAP Committee on Infectious Diseases. Technical report: reduction of the influenza burden in children. *Pediatrics* 2002;110:e80.

Section IX: Meningococcal polysaccharide conjugate

Balmer P, Borrow R, Miller E. Impact of meningococcal C conjugate vaccine in the UK. *J Med Microbiol* 2002;51:717–722.

Borrow R, Goldblatt D, Andrews N, et al. Influence of prior meningococcal C polysaccharide vaccination on the response and generation of memory after meningococcal C conjugate vaccination in young children. *J Infect Dis* 2001;184:377–380.

Campbell JD, Edelman R, King JC, et al. Safety, reactogenicity, and immunogenicity of a tetravalent meningococcal polysaccharide-diphtheria toxoid conjugate vaccine given to healthy adults. *J Infect Dis* 2002; 186:1848–1851.

Lakshman R, Jones I, Walker D, et al. Safety of a new conjugate meningococcal C vaccine in infants. *Arch Dis Child* 2001;85:391–397.

MacDonald NE, Halperin SA, Law BJ, et al. Induction of immunologic memory by conjugated vs plain meningococcal C polysaccharide vaccine in toddlers. *JAMA* 1998;280:1685–1689.

MacLennan JM, Shackley F, Heath PT, et al. Safety, immunogenicity, and induction of immunologic memory by a serogroup C meningococcal conjugate vaccine in infants. *JAMA* 2000;283:2795–2801.

MacLennan J. Meningococcal group C conjugate vaccines. *Arch Dis Child* 2001;84:383–386.

Rosenstein NE, Fischer M, Tappero JW. Meningococcal vaccines. *Infect Dis Clin North Am* 2001;15:155–169.

Soriano-Gabarro M, Stuart JM, Rosenstein NE. Vaccines for the prevention of meningococcal disease in children. *Semin Pediatr Infect Dis* 2002;13:182–189.

Section X: Increased valency pneumococcal polysaccharide conjugates

Dagan R, Sikuler-Cohen M, Zamir O, et al. Effect of a conjugate pneumococcal vaccine on the occurrence of respiratory infections and antibiotic use in day-care center attendees. *Pediatr Infect Dis J* 2001;20:951–958.

Dagan R, Givon-Lavi N, Zamir O, et al. Reduction of nasopharyngeal carriage of *Streptococcus pneumoniae* after administration of a 9-valent pneumococcal conjugate vaccine to toddlers attending day care centers. *J Infect Dis* 2002;185:927–936.

Hausdorff WP, Bryant J, Paradiso PR, et al. Which pneumococcal serogroups cause the most invasive disease: implications for conjugate vaccine formulation and use, Part I. *Clin Infect Dis* 2000;30:100–121.

Mbelle N, Huebner RE, Wasas AD, et al. Immunogenicity and impact on nasopharyngeal carriage of a nonavalent pneumococcal conjugate vaccine. *J Infect Dis* 1999;180:1171–1176.

Puumalainen T, Zeta-Capeding R, Kayhty H, et al. Antibody response to an eleven valent diphtheria- and tetanus-conjugated pneumococcal conjugate vaccine in Filipino infants. *Pediatr Infect Dis J* 2002;21:309–314.

Robinson KA, Baughman W, Rothrock G, et al. Epidemiology of invasive *Streptococcus pneumoniae* infections in the United States, 1995–1998: opportunities for prevention in the conjugate vaccine era. *JAMA* 2001; 285:1729–1735.

Wuorimaa T, Dagan R, Eskola J, et al. Tolerability and immunogenicity of an eleven-valent pneumococcal conjugate vaccine in healthy toddlers. *Pediatr Infect Dis J* 2001;20:272–277.

Section XI: Parainfluenza virus

Hurwitz JL, Soike KF, Sangster MY, et al. Intranasal Sendai virus vaccine protects African green monkeys from infection with human parainfluenza virus-type one. *Vaccine* 1997;15:533–540.

Karron RA, Wright PF, Hall SL, et al. A live attenuated bovine parainfluenza virus type 3 vaccine is safe, infectious, immunogenic and phenotypically stable in infants and children. *J Infect Dis* 1995;171:1107–1114.

Karron RA, Wright PF, Newman FK, et al. A live human parainfluenza type 3 virus vaccine is attenuated and immunogenic in healthy infants and children. *J Infect Dis* 1995;172:1445–1450.

Karron RA, Makhene M, Gay K, et al. Evaluation of a live attenuated bovine parainfluenza type 3 vaccine in two- to six-month-old infants. *Pediatr Infect Dis J* 1996;15:650–654.

Lee M, Greenberg DP, Yeh SH, et al. Antibody responses to bovine parainfluenza virus type 3 (PIV3) vaccination and human PIV3 infection in young infants. *J Infect Dis* 2001;184:909–913.

Skiadopoulos MH, Tatem JM, Surman SR, et al. The recombinant chimeric human parainfluenza virus type 1 vaccine candidate, rHPIV3-1cp45, is attenuated, immunogenic, and protective in African green monkeys. *Vaccine* 2002;20:1846–1852.

Tao T, Davoodi F, Surman SR, et al. Construction of a live-attenuated bivalent vaccine virus against human parainfluenza virus (PIV) types 1 and 2 using a recombinant PIV3 backbone. *Vaccine* 2001;19:3620–3631.

Section XII: Respiratory syncytial virus

Collins PL, Murphy BR. Respiratory syncytial virus: reverse genetics and vaccine strategies. *Virology* 2002;296:204–211.

Crowe JE. Respiratory syncytial virus vaccine development. *Vaccine* 2002;20:S32–S37.

Dudas RA, Karron RA. Respiratory syncytial virus vaccines. *Clin Microbiol Rev* 1998;11:430–439.

Kahn JS. Respiratory syncytial virus vaccine development. *Curr Opin Pediatr* 2000;12:257–262.

Piedra PA. Future directions in vaccine prevention of respiratory syncytial virus. *Pediatr Infect Dis J* 2002;21:482–487.

Power UF, Nguyen TN, Rietveld E, et al. Safety and immunogenicity of a novel recombinant subunit respiratory syncytial virus vaccine (BBG2Na) in healthy young adults. *J Infect Dis* 2001;184:1456–1460.

Schmidt AC, McAuliffe JM, Murphy BR, et al. Recombinant bovine/human parainfluenza virus type 3 (B/HPIV3) expressing the respiratory syncytial virus (RSV) G and F proteins can be used to achieve simultaneous mucosal immunization against RSV and HPIV3. *J Virol* 2001;75:4594–4603.

Shay DK, Holman RC, Roosevelt GE, et al. Bronchiolitis-associated mortality and estimates of respiratory
syncytial virus-associated deaths among U.S. children, 1979–1997. *J Infect Dis* 2001;183:16–22.

Section XIII: Rotavirus

Bernstein DI, Sack DA, Reisinger K, et al. Second-year
follow-up evaluation of live, attenuated human
rotavirus vaccine 89–12 in healthy infants. *J Infect
Dis* 2002;186:1487–1489.

Chang HG, Smith PF, Ackelsberg J, et al. Intussusception, rotavirus diarrhea, and rotavirus vaccine use
among children in New York State. *Pediatrics* 2001;
108:54–60.

Clark HF, Offit PA, Ellis RW, et al. The development of
multivalent bovine rotavirus (strain WC3) reassortant
vaccine for infants. *J Infect Dis* 1996;174:S73–S80.

Clements-Mann ML, Dudas R, Hoshino Y, et al. Safety
and immunogenicity of live attenuated quadrivalent
human-bovine (U.K.) reassortant rotavirus vaccine
administered with childhood vaccines to infants. *Vaccine* 2001;19:4676–4684.

Cunliffe NA, Bresee JS, Hart CA. Rotavirus vaccines:
development, current issues and future prospects. *J
Infect* 2002;45:1–9.

Joensuu J, Koskenniemi E, Pang X-L, et al. Randomised
placebo-controlled trial of rhesus-human reassortant
rotavirus vaccine for prevention of severe rotavirus
gastroenteritis. *Lancet* 1997;350:1205–1209.

Offit PA. The future of rotavirus vaccines. *Semin Pediatr Infect Dis* 2002;13:190–195.

Pérez-Schael I, Guntiñas MJ, Pérez M, et al. Efficacy of
the rhesus rotavirus-based quadravalent vaccine in
infants and young children in Venezuela. *N Engl J
Med* 1997;337:1181–1187.

Rennels MB, Glass RI, Dennehy PH, et al. Safety and
efficacy of high-dose rhesus-human reassortant rotavirus vaccines: report of the National Multicenter Trial.
Pediatrics 1996;97:7–13.

Section XIV: Group A streptococcus

AAP. Severe invasive group A streptococcal infections: a
subject review. *Pediatrics* 1998;101:136–140.

Bisno AL, Stevens DL. Streptococcal infections of skin
and soft tissues. *N Engl J Med* 1996;334:240–245.

Bisno AL. Acute pharyngitis. *N Engl J Med* 2001;344:
205–211.

Dale JB. Group A streptococcal vaccines. *Infect Dis Clin
North Am* 1999;13:227–243.

Davies HD, Schwartz B. Invasive group A streptococcal
infections in children. *Adv Pediatr Infect Dis*
1999;14:129–145.

Markowitz M. Changing epidemiology of group A streptococcal infections. *Pediatr Infect Dis J* 1994;13:557–560.

Stevens DL. Streptococcal toxic-shock syndrome: spectrum of disease, pathogenesis, and new concepts in treatment. *Emerg Infect Dis* 1995;1:69–78.

Stevens DL. Invasive group A streptococcal disease. *Infect Agent Dis* 1996;5:157–166.

Section XV: Group B streptococcus

Baker CJ, Rench MA, Edwards MS, et al. Immunization of pregnant women with a polysaccharide vaccine of group B streptococcus. *N Engl J Med* 1988;319:1180–1185.

Baker CJ. Vaccine prevention of group B streptococcal disease. *Pediatr Ann* 1993;22:711–714.

Baker CJ, Paoletti LC, Wessels MR, et al. Safety and immunogenicity of capsular polysaccharide–tetanus toxoid conjugate vaccines for group B streptococcal types Ia and Ib. *J Infect Dis* 1999;179:142–150.

Baker CJ, Paoletti LC, Rench MA, et al. Use of capsular polysaccharide–tetanus toxoid conjugate vaccine for type II group B streptococcus in healthy women. *J Infect Dis* 2000;182:1129–1138.

CDC. Prevention of perinatal group B streptococcal disease: revised guidelines from CDC. *MMWR* 2002;51 (RR-11):1–22.

Coleman RT, Sherer DM, Maniscalco WM. Prevention of neonatal group B streptococcal infections: advances in maternal vaccine development. *Obstet Gynecol* 1992;80:301–309.

Schrag SJ, Zywicki S, Farley MM, et al. Group B streptococcal disease in the era of intrapartum prophylaxis. *N Engl J Med* 2000;342:15–20.

Schrag SJ, Zell ER, Stat M, et al. A population-based comparison of strategies to prevent early-onset group B streptococcal disease in neonates. *N Engl J Med* 2002;347:233–239.

Schuchat A. Group B streptococcus. *Lancet* 1999;353:51–56.

Schwartz B, Schuchat A, Oxtoby MJ, et al. Invasive group B streptococcal disease in adults: a population-based study in metropolitan Atlanta. *JAMA* 1991;266:1112–1114.

Chapter 11: Passive immunization
Section I: Cytomegalovirus immune globulin intravenous

Sia IG, Patel R. New strategies for prevention and therapy of cytomegalovirus infection and disease in solid-organ transplant recipients. *Clin Microbiol Rev* 2000;13:83–121.

Snydman DR, Werner BG, Heinze-Lacey B, et al. Use of cytomegalovirus immune globulin to prevent cytomegalovirus disease in renal-transplant recipients. *N Engl J Med* 1987;317:1049–1054.

Snydman DR, Werner BG, Dougherty NN, et al. Cytomegalovirus immune globulin prophylaxis in liver transplantation: a randomized, double blind, placebo-controlled trial. *Ann Intern Med* 1993;10:984–991.

van der Meer JTM, Drew WL, Bowden RA, et al. Summary of the International Symposium on Advances in the Diagnosis, Treatment and Prophylaxis of Cytomegalovirus Infection. *Antiviral Res* 1996;32:119–140.

Wittes JT, Kelly A, Plante KM. Meta-analysis of CMVIG studies for the prevention and treatment of CMV infection in transplant patients. *Transplant Proc* 1996;28(6 Suppl 2):17–24.

Section II: Hepatitis B immune globulin

CDC. Updated U.S. Public Health Service guidelines for the management of occupational exposures to HBV, HCV, and HIV and recommendations for postexposure prophylaxis. *MMWR* 2001;50(RR-11):1–52.

CDC. Sexually transmitted diseases treatment guidelines 2002. *MMWR* 2002;51(RR-6):1–78.

Section III: Immune globulin

AAP. Passive immunization. In: Pickering LK, ed. *Red book: 2003 report of the Committee on Infectious Diseases*, 26th ed. Elk Grove Village, IL: American Academy of Pediatrics; 2003:53–66.

Anderson MS. Intravenous gammaglobulin for pediatric infectious diseases. *Pediatr Ann* 1999;28:499–506.

Mofenson LM, Moye J, Bethel J, et al. Prophylactic intravenous immunoglobulin in HIV-infected children with CD4+ counts of 0.02×10^9/L or more: effect on viral, opportunistic, and bacterial infections. *JAMA* 1992;268:483–488.

Mofenson LM, Moye J, Korelitz J, et al. Crossover of placebo patients to intravenous immunoglobulin confirms efficacy for prophylaxis of bacterial infections and reduction of hospitalizations in human immunodeficiency virus-infected children. *Pediatr Infect Dis J* 1994;13:477–484.

Seigel J. Intravenous immune globulins: therapeutic, pharmaceutical, and cost considerations. *Pharm Pract News* 2002;29:13–15.

Spector SA, Gelber RD, McGrath N, et al. A controlled trial of intravenous immune globulin for the prevention of serious bacterial infections in children receiving zidovudine for advanced human immunodeficiency virus infection. *N Engl J Med* 1994;331:1181–1187.

Stiehm ER. Human intravenous immunoglobulin in primary and secondary antibody deficiencies. *Pediatr Infect Dis J* 1997;16:696–707.

The National Institute of Child Health and Human Development Intravenous Immunoglobulin Study Group. Intravenous immune globulin for the prevention of bacterial infections in children with symptomatic human immunodeficiency virus infection. *N Engl J Med* 1991;325:73–80.

Section IV: Palivizumab [humanized murine monoclonal antibody to RSV (RSV-mAb)] and RSV immune globulin intravenous (RSV-IGIV)

AAP. Respiratory syncytial virus immune globulin intravenous: indications for use. *Pediatrics* 1997;99:645–650.

AAP. Prevention of respiratory syncytial virus infections: indications for the use of palivizumab and update on the use of RSV-IGIV. *Pediatrics* 1998;102:1211–1216.

AAP. Respiratory syncytial virus. In: Pickering LK, ed. *Red book: 2003 report of the Committee on Infectious Diseases*, 26th ed. Elk Grove Village, IL: American Academy of Pediatrics; 2003:523–528.

DeVincenzo J. Prevention and treatment of respiratory syncytial virus infections. *Adv Pediatr Infect Dis* 1998;13:1–47.

Hall CB. Respiratory syncytial virus and parainfluenza virus. *N Engl J Med* 2001;344:1917–1928.

Sanchez PJ. Immunoprophylaxis for respiratory syncytial virus. *Pediatr Infect Dis J* 2002;21:473–478.

Shay DK, Holman RC, Newman RD, et al. Bronchiolitis-associated hospitalizations among U.S. children, 1980–1996. *JAMA* 1999;282:1440–1446.

The IMpact-RSV Study Group. Palivizumab, a humanized respiratory syncytial virus monoclonal antibody, reduces hospitalization from respiratory syncytial virus infection in high-risk infants. *Pediatrics* 1998;102:531–537.

The PREVENT Study Group. Reduction of respiratory syncytial virus hospitalization among premature infants and infants with bronchopulmonary dysplasia using respiratory syncytial virus immune globulin prophylaxis. *Pediatrics* 1997;99:93–99.

Section V: Rabies immune globulin [see Chapter 8(VIII)]

Section VI: Tetanus immune globulin [see Chapter 5(I)]

Section VII: Varicella-zoster immune globulin [see also Chapter 5(VII)]

Feldman S, Lott L. Varicella in children with cancer: impact of antiviral therapy and prophylaxis. *Pediatrics* 1987;80:465–472.

Orenstein WA, Heymann DL, Ellis RJ, et al. Prophylaxis of varicella in high-risk children: dose-response effect of zoster immune globulin. *J Pediatr* 1981;98:368–373.

Zaia JA, Levin MJ, Preblud SR, et al. Evaluation of varicella-zoster immune globulin: protection of immunosuppressed children after household exposure to varicella. *J Infect Dis* 1983;147:737–743.

Section VIII: Human botulinum immune globulin and equine botulinum antitoxin

AAP. Botulism and infant botulism. In: Pickering LK, ed. *Red book: 2003 report of the Committee on Infec-*

tious Diseases, 26th ed. Elk Grove Village, IL: American Academy of Pediatrics; 2003:243–246.

Donadio JA, Gangarosa EJ, Faich GA. Diagnosis and treatment of botulism. *J Infect Dis* 1971;124:108–111.

Hatheway CH, Snyder JD, Seals JE, et al. Antitoxin levels in botulism patients treated with trivalent equine botulism antitoxin to toxin types A, B, and E. *J Infect Dis* 1984;150:407–412.

Long SS. Infant botulism. *Pediatr Infect Dis J* 2001;20:707–709.

Mayers CN, Holley JL, Brooks R. Antitoxin therapy for botulinum intoxication. *Rev Med Microbiol* 2001;12:29–37.

Middlebrook JL, Brown JE. Immunodiagnosis and immunotherapy of tetanus and botulism neurotoxins. *Curr Top Microbiol Immunol* 1995;195:89–122.

Schwarz PJ, Arnon SS. Botulism immune globulin for infant botulism arrives—One year and a Gulf War later. *West J Med* 1992;156:197–198.

Tacket CO, Shandera WX, Mann JM, et al. Equine antitoxin use and other factors that predict outcome in type A foodborne botulism. *Am J Med* 1984;76:794–798.

Section IX: Equine diphtheria antitoxin

AAP. Diphtheria. In: Pickering LK, ed. *Red book: 2003 report of the Committee on Infectious Diseases*, 26th ed. Elk Grove Village, IL: American Academy of Pediatrics; 2003:263–266.

CDC. Diphtheria, tetanus, and pertussis: recommendations for vaccine use and other preventive measures: recommendations of the Immunization Practices Advisory Committee (ACIP). *MMWR* 1991;40(RR-10):1–28.

Chapter 12: Vaccination in special circumstances
Section I: Impaired immunity

AAP. Immunocompromised children. In: Pickering LK, ed. *Red book: 2003 report of the Committee on Infectious Diseases*, 26th ed. Elk Grove Village, IL: American Academy of Pediatrics; 2003:69–81.

CDC. Recommendations of the Advisory Committee on Immunization Practices (ACIP): use of vaccines and immune globulins in persons with altered immunocompetence. *MMWR* 1993;42(RR-4):1–19.

CDC. Guidelines for preventing opportunistic infections among hematopoietic stem cell transplant recipients: recommendations of CDC, the Infectious Disease Society of America, and the American Society of Blood and Marrow Transplantation. *MMWR* 2000;49(RR-10):1–128.

CDC. General recommendations on immunization: recommendations of the Advisory Committee on Immunization Practices (ACIP) and the American Academy of Family Physicians. *MMWR* 2002;51(RR-2):1–36.

McFarland E. Immunizations for the immunocompromised child. *Pediatr Ann* 1999;28:487–496.

Moss W, Lederman H. Immunization of the immunocompromised host. In: *Clinical Focus on Primary Immune Deficiencies*. Towson, MD: Immune Deficiency Foundation; 1998:1.

Pirofski L-A, Casadevall A. Use of licensed vaccines for active immunization of the immunocompromised host. *Clin Microbiol Rev* 1998;11:1–26.

Puck JM. Primary immunodeficiency diseases. *JAMA* 1997;278:1835–1841.

Section II: Pregnancy and breast-feeding
CDC. Guidelines for vaccinating pregnant women (updated November 2002). www.cdc.gov/nip/home-hcp.htm (accessed 01/26/03).

Section IV: Health care personnel
Poland AG, Schaffner W, Pugliese G, eds. Immunizing Healthcare Workers: A Practical Approach. Thorofare, NJ: The Society for Healthcare Epidemiology of America, Slack Inc., 2000.

Chapter 13: Vaccine regulation, policy, and safety
Section III.A: The vaccine safety net: Vaccine Adverse Event Reporting Systems (VAERS)
CDC. Surveillance for safety after immunization: Vaccine Adverse Event Reporting System (VAERS)—United States, 1991–2001. *MMWR* 2003;52(SS-1):1–24.

Chen RT, Rastogi SC, Mullen JR, et al. The Vaccine Adverse Event Reporting System (VAERS). *Vaccine* 1994;12:542–550.

Singleton JA, Lloyd JC, Mootrey GT, et al. An overview of the vaccine adverse event reporting system (VAERS) as a surveillance system. *Vaccine* 1999;17:2908–2917.

Section III.B: The vaccine safety net: the Vaccine Safety Datalink
Chen RT, Glasser JW, Rhodes PH, et al. Vaccine Safety Datalink Project: a new tool for improving vaccine safety monitoring in the United States. *Pediatrics* 1997;99:765–773.

Section III.E: The vaccine safety net: Task Force on Safer Childhood Vaccines
National Institute of Allergy and Infectious Diseases. Task Force on Safer Childhood Vaccines: Final Report and Recommendations. www.niaid.nih.gov/publications/Vaccine/safervacc.htm (accessed 10/23/02).

Section III.F: The vaccine safety net: the safety net in action
AAP Committee on Infectious Diseases. Prevention of rotavirus disease: guidelines for use of rotavirus vaccine. *Pediatrics* 1998;102:1483–1491.

CDC Advisory Committee on Immunization Practices. Rotavirus vaccine for the prevention of rotavirus gastroenteritis among children. *MMWR* 1999:48(RR-2):1–20.

CDC. Intussusception among recipients of rotavirus vaccine—United States, 1998–1999. *MMWR* 1999;48:577–581.

Murphy TV, Gargiullo PM, Massoudi M, et al. Intussusception among infants given an oral rotavirus vaccine. *N Engl J Med* 2001;344:564–572.

Peter G, Myers MG. Intussusception, rotavirus, and oral vaccines: summary of a workshop. *Pediatrics* 2002;110:e67.

Section IV.B: Current public concerns about vaccines: do children get too many vaccines at one time?

Offit PA, Quarles J, Gerber MA, et al. Addressing parents' concerns: do multiple vaccines overwhelm or weaken the infant's immune system? *Pediatrics* 2002;109:124–129.

Section IV.C: Current public concerns about vaccines: do vaccines weaken the immune system?

Black SB, Cherry JD, Shinefield HR, et al. Apparent decreased risk of invasive bacterial disease after heterologous childhood immunization. *Am J Dis Child* 1991;145:746–749.

Davidson M, Letson W, Ward JI, et al. DTP immunization and susceptibility to infectious diseases: is there a relationship? *Am J Dis Child* 1991;145:750–754.

Laupland KB, Davies HD, Low DE, et al. Invasive group A streptococcal disease in children and association with varicella-zoster virus infection. *Pediatrics* 2000;105:e60.

O'Brien KL, Walters MI, Sellman J, et al. Severe pneumococcal pneumonia in previously healthy children: the role of preceding influenza infection. *Clin Infect Dis* 2000;30:784–789.

Otto S, Mahner B, Kadow I, et al. General non-specific morbidity is reduced after vaccination within the third month of life—the Greifswald study. *J Infect* 2000;41:172–175.

Storsaeter J, Olin P, Renemar B, et al. Mortality and morbidity from invasive bacterial infections during a clinical trial of acellular pertussis vaccines in Sweden. *Pediatr Infect Dis J* 1988;7:637–645.

Section IV.D: Current public concerns about vaccines: do vaccines cause autism?

Dales L, Hammer SJ, Smith NJ. Time trends in autism and in MMR immunization coverage in California. *JAMA* 2001;285:1183–1185.

Farrington CP, Miller E, Taylor B. MMR and autism: further evidence against a causal association. *Vaccine* 2001;19:3632–3635.

Fombonne E, Chakrabarti S. No evidence for a new variant of measles-mumps-rubella-induced autism. *Pediatrics* 2001;108:e58.

Kaye JA, Melero-Montes M, Jick H. Mumps, measles, and rubella vaccine and the incidence of autism recorded by general practitioners: a time trend analysis. *BMJ* 2001;322:460–463.

Madsen KM, Hviid A, Vestergaard M, et al. A population-based study of measles, mumps, and rubella vaccination and autism. *N Engl J Med* 2002;347:1477–1482.

Taylor B, Miller E, Farrington P, et al. Autism and measles, mumps, and rubella vaccine: no epidemiologic evidence for a causal association. *Lancet* 1999;353:2026–2029.

Taylor B, Miller E, Lingam, et al. Measles, mumps, and rubella vaccination and bowel problems or developmental regression in children with autism: population study. *BMJ* 2002;324:393–396.

Wakefield AJ, Murch SH, Anthony A, et al. Ileal-lymphoid-nodular hyperplasia, non-specific colitis, and pervasive developmental disorder in children. *Lancet* 1998;351:637–641.

Section IV.E: Current public concerns about vaccines: did the whole-cell pertussis vaccine cause permanent brain damage?

Cody CL, Baraff LJ, Cherry JD, et al. Nature and rates of adverse reactions associated with DTP and DT immunizations in infants and children. *Pediatrics* 1981;68:650–660.

Gale JL, Thapa PB, Wassilak SGF, et al. Risk of serious acute neurological illness after immunization with diphtheria-tetanus-pertussis vaccine: a population-based case-control study. *JAMA* 1994;271:37–41.

Golden GS. Pertussis vaccine and injury to the brain. *J Pediatr* 1990;116:854–861.

Griffin MR, Ray WA, Schaffner W, et al. Risk of seizures and encephalopathy after immunization with diphtheria-tetanus-pertussis vaccine. *JAMA* 1990;263:1641–1645.

Kulenkampff M, Schwartzman JS, Wilson J. Neurological complications of pertussis inoculation. *Arch Dis Child* 1974;49:46–49.

Pollock TM, Morris J. A 7-year survey of disorders attributed to vaccination in Northwest Thames Region. *Lancet* 1983;1:753–757.

Shields WD, Nielsen C, Buch D, et al. Relationship of pertussis immunization to the onset of neurologic disorders. *J Pediatr* 1988;113:801–805.

Section IV.G: Current public concerns about vaccines: are vaccines made from fetal tissue?

Grabenstein JD. On the moral acceptability of certain viral vaccines. *Catholic Pharmacist* 1996;29:2–4.

Hayflick L. The limited in vitro lifetime of human diploid cell strains. *Exp Cell Res* 1963;37:614–636.

Section IV.H: Current public concerns about vaccines: do vaccines cause allergies?

Anderson HR, Poloniecki JD, Strachan DP, et al. Immunization and symptoms of atopic disease in children: results from the international study of asthma and allergies in children. *Am J Public Health* 2001;91:1126–1129.

DeStefano F, Gu D, Kramarz P, et al. Childhood vaccinations and the risk of asthma. *Pediatr Infect Dis J* 2002;21:498–504.

Gruber C, Kulig M, Bergmann R, et al. Delayed hypersensitivity to tuberculin, total immunoglobulin E, specific sensitization, and atopic manifestations in longitudinally followed early Bacille Calmette-Guérin-vaccinated and nonvaccinated children. *Pediatrics* 2001;107:e36.

Kramarz P, DeStefano F, Gargiullo PM, et al. Does influenza vaccination exacerbate asthma? *Arch Fam Med* 2000;9:617–623.

Nicholson KG, Nguyen-Van-Tam JS, Ahmed AH, et al. Randomised placebo-controlled crossover trial on effect of inactivated influenza vaccine on pulmonary function in asthma. *Lancet* 1998;351:326–331.

Nilsson L, Kjellman N, Bjorksten B. A randomized controlled trial of the effect of pertussis vaccines on atopic disease. *Arch Pediatr Adolesc Med* 1998;152:734–738.

Reid DW, Bromly CL, Stenton SC, et al. A double-blind placebo-controlled study of the effect of influenza vaccination on airway responsiveness in asthma. *Resp Med* 1998;92:1010–1011.

Wickens K, Crane J, Kemp T, et al. A case-control study of risk factors for asthma in New Zealand children. *Aust NZ Public Health* 2001;25:44–49.

Section IV.I: Current public concerns about vaccines: do vaccines cause diabetes mellitus?

Black SB, Lewis E, Shinefield H, et al. Lack of association between receipt of conjugate *Haemophilus influenzae* type b vaccine (HbOC) in infancy and risk of type 1 (juvenile onset) diabetes: long term follow-up of the HbOC efficacy trial cohort. *Pediatr Infect Dis J* 2002;21:568–569.

DeStefano F, Mullooly JP, Okoro CA, et al. Childhood vaccinations, vaccination timing, and risk of type 1 diabetes mellitus. *Pediatrics* 2001;108:e112.

Graves PM, Barriga KJ, Norris JM, et al. Lack of association between early childhood immunizations and β-cell autoimmunity. *Diabetes Care* 1999;22:1694–1697.

Heijbel H, Chen RT, Dahlquist G. Cumulative incidence of childhood-onset IDDM is unaffected by pertussis immunization. *Diabetes Care* 1997;20:173–175.

Hummel M, Fuchtenbusch M, Schenker M, et al. No major association between breast-feeding, vaccinations, and childhood viral diseases with early islet autoimmunity in the German BABYDIAB study. *Diabetes Care* 2000;23:969–974.

Section IV.J: Current public concerns about vaccines: do vaccines cause multiple sclerosis?

Ascherio A, Zhang SM, Hernan MA, et al. Hepatitis B vaccination and the risk of multiple sclerosis. *N Engl J Med* 2001;344:327–332.

Confavreux C, Suissa S, Saddier P, et al. Vaccinations and the risk of relapse in multiple sclerosis. *N Engl J Med* 2001;344:319–326.

De Keyser J, Zwanikken C, Boon M. Effects of influenza vaccination and influenza illness on exacerbations in multiple sclerosis. *J Neurol Sciences* 1998;159:51–53.

Fourrier A, Touze E, Alperovitch A, Begaud B. Association between hepatitis B vaccine and multiple sclerosis: a case-control study. *Pharmacoepidemiol Drug Saf* 1999;8(Suppl):S140–S141.

Hall A, Kane M, Roure C, Meheus A. Multiple sclerosis and hepatitis B vaccine? *Vaccine* 1999;17:2473–2475.

Miller AE, Morgante LA, Buchwald LY, et al. A multicenter, randomized, double-blind, placebo-controlled trial of influenza immunization in multiple sclerosis. *Neurology* 1997;48:312–314.

Moriabadi NF, Niewiesk S, Kruse N, et al. Influenza vaccination in MS: absence of T-cell response against white matter proteins. *Neurology* 2001;56:938–943.

Sturkenboom MCJM, Abenhaim L, Wolfson C, et al. Vaccinations, Demyelination, and Multiple Sclerosis Study (VDAMS): a population-based study in the UK. *Pharmacoepidemiol Drug Saf* 1999;8:(Suppl):S170–S171.

Touze E, Gout O, Verdier-Taillefer MH, et al. Premier episode de demyelinisation du systeme nerveux central et vaccination contre l'hepatite B: etude cas-temoins pilote. *Rev Neurol (Paris)* 2000;156:242–246.

Section IV.K: Current public concerns about vaccines: did the thimerosal in some vaccines cause harm?

Ball LK, Ball R, Pratt RD. An assessment of thimerosal use in childhood vaccines. *Pediatrics* 2001;107:1147–1154.

CDC. Summary of the joint statement on thimerosal in vaccines. *MMWR* 2000;49:622–631.

Freed GL, Andreae MC, Cowan AE, et al. The process of public policy formulation: the case of thimerosal in vaccines. *Pediatrics* 2002;109:1153–1159.

Halsey NA. Limiting infant exposure to thimerosal in vaccines and other sources of mercury. *JAMA* 1999;282:1763–1766.

Pichichero ME, Cernichiari E, Lopreiato J, et al. Mercury concentrations and metabolism in infants receiving vaccines containing thiomersal: a descriptive study. *Lancet* 2002;360:1737–1741.

Section IV.L: Current public concerns about vaccines: do vaccines contain the agent associated with "mad cow disease"?

Centers for Biologics Evaluation and Research. Bovine spongiform encephalopathy (BSE). www.fda.gov/cber/bse/bse.htm#tran (accessed 10/22/02).

Centers for Biologics Evaluation and Research. Transmissible Spongiform Encephalopathy Advisory Committee. www.fda.gov/cber/advisory/tse/tsemain.htm (accessed 10/22/02).

CDC. Public health service recommendations for the use of vaccines manufactured with bovine-derived materials. *MMWR* 2000;49:1137–1138.

Section IV.M: Current public concerns about vaccines: do vaccines cause cancer?

Ferber D. Monkey virus links to cancer grow stronger. *Science* 2002;296:1012–1015.

Section IV.N: Current public concerns about vaccines: did the polio vaccine start the AIDS epidemic?

Berry N, Davis C, Jenkins A, et al. Analysis of oral polio vaccine CHAT stocks. *Nature* 2001;410:1046–1047.

Blancou P, Vartanian J-P, Christopherson C, et al. Polio vaccine samples not linked to AIDS. *Nature* 2001;410:1045–1046.

Korber B, Muldoon M, Theiler J, et al. Timing the ancestor of the HIV-1 pandemic strains. *Science* 2000;288:1789–1796.

Poinar H, Kuch M, Pääbo S. Molecular analysis of oral polio vaccine samples. *Science* 292:743–744, 2001.

Rambaut A, Robertson DL, Pybus OG, et al. Phylogeny and the origin of HIV-1. *Nature* 2001;410:1047–1048.

Section IV.O: Current public concerns about vaccines: do vaccines cause sudden infant death syndrome (SIDS)?

Fleming PJ, Blair PS, Platt MW, et al. The U.K. accelerated immunization program and sudden unexpected death in infancy: case-control study. *BMJ* 2001;322:822–825.

Griffin MR, Ray WA, Livengood JR, et al. Risk of sudden infant death syndrome after immunization with the diphtheria-tetanus-pertussis vaccine. *N Engl J Med* 1988;319:618–623.

Niu MT, Salive ME, Ellenberg SS. Neonatal deaths after hepatitis B vaccine: the vaccine adverse event reporting system, 1991–1998. *Arch Pediatr Adolesc Med* 1999;153:1279–1282.

Abbreviations

AAFP	American Academy of Family Physicians
AAP	American Academy of Pediatrics
ACCV	Advisory Commission on Childhood Vaccines
ACHA	American College Health Association
ACIP	Advisory Committee on Immunization Practices
ACOG	American College of Obstetricians and Gynecologists
ACP-ASIM	American College of Physicians–American Society of Internal Medicine
AIDS	Acquired immune deficiency syndrome
ANA	American Nurses Association
APhA	American Pharmaceutical Association
APHA	American Public Health Association
ARF	Acute rheumatic fever
ASD	Autistic spectrum disorder
ATPM	Association of Teachers of Preventive Medicine
AVG	Allied Vaccine Group
BCG	Bacille Calmette-Guérin vaccine (for tuberculosis)
BIG	Botulinum immune globulin, human (human-derived botulinum antitoxin)
BRFSS	Behavioral Risk Factor Surveillance System
CASA	Clinical Assessment Software Application
CBER	Centers for Biologics Evaluation and Research
CDC	Centers for Disease Control and Prevention
CHD	Congenital heart disease
CISA	Clinical Immunization Safety Assessment
CLD	Chronic lung disease (bronchopulmonary dysplasia)
CMS	Centers for Medicare and Medicaid Services, formerly known as the Health Care Financing Administration
CMV	Cytomegalovirus
CMV-IGIV	Cytomegalovirus immune globulin intravenous, human
CNS	Central nervous system
COID	Committee on Infectious Diseases
CRM_{197}	Cross-reactive material, a mutant diphtheria toxin
CSF	Cerebrospinal fluid
CTL	Cytotoxic T lymphocyte
DT	Diphtheria and tetanus vaccine for pediatric use
DTP	Diphtheria, tetanus, and whole-cell pertussis vaccine
DTaP(n)	Diphtheria, tetanus, and acellular pertussis vaccine (number of pertussis antigens in the vaccine)
DU	D-antigen units
EBV	Epstein-Barr virus
EEG	Electroencephalogram

EPA	Environmental Protection Agency
FDA	U.S. Food and Drug Administration
FHA	Filamentous hemagglutinin
FIM	Fimbriae (agglutinogens)
GAS	Group A streptococcus
GBS	Group B streptococcus
GMP	Good Manufacturing Practices
HBIG	Hepatitis B immune globulin, human
HbOC	Polyribosylribotol phosphate (the capsular polysaccharide of *Haemophilus influenzae* type b) conjugated to mutant diphtheria protein CRM_{197}
HBsAg	Hepatitis B virus surface antigen
HCFA	Health Care Financing Administration, now known as the Centers for Medicare and Medicaid Services
HEDIS	Health Plan Employer Data and Information Set
Hep-B	Hepatitis B vaccine
Hib	*Haemophilus influenzae* type b
Hep-A	Hepatitis A vaccine
HIV	Human immunodeficiency virus
HPV	Human papilloma virus
HSV	Herpes simplex virus
IAC	Immunization Action Coalition
IDSA	Infectious Diseases Society of America
IGIM	Polyclonal immune globulin for intramuscular administration
IGIV	Polyclonal immune globulin for intravenous administration
IOM	Institute of Medicine
IPV	Inactivated poliovirus vaccine
ITP	Immune-mediated thrombocytopenic purpura
JEV	Japanese encephalitis virus
LAIV	Live-attenuated influenza vaccine
Lf	Limit of flocculation
LRI	Lower respiratory infection
LTBI	Latent tuberculous infection
MCD	Mad cow disease
MCV	Meningococcal conjugate vaccine
Men-PS	Meningococcal polysaccharide vaccine
MMR	Measles, mumps, and rubella vaccine
MMRV	Measles, mumps, rubella, and varicella vaccine
MRI	Magnetic resonance imaging
MS	Multiple sclerosis
NCVIA	National Childhood Vaccine Injury Act
NIAID	National Institute of Allergy and Infectious Diseases
NIH	National Institutes of Health
NIP	National Immunization Program
NIS	National Immunization Survey
NNDSS	National Notifiable Disease Surveillance System
NNii	National Network for Immunization Information
NVAC	National Vaccine Advisory Committee
NVPO	National Vaccine Program Office

OPV	Oral poliovirus vaccine
OspA	Outer surface protein
PAHO	Pan American Health Organization
PCV-7	Pneumococcal polysaccharide conjugated to mutant diphtheria protein CRM_{197} (7-valent)
PFP	Purified F protein
PIV	Parainfluenza virus
Pne-PS	Pneumococcal polysaccharide vaccine
PRN	Pertactin
PRP-OMP	Polyribosylribotol phosphate (the capsular polysaccharide of *Haemophilus influenzae* type b) conjugated to the outer membrane protein of *Neisseria meningitidis*
PRP-T	Polyribosylribotol phosphate (the capsular polysaccharide of *Haemophilus influenzae* type b) conjugated to tetanus protein
PS	Polysaccharide (capsular)
PSGN	Post-streptococcal glomerulonephritis
PT	Pertussis toxin
PTLD	Posttransplant lymphoproliferative disease
QALY	Quality-adjusted life year
RBC	Red blood cell
RET	Reportable Events Table
RIG	Rabies immune globulin, human
rOspA	Recombinant outer surface protein A (*Borrelia burgdorferi*)
RRV-TV	Rhesus-human reassortant rotavirus vaccine, tetravalent
RSV	Respiratory syncytial virus
RSV-IGIV	RSV immune globulin intravenous, human
RSV-mAb	Humanized murine monoclonal antibody to RSV (palivizumab)
SCHIP	State Children's Health Insurance Program
SEM	Skin, eye, and mucous membrane
SIV	Simian immunodeficiency virus
TCID	Tissue culture–infective dose
Td	Diphtheria and tetanus vaccine for adult use
TIG	Tetanus immune globulin, human
TST	Tuberculin skin test, formerly referred to as PPD (purified protein derivative)
TT	Tetanus toxoid
Ty-ViPS	Typhoid Vi polysaccharide
URI	Upper respiratory infection
USAMRIID	U.S. Army Medical Research Institute of Infectious Diseases
VAERS	Vaccine Adverse Event Reporting System
vCJD	Variant Creutzfeldt-Jakob disease
VCTU	Vaccine Clinical Trials Unit
VFC	Vaccines for Children
VICP	Vaccine Injury Compensation Program
VIG	Vaccinia immune globulin
VIT	Vaccine Injury Table

VLP	Viruslike particle
VRBPAC	Vaccine and Related Biological Products Advisory Committee
VSD	Vaccine Safety Datalink
VZIG	Varicella-zoster immune globulin, human
WBC	White blood cell
WHO	World Health Organization
WIC	Department of Agriculture's Special Supplemental Nutrition Program for Woman, Infants, and Children
YF	Yellow fever

Index

Page numbers followed by *f* indicate figures; page numbers followed by *t* indicate tables.